Heal Your Heart

5-5-02

To my precious sons ~

I hope that you will read this and maybe get your own copy as you pass it along. Some of it is written for doctors, but much of it is quite readable. Dr. Merhige was recommended to me via the Scripps Center in La Jolla. He has given me a number of tests, and I will see him again July 2nd.

Dad

Heal Your Heart

HOW YOU CAN PREVENT OR REVERSE HEART DISEASE

K. Lance Gould, M.D.

Rutgers University Press
New Brunswick, New Jersey, and London

Library of Congress Cataloging-in-Publication Data

Gould, K. Lance.
    Heal your heart : how you can prevent or reverse heart disease /
K. Lance Gould.
        p.   cm.
    Includes bibliographical references and index.
    ISBN 0-8135-2523-3 (cloth) — ISBN 0-8135-2896-8 (pbk.)
    1. Coronary heart disease—Popular works.   2. Coronary heart
disease—Prevention.   3. Coronary heart disease—Diet therapy.
4. Coronary heart disease—Exercise.   I. Title.
RC685.C6G686   1998
616.1′23—dc21   97-39172
                                                                      CIP

British Cataloging-in-Publication data for this book is available from the
British Library

First paperback printing, 2000

Manufactured in Canada

To Lenja

Contents

PART 3

Steering through the Medical Maze   75

PART 4

The Gould Guidelines to Prevent or Reverse Vascular and Coronary Heart Disease   127

List of Figures and Tables

Figures

Tables

Preface

The Second World War had ended two years earlier. I was nine years old. It was deep rural, South Alabama and getting dark. The heat was gone, and I could rest my feet on the metal floor of the open jeep without burning them. The chuck-wills'-widows were flitting through the shadows, their calls clear above the grinding motor as we lurched along the rutted road under loblolly pines. My father was driving. Our passenger was having a lot of chest pain, sweat pouring off him. He moaned some, in a daze, intermittently wide awake, sick to his stomach. We arrived at the small hospital that my father had built, the only medical facility within fifty miles. After getting a shot of morphine, the man slept. At home over supper conversation, I gathered that he might not live. While I did not quite understand what was going on, I liked his family. My brother and I would take off on Saturdays and chase rabbits with his kids. The man lived through his heart attack. He said a black family without a man didn't do very well, so he had better stay alive. Later he got stronger, and I would see him walking fast somewhere or really pushing his mules behind a plow. He said my daddy told him to stop eating fat, get out and do things; that staying in shape by hard physical work was good for him.

My father explained how the heart works, how blood carries oxygen, what causes infection, and told a myriad of other medical "stories" on endless house calls in that jeep.

Later, when I was an adult, my father told me that his medical colleagues thought he was crazy to push his heart patients to do regular physical activity and stay lean. I remember some of them did look pretty thin. My father said he felt better himself when he was lean and fit, and that his patients did too. Without knowing why, against medical tradition and without much fanfare, he was the first doctor I ever heard about to treat heart patients that way—the first heart disease reversal program. Perhaps those evenings in the jeep affected something in my subconscious. At least, that is one explanation for the odyssey from rural meanderings to intense scientific research, from physics to medicine, from my father's physiology stories in a rattly old jeep to this book.

Heal Your Heart describes the principles and practical steps for preventing, stabilizing, or reversing coronary heart disease and associated atherosclerosis throughout the body. It is a pictorial guide for everyone who wants to prevent or reverse vascular disease. The treatment program presented in this book follows the advice my father gave to his patients: cut down on fatty foods, stay lean, exercise, stop smoking, reduce stress, and work as an equal partner with your doctor to overcome heart disease. These fundamentals for preventing or reversing cardiovascular disease are based on extensive scientific publications, as well as my own research and personal experience from my clinical practice of cardiovascular medicine over the past thirty years.

Perhaps my training in cardiology began with those childhood experiences in rural Alabama, However, medicine was remote, separate from me, something my father did. In college, I studied physics and avoided biology courses, wanting no part of medicine. Viewed in retrospect, I was scared of all that I would need to know to be a doctor. In my senior year, I took a required biology course in order to graduate with a degree in physics. Something clicked in that course, and I applied to Western Reserve Medical School in Cleveland, Ohio. There, my physics background made biophysics come alive. The heart, nerve transmission, muscle contraction, electrocardiograms, fluid dynamics, blood flow, the pumping heart chambers, control of blood pressure—all of this became a passion for me.

In medical school, my uncle, Dr. Dick Hallaran, a cardiologist in private practice in Cleveland, Ohio, and Dr. Herman Hellerstein taught me to read electrocardiograms (ECGs). Dr. Hellerstein had a tough way of teaching. In the lecture amphitheater of the hospital, he would literally throw an ECG tracing, mounted on a cardboard sheet, at one of the students. We students sat in the first row, with twenty to thirty residents or graduate fellows in the seats behind us. The student had to catch it and interpret it in front of everyone while Dr. Hellerstein counted to ten. If the student gave an incorrect answer, Dr. H. would take the sheet away and flip it to the next student, along with some biting comment about mental capacity. My six-foot, six-inch frame was a target that was hard to overlook. At first, this teaching style was traumatic, but I soon learned how to read ECGs at a glance, like speed reading. Then we both had fun with it. Could he find some ECG that I couldn't read? No, he never could.

Like my father, Dr. Hellerstein was a prophetic proponent of cardiovascular rehabilitation and management of risk factors. He used his razor-sharp mind and tongue to convince his patients and a few colleagues of the value of low-cholesterol foods and exercise. However, my physics training in the "hard sciences" made me skeptical, since the data then available in support of his position were meager and unconvincing. I kept my focus elsewhere, on the workings of the heart and vascular system; I was fascinated with how the heart pumps, how blood flows in the coronary arteries. I played with the physical principles in my mind, melding my training in physics and physiology into a functional intuition, a way of thinking about blood flow in arteries that guided my life of research.

Dr. Claude Beck, another of my mentors, was a terror to students. On my surgical rotation, I had to assist him during heart surgery. In those days (the early sixties), operating on the heart was not well established, and Dr. Beck was one of the early pioneers. He opened up the thin, membranous sac surrounding the heart while I held the retractors. He would then make a small channel in the heart muscle and insert an artery from the chest wall, called the internal mammary artery, into the channel. The idea was that the artery would grow branches that fed the heart muscle of patients whose coronary arteries were blocked with atherosclerosis. He also sprinkled asbestos in the pericardial sac to stimulate inflammation and the growth of new blood vessels, called collaterals. These collaterals were supposed to bring new blood to the heart muscle to save "hearts too good to die." Although these early surgical methods are now considered crude and unsuccessful, the patients usually survived the surgery. They even improved sometimes, probably because of the psychological belief that they should be better after such a dramatic and painful surgical experience.

To me as a young medical student, watching the beating heart and its arteries flexing, alive, was fascinating, hypnotic, like seeing life itself. Dr. Beck didn't talk much to students. He just slapped my hands with forceps when I didn't hold something right or he wanted something changed. In a fog of sleeplessness, learning by seeing one operation after another, chrome instruments in a red field burned into my vision, watching the miracle of hearts that pumped and those that didn't, feeling the ebb and flow of life, I didn't realize I was living through the origins of heart surgery, the beginning of a new medical era.

In the sixties, the first heart-lung bypass machines were developed in Cleveland. By now, I was a student in surgery at another hospital in that city, again holding retractors. I was scrubbed for the third or fourth bypass operation done there. The heart-lung bypass machines were still experimental, and the procedures weren't well developed. Yet, this operation seemed to be going well. The heart was arrested, the grafts were being placed, the surgeon hummed to himself. Everything seemed fine. Then the heart-lung machine stopped. It just stopped. Nobody could get it going. The lessons were sinking in. Pay attention to details, check things out, anticipate trouble, little mechanical details can get you, never take anything for granted.

He was a circus barker, a solidly built, good-looking man with deep creases, great stories, and a stunning younger girlfriend. When I first saw him in the emergency room in my first-year internship in 1964 at the King County

Hospital in Seattle, he was in bad shape. Like the passenger in our jeep when I was a kid, this fellow was having bad chest pain, sweating, sick to his stomach, pale, with that terrible fear in his face, the fear that death was close. He had an abnormal heartbeat, the kind that can stop the heart instantly.

We didn't have specialized coronary care units in those days, no specialized nurses, no alarm systems to warn about lethal heart irregularities. All we had were crude ECG monitors that sat by the bedside. We had only one or two drugs for this kind of heart irregularity and used electrical paddles on the chest to shock the heart into a safer rhythm. If there was a working heart monitor available, and if you could make it work (my physics background really helped), if you could stay awake, if you had a buddy to cover your other duties for a while, you sat in front of the monitor for a day or so and zapped the patient with paddles every time the heart rhythm deteriorated. If there was a warning buildup of extra heartbeats, sometimes you could give intravenous drugs to slow the heart down before having to use the paddles.

It took three days and two nights, but the circus barker made it. Without knowing why, I told him what my father had said about not eating fat and staying in good physical shape. For many years, he called me long distance from his circus travels to tell me how he was doing. But eventually the calls stopped. The circus barker taught me that patients are individuals, all different, interesting, responsive to caring. Medicine is not the same as business. It is a mutual effort to improve life and survival.

Back then, King County Hospital in Seattle was a medical battlefield. The call schedule was three days and two nights on call, one night off. Four to six new admissions hit each intern every night. We did all of the lab work on our new patients: blood counts, urinalysis, bacterial cultures, chemistry, spinal fluid analysis, X rays, everything. We gave all of the intravenous medications to each of our patients. The diagnostic work, the initial treatment, and the chart on each new hospital admission had to be complete by morning rounds. The usual four to six admissions of acutely ill patients per night meant working through the night. Sometimes, at three or four in the morning I would fall asleep over the microscope. My head would fall forward and bang the eyepiece, leaving black-and-blue spots around my eyes. In moments of sleep, I had a recurring nightmare that I dozed off on a patient's bed, straight through to morning rounds.

The hospital and the interns' clinical laboratory were on a hill overlooking the city and harbor immediately below. As I finished the night's work at the microscope, the early morning sun would reflect off the water, silhouetting the shadowed city buildings. The sunrise and first mewing gulls indicated two hours left to complete work before morning rounds. The beauty of these scenes fused with the sleepless intensity of the work powerfully reacted with my visually oriented thinking. Visual impressions are intensely intertwined with medicine in my mind, like the illustrations in this book.

Our equipment then was fairly primitive, like the old vertical, single brass tube microscopes that required hunching over for half the night. We got no pay for the "privilege of training." By threatening a strike, we finally received $1,500 per year and new slanted, sleek binocular microscopes with a light brightness control that made the colors in the microscopic slides really light up. In short, we learned technical medicine, how to deal with the worst medical problems, how to get things done, how to focus hard on keeping somebody alive no matter what the conditions or how tired we were.

These years served to develop a focus on the ebb and flow of life itself, on the processes of medicine and of survival, one's own and the patients'. In the crazy scramble of seeing patients, doing lab work, carrying out procedures, giving critical intravenous medications, I learned to focus on the essentials, on the key pieces of information, the clues—something in the medical history, a finding on a physical exam, an odd lab value, an unexpected response to treatment. No matter what the myriad tasks I was doing, no matter how busy or tired I was, no matter what the emergency, I learned to stay focused on the few central issues that meant life and death to my patients. Later on, as this book illustrates, that lesson translated into finding the basic or essential concepts buried in a mass of conflicting, confusing scientific or medical data, into extracting a pattern from disjointed information, no matter how long it takes. Consequently, I often forget meetings or am frequently late. When I operate in this mode, my wife says I'm on cardiology time, not real time.

In my final year of general medicine residency in 1966, I had a patient I'll never forget. She was a flaming redhead in her early forties, with great wit and appeal. She really made me laugh on morning rounds. Her problem was some kind of atypical chest pain unlike the exertional angina that men get with coronary heart disease. She had been relatively healthy, except for a hysterectomy, and she smoked

At first, the attending cardiologist thought she was just hysterical, that her pain was due to some nonmedical cause. Finally the cardiologist decided to do a coronary arteriogram, a new procedure that had just been introduced into this hospital that year, but only in order to support his contention that she had no real heart disease and should see a psychiatrist.

I remember going down to the cardiac procedure lab with her to watch the coronary arteriogram. I remember watching her heart beat on the fluoroscopy screen with the catheter tubes in place. With the first injection of the X-ray dye into her coronary arteries, the X-ray dye on the fluoroscopic screen trickled slowly like a thread down the front part of her heart in what was supposed to be the big coronary artery there. Then even this thin trickle stopped. At that moment, the heart silhouette on the fluoroscopy stopped beating. It just stopped. I looked at her to see what was going on. She was very still. Nothing helped after that. Nobody did anything wrong. She just died.

Nowadays, coronary arteriograms are quite safe, with new X-ray dyes, new technology for people with severe diffuse coronary heart disease—the condition responsible for the redhead's chest pain. We also understand more about coronary heart disease in women and how it differs from heart disease in men. The lessons then were rammed home—life is fragile, treat it carefully, never assume anything, listen to your patients, anticipate trouble.

I would spend thirty years developing techniques to quantify the extent of coronary artery disease seen on coronary arteriograms. I wrote the first and only book on quantitative analysis of coronary arteriograms and effects of narrowing of the arteries on coronary blood flow. Humbled by its miraculous intricacy, I would come to understand something about blood flow in the coronary arteries, about what atherosclerotic narrowing does to them. When one studies the heart for a long time, thinks intensely about it from all angles, lives with it day and night, its behavior tells the story of how it works.

The search for the essential clue, the timelessness of pursuing some scientific truth, the total commitment, the attention to detail, the understanding of physical and biological processes—all of this led me to change direction in my last year of residency. I shifted my focus from learning medicine, from the ebb and flow of patients' lives, to the scientific unknown. What causes the narrowings in some places in the coronary arteries but not others? How does one measure these narrowings? How does narrowing affect blood flow through the artery? What can one do about it?

Dr. Robert Bruce, a tall, lean, taciturn man with a flat East Coast accent, developed the treadmill stress test during my training years in cardiology in the late sixties; it's called the Bruce treadmill test. I did a lot of treadmill testing on patients with him in Seattle. Dr. Bruce viewed the treadmill test correctly as another risk factor for coronary heart disease. Like measuring cholesterol, or smoking, the treadmill test serves as an epidemiologic marker of cardiovascular risk, not a specific diagnostic test. Later, as used by others, treadmill stress assumed the status of diagnostic testing despite its limited accuracy for identifying heart disease in an individual. My experience with Dr. Bruce and the limitations of the treadmill test emphasized the need for more accurate, noninvasive ways of examining the heart, measuring its blood flow directly, and evaluating the effects of coronary heart disease. As treadmill testing became more widespread and popular, I became more skeptical about its value.

By the end of my training in clinical cardiology in the early seventies, treadmill testing, coronary arteriography, and coronary bypass surgery were well established. They were the only effective treatment for coronary heart disease. The coronary arteries affected by atherosclerosis were considered rigid tubes, partially blocked by buildup of cholesterol, scarring, and calcium that required new surgically implanted tubes to carry blood to the heart muscle. It was the era of cardiovascular plumbing. However, there was no understanding of how to quantify or measure severity of the narrowings seen on coronary arteriograms. There was little understanding of blood flow through the coronary arteries and how to measure it. As far as I could tell, few people cared about these topics. The clinical approach to the problem was fairly standard: take an X ray or arteriographic picture of the coronary arteries, look at it, and operate; problem solved. Later, of course, that approach turned out to be wrong since it did not solve the problem. In this book, I explain why.

At the time, I saw patients, cared for them, did the coronary arteriograms, and recommended them for surgery, just as other cardiologists did. But my mind was preoccupied with the experiments I was conducting on coronary blood flow and the effect of narrowings on the coronary arteries. Coronary arteriograms often showed severe narrowing in patients who were not limited in their physical activity and had little or no chest pain. This observation led to a series of questions: How could the severe narrowings be present without continuously impairing blood flow through the coronary arteries to the heart muscle? How did the narrowings in the coronary artery relate to blood flow through it? How should the narrowing be measured quantitatively? Did severity of narrowing indicate who needed bypass surgery and who didn't, who died, who didn't? Were the narrowings in the coronary arteries reversible? This book gives the answers to those questions, but back then, no one knew.

One late Monday afternoon, I was gazing through my open lab window at the sun setting over Puget Sound. The Olympic mountain range was hazy above the water, late summer snow left on the highest peaks, gulls riding the evening wind over the harbor. I could hear hooting of the ferries as they broke the sun's reflection in the water. I had just finished an interesting experiment that had finally worked after three years of building and repairing old research equipment, after many failures and many mistakes. I had developed a certain kind of difficult experimental heart surgery for implanting measurement devices in the heart to measure blood flow and pressure beyond experimentally produced narrowings of the coronary arteries. It had taken nearly two years just to get the surgical preparation down in order to do the experiment. But finally, we had our first results.

While idly staring at the evening light glittering on the water, I realized that we had discovered a way of quantifying the functional severity of coronary artery narrowing. Although the narrowings did not reduce coronary blood flow until it was nearly completely blocked, these narrowings reduced the capacity for increasing blood flow during physical exertion or corresponding pharmacologic stress. Normally, there is tremendous reserve capacity for increasing blood flow in the arteries to the heart muscle, which I called coronary flow reserve, to meet the work demands of the heart during exercise or stress. Our new results indicated that narrowing of the coronary arteries reduced or limited this coronary flow reserve capacity long before affecting coronary flow at resting conditions. I was happy and excited about these findings. Every experiment after that showed the same results.

Still, this research raised a lot of questions in my mind. There was no way of knowing then that answering these questions about my discovery of coronary flow reserve would consume the next twenty-eight years of my research, would culminate in the writing of this book, and would be recognized throughout the world as the standard for assessing the functional severity of coronary artery narrowing.

The next step was to relate this newly discovered concept of coronary flow reserve to the detailed shape of narrowings in the coronary arteries—their length, absolute diameter, relative degree of narrowing, and fluid dynamic streamlining. One set of experiments gave really disturbing results, suggesting that my fundamental understanding and equations relating coronary blood flow to the geometric shape and dimensions of the arterial narrowings were incorrect. I repeated experiments, made better measurements, rechecked theoretical equations—always with the same disturbing results. A sinking, empty feeling of failure took hold of me. Finally, I noticed that the relative severity of the narrowings of the coronary arteries was worse at the higher levels of blood flow found during the measurements of coronary flow reserve. The coronary size and narrowings were not rigid, partially plugged pipes. Rather, the arteries changed their shape and their size *dynamically* when the blood flow was high. When this dynamically changing narrowing of the coronary arteries was accounted for, the measurements fit the theoretical equations perfectly.

Although relieved, I was in a dilemma. Should I redirect all of my efforts into examining the mechanism of this new phenomenon of the normal coronary artery dilating to a larger size at high coronary blood flows? It was an important new observation, but the mechanism was unknown. Studying it would require completely different experimental methods and several more years of delay before my findings could be applied to care of patients. My first articles on the concept of coronary flow reserve had been well received. I published the first article showing dynamic changes in coronary arteries and the transient increase in arterial size associated with high blood flow. However, I decided against follow-up experiments to define the mechanism of this observation in order to pursue my studies of coronary flow reserve.

Later, many other scientists in different types of experiments also observed these dynamic changes in the size of coronary arteries in relation to their blood flow and identified the mechanisms. Their work was instrumental in evolving the new field of vascular biology. I have half jokingly concluded that I missed a major basic scientific discovery by deciding against further study of this early observation. But my intense focus on my primary scientific goal of understanding effects of narrowing on blood flow in the coronary arteries, without deflection by "incidental" observations en route, did prove to be fruitful: I came to understand coronary artery narrowing and coronary flow reserve fairly well.

My next step was to demonstrate that coronary flow reserve for measuring severity of coronary artery narrowings was applicable to patients with coronary heart disease. I proved the concept in patients while obtaining clinically necessary X-ray arteriographic pictures of their coronary arteries. In the first set of studies, I injected X-ray dye for coronary arteriograms through small tubes inserted into a patient's arteries using an invasive surgical technique. But, in order to avoid this invasive method which has some risk of complications, I developed the concept of noninvasive pharmacologic stress using an intravenous drug called dipyridamole. This medication, given intravenously, is ideal for assessing coronary flow reserve because it causes coronary blood flow to increase four times above resting levels, more than the increase produced by exercise or X-ray dye. After testing the proper dose on myself, I administered it to patients and observed the flow of blood through the coronary arteries.

Pictures of blood flow in the heart muscle during dipyridamole stress were obtained by using a scanner or camera that takes pictures of a radionuclide tracer. This radiotracer is given intravenously and tracks the blood flow in the heart. In areas of narrowed coronary arteries, as shown in this book, the coronary flow reserve is restricted and blood flow to the heart muscle cannot increase normally in response to dipyridamole. At the peak blood flow after dipyridamole, the radiotracer is given intravenously and tracks the blood flow in the heart. Any narrowing of the artery causes a defect or abnormality in the blood flow pictures of the heart obtained by scanning the radionuclide tracer. The size and the severity of this blood flow abnormality on the blood flow pictures indicate the extent and severity of the narrowed coronary arteries. As I later discovered, and show in this book, this abnormal blood flow in the hearts of people with coronary heart disease markedly improves after reversal treatment.

Standard nuclear imaging of radionuclide tracers in the heart is limited by several technical problems, apparent to me even then. Therefore, my next step was to obtain pictures of coronary flow reserve in the heart by using more accurate tomographic imaging planes, or slices. This tomographic form of imaging makes pictures as if slicing up the heart like a loaf of bread, by computer of course, using a very accurate technology called positron emission tomography (PET). The visual slices, or planes, provide three-dimensional views of blood flow in the heart. After a series of preliminary experiments to prove the potential of this approach, my laboratory crew, equipment, and I flew to the then new PET laboratory at the University of California at Los Angeles.

In our initial studies using the prototype PET scanner and radionuclide tracers made in the cyclotron at UCLA, my colleague there, Dr. Heinrich

Schelbert, and my lab team did the first studies on PET imaging of coronary flow reserve. The studies took four hectic weeks. We showed that PET imaging could identify mild, early coronary artery narrowing and could noninvasively quantify more severe narrowings with much greater accuracy than reported for standard nuclear imaging of the heart. On the last day of the study, a power supply blew and the PET scanner went down, a sign that it was time to write up the results. I worked all night analyzing the preliminary results and writing an article to meet the next day's submission deadline, competing for an international prize for research in nuclear medicine. That article won the George von Hevesy prize, one of the highest honors awarded for research in nuclear medicine, at the Second World Congress for Nuclear Medicine in Washington, D.C., in 1978.

As a result of winning the von Hevesy prize, I moved from Seattle to the University of Texas Medical School in Houston, Texas, in 1979 to establish the world's first major clinical PET imaging center and serve as its chief of cardiology. While waiting for construction of the cyclotron and its building, my team built the first PET scanner with complete multiple rings of radiation detectors that could take pictures of the whole heart, a design that is now standard. In parallel, my laboratory worked with a commercial company to show the feasibility of clinical PET imaging of the heart using another source of a positron radiotracer called rubidium. Because rubidium did not require the expense and complexity of a cyclotron to make the radiotracers necessary for imaging the heart, PET imaging could become more widely used in clinics outside of university research centers.

The results of the first 1,500 clinical heart studies at the Houston PET Center indicated that PET was identifying early coronary heart disease as well as advanced, severe disease in people who had only mild or no symptoms, often years before a heart attack or the need for bypass surgery. But what were we to do with these people who felt well but who were likely to suffer a heart attack sometime in the future?

A new procedure involving dilation of coronary artery narrowings with a balloon on a catheter had just been introduced. It promised a therapeutic solution without heart surgery. A number of my patients had advanced, severe narrowing of the coronary arteries found by PET imaging but no symptoms. They underwent the new balloon procedure with the idea that it would prevent trouble later. Unfortunately, balloon dilation of the narrowings in the coronary arteries frequently did not solve the problem. The narrowings often recurred, sometimes worse than before, causing symptoms that then required bypass surgery. As reviewed in this book, later data showed that there is a high recurrence of narrowings after balloon dilation; furthermore, balloon dilation and bypass surgery failed to prevent deaths or heart attacks.

My dilemma was acute: how should I treat people who had coronary heart disease but no symptoms? They felt well. Without their PET scan, they would not have known that they were walking time bombs, primed for a heart attack. Knowing the limitations of balloon dilation and bypass surgery, I searched for good alternatives. Previous studies of cholesterol lowering were disappointing; it was found to be ineffective in preventing heart attacks or death. The 20 to 30 percent fat diet recommended by the American Heart Association and the National Cholesterol Education Program failed to reliably prevent progression, heart attacks, or deaths in individuals with coronary heart disease.

Two recent medical advances offered a solution to my dilemma. The first was demonstration by our PET studies that a very low-fat diet, lower than that recommended by the American Heart Association, improved blood flow in the hearts of patients with coronary heart disease. These studies were carried out as part of the Lifestyle Heart Trial, done with Dr. Dean Ornish, for which I was the senior clinical scientist responsible for measuring the severity of coronary artery narrowings on arteriograms and for obtaining PET images of blood flow in the heart. As shown in this book, noninvasive PET imaging proved to be as accurate or more accurate than invasive coronary arteriograms for assessing the progression or regression of coronary heart disease.

However, later, after more experience with PET and additional medical evidence, I found that the vegetarian, high-carbohydrate diet was not achieving the clinical results that I sought in many patients. The commercial version of this diet recommended very low fat consumption but also high levels of carbohydrate-rich food for adequate dietary protein. The high-carbohydrate content of this vegetarian diet often causes a detrimental change in other fats found in the blood, called triglycerides, and in the balance of good-bad cholesterol levels associated with high risk of heart attacks. Although the risks of death and heart attack were decreased somewhat by this low-fat diet, these risks remained too high to be acceptable to me, and the study was simply too small to draw generalized conclusions about decreasing the incidence of deaths or heart attacks

Consequently, I abandoned the high-carbohydrate vegetarian version of the very low-fat diet and replaced it with a more advanced, low-carbohydrate, very low-fat diet, adequate in protein. This new food plan is more flexible, easier to use, and more effective in achieving the necessary balance of triglycerides and good-bad cholesterol levels. In this book, I discuss this new approach to low-fat food in detail and provide sample menus.

The second medical advance resulted from several clinical studies of a new class of cholesterol-lowering drugs called statins. In large medical trials done at other centers, these cholesterol-lowering drugs caused a 30 to 75 percent decrease in the frequency of heart attacks, deaths, bypass surgery, or balloon dilation in patients with coronary heart disease. (Readers will find a review of these studies in this book.) Good scientific data suggested that the combination of a very low-fat diet plus these cholesterol-lowering drugs had independent additive effects. My subsequent clinical experience indicated that the combination of very low-fat, low-calorie foods and cholesterol-lowering drugs produces a 90 percent or greater decrease in deaths, heart attacks, bypass surgery, or balloon dilation in people with stable coronary heart disease.

Not only did I have the solution to my dilemma, but I also had a comprehensive new approach to the primarily noninvasive management of coronary heart disease. PET imaging replaced treadmill exercise stress testing and invasive coronary arteriography; reversal treatment using my modern, very low-fat food plan, combined with cholesterol-lowering medications, replaced balloon dilation and bypass surgery. Thus, my approach largely avoided coronary arteriography, balloon dilation, and bypass surgery—the bread and butter of cardiovascular medicine. It also incurred much lower costs with better results: higher survival rates and fewer heart attacks.

Reversal treatment of coronary heart disease utilizing very low-fat foods and cholesterol-lowering drugs is based on more sound medical studies including more patients studied than any other treatment, particularly in comparison to bypass surgery and balloon dilation. While the medical profession is influenced by good scientific medical trials, it is curious that the most prevalent procedure for coronary heart disease now, balloon dilation, called balloon angioplasty, has never been tested by proper scientific trial until recently, with negative results on preventing heart attacks or deaths. The data, graphically shown in this book, demonstrate that balloon angioplasty does not prevent heart attacks or deaths. However, this procedure is an accepted, widespread, first approach to the management of coronary heart disease. In contrast, only 25 percent or less of people with known coronary heart disease are treated adequately with cholesterol lowering despite at least twenty-five major clinical trials showing the benefits. As a clinician and scientist, I concluded that the economic incentives for invasive procedures like coronary arteriography, balloon dilation, and bypass surgery strongly influence their widespread use.

Therefore, the next step of my odyssey was a practical demonstration in clinical practice of my noninvasive approach for managing coronary heart disease by reversal treatment. Hence, this book. It is the outcome of a voyage of discovery from a rattly old jeep with its heart attack passenger to the most advanced medical technology, pharmacology, and psychology for stabilizing or reversing coronary heart disease. This book provides the guidelines for preventing and reversing the cholesterol buildup of vascular disease everywhere in the body by a practical combination of do-it-yourself steps, effective safe cholesterol-lowering medications, and how-to-manage-your-doctor advice.

Formerly, I was a founding director and consultant to Positron Corporation, which now holds my patent on PET technology. I was also a consultant to Siemens Medical Systems, Philips Medical Systems, Boerhinger Mannheim,

R. P. Kincheloe Co., Bristol-Myers Squibb, Novartis, and Merck & Co. I currently hold no stock and have no position or personal financial ties to, or consulting agreements with, any corporation or business involved with medical technology, pharmaceuticals, food, or any products or procedures discussed in this book.

I am publishing a companion scientific-medical textbook for physicians and cardiovascular scientists entitled *Coronary Artery Stenosis and Reversing Heart Disease*, second edition, with Lippincott Raven, Philadelphia. It provides the detailed scientific data and basis for preventing, stabilizing, or reversing heart and vascular disease which has been simplified and summarized for the general nonmedical reader in *Heal Your Heart*.

I would like to thank Lenja Gould, my wife, for guidance on the visual layout of illustrations and on simplifying concepts for nonmedical readers; Bob Boeye for creative computer graphics, Mary Jane Hess, R.N., Mary Haynie, R.N., M.B.A., Ro Edens, Ph.D., Patsy Kleypas, Sherri Richmond, Dilip Patel, R.T., Kathy McCormick, R.T., Nizar Mullani, Ross Hartz, Richard Kirkeeide, Ph.D., Yvonne Stuart, R.T., Neal Parker, M.S., Jennie Li, M.S., Leonard Bolomcy, Frank Dobbs, Ph.D., Aamir Siddiqui, Nancy Haberman, and Faye Pryor for their talented professional services in this program for preventing or reversing vascular and coronary heart disease; Patsy Kleypas for manuscript preparation; the many participants with coronary heart disease whose insight, commitment, and success in healthy living make my work worthwhile; my first two professors, Kenneth N. Gould, M.D., and Elizabeth B. Gould. I also thank the following for research or educational funding support since 1960: National Institutes of Health, American Heart Association, Veterans Administration Career Development, M. D. Anderson Foundation, Houston Endowment, George von Hevesy Foundation, Albert and Celia Weatherhead of the Weatherhead Foundation and founders of the Weatherhead PET Center for Reversing and Preventing Atherosclerosis at the University of Texas Medical School, Houston; Mr. C. W. Wellen, current president, and Mr. W. T. Launius, former president, of the Clayton Foundation; M. David Low, M.D., Ph.D., president of the University of Texas Health Science Center-Houston; Thomas F. Burks, Ph.D., vice president for academic affairs, L. Maximilian Buja, M.D., dean of the University of Texas Medical School; James T. Willerson, M.D., chairman of the Department of Medicine, S. Ward Casscells III, M.D., director, Division of Cardiology, John Porretto, executive vice president for administration and finance, University of Texas Health Science Center-Houston; Gary Wood, Ph.D., president and chairman of the board, Positron Corporation; Doreen Valentine, Ph.D., acquiring editor for the sciences of Rutgers University Press; and the following corporations: Boehringer Mannheim; Bristol-Myers Squibb; Merck & Co.; Sandoz; Enron Corporation; Positron Corporation; Philips Medical Systems; Siemens Medical Systems. Numerous private donors made a significant contribution as well. Finally, I would like to acknowledge the following present or former colleagues, teachers, assistants, students, or associates:

John Adamson, M.D.
Steve Adler, Ph.D.
Ellen Aldrich, R.N.
Thomas Andreoli, M.D.
Max Anliker, M.D., Ph.D.
Chris Baca
Claude Beck, M.D.
Ben Bendriem, Ph.D.
Marc Berridge, Ph.D.
Edwin Bierman, M.D.
John Blackmon, M.D.
Eugene Braunwald, M.D.
David Bristow, M.S.
Gregg Brown, M.D.
Robert Bruce, M.D.
John Brunzell, M.D.
Martin Buchi, M.D.
Roger Bulger, M.D.
Bob Catlin
Jack Caughey, M.D.
Denton Cooley, M.D.
Simon Dack, M.D.
Linda Demer, M.D., Ph.D.
Harold Dodge, M.D.
Lauren Enck
Bud Evans, M.D.
Eric Feigl, M.D.
Cathy Felgar
Claire Finn
Mark Franceschini
O. Howard Frazier, M.D.
Paula Freeman
Greg Freund, M.D.
Jay Gaeta, M.S.
Rick Gaines
Dahlia Garza, M.D.
Richard Goldstein, M.D.
Antonio Gotto, M.D.
Bob Guezuraga

Dick Hallaran, M.D.
Glen Hamilton, M.D.
William Hazzard, M.D.
Hermann Hellerstein, M.D.
Alan Herd, M.D.
David Hess, M.D.
Kerri Hicks, M.S.
Dick Hitchens, M.S.
Julien Hoffman, M.D.
Rick Holmes
Dick Johnson
Katharine Kelley, M.D.
Ward Kennedy, M.D.
David Kuhl, M.D.
Janice Kuhn, R.N.
David Kusnerik
Claude Lenfant, M.D.
Alex Langmuir, M.D.
Dennis Lee
Kirk Lipscomb, M.D.
Kathy Lovgren
Spencer McCallie, Ph.D.
Zena McCallum
Salma Marani, M.S.
Marge Matthews, R.N.
Kenneth Melmon, M.D.
Michael Merhige, M.D.   AMHERST N.Y
Keiichi Nakagawa, M.D.
Yuko Nakagawa, M.D.
Robert Oppermann
Dean Ornish, M.D.
David Page
Joan Goldstein Parker
William Parmley, M.D.
Linda Parsel, R.T.
Robert Petersdorf, M.D.
Michael Phelps, Ph.D.
Eddie Philippe, Ph.D.
Veronica Pina, M.D.

Michael Ter Porgossian, Ph.D.
Daniel Porte, M.D.
Kathryn Rainbird
C. H. Rammelkamp, M.D.
Jackie Raymond
Larry Reduto, M.D.
Victoria Reeders
T. Joseph Reeves, M.D.
Fredrick Robbins, M.D.
Russell Ross, M.D.
Robert Rushmer, M.D.
Heinrich Schelbert, M.D.
David Sease, M.D.
Christian Seiler, M.D.
Richard Smalling, M.D., Ph.D.
Nick Spirelakis, Ph.D.
Eugene Strandness, M.D.
Michael Sweeney, M.D.

Heinrich Taegtmeyer, M.D.,
  Ph.D.
Tim Tewson, Ph.D.
Elmerice Traks, M.D.
Henny Van Dyke
Nora Volkow, M.D.
Henry Wagner, Jr., M.D.
Lynn Walts, Dr.P.H.
Albert Weatherhead
Frank Webber, M.D.
Stewart West, Ph.D.
Byron Williams, M.D.
Katherine Wingate, Ph.D.
Gary Wong, Ph.D.
Eddie Xu, Ph.D.
Bryan Yeoman
Katsuya Yoshida, M.D.

How to Use This Book

The contents are organized into four sections. The first describes how the heart works, what happens when cholesterol builds up in the arteries of the heart, how blood flow through the coronary arteries carrying blood to the heart muscle is affected, how heart attacks occur, what happens with a damaged heart. The second part addresses the questions of who gets heart disease and why, what are risk factors for coronary heart disease and how can it be prevented or reversed. The third part reviews the traditional approach to diagnosing and treating coronary heart disease, its risks and limitations, how to steer through the medical maze as you take charge of your heart health, and how to manage your doctor in this undertaking. The fourth part presents my lifestyle guidelines integrated with cholesterol-lowering medications. Separate sections outline every step for integrating daily healthy living habits with cholesterol-lowering or cardiovascular drugs as needed.

This reversal program attacks the root of the problem—atherosclerosis. It goes beyond the traditional active-physician, passive-patient relation which characterizes surgical or catheter procedures. It reaches for more definitive solutions than the short-term effects of coronary bypass surgery or balloon dilation. Its goals are better survival and improved health.

Designed for the general reader, the book serves as a manual for preventing or reversing cardiovascular disease, a take-charge guide for optimally integrating a healthy lifestyle with lifesaving cholesterol-lowering medications and for actively managing one's physician as a consultant or equal partner in achieving a healthy heart. For the health care executive, it provides the basis for comprehensive, managed cardiovascular medicine at substantially reduced costs.

The scientific information and practical guidelines are presented in nontechnical language incorporating the most recent medical knowledge. Accompanying the text are an abundance of simple illustrations, summary graphs, and tables. For the critical reader, each conclusion is documented by extensive scientific references at the end of the book.

The principles of reversing cardiovascular disease used in this program may be adapted to various lifestyles, habits, tastes, time constraints, and personalities. The program can benefit people from all walks of life: the tightly scheduled professional with little time, the executive with frequent business lunches and travel, the truck driver on the road with a deadline, the construction worker doing heavy labor, the retired couple with plenty of time, the young or middle-aged couple with premature heart disease or high risk factors and children at home, fast-food freaks, steak-and-potatoes people, the more or less well-to-do.

There is no single, unique regimen, diet, or method to which all these individuals must conform. Each needs an individualized, flexible program incorporating the fundamental steps into their daily routines. This program avoids multiple medical consultations, special facilities or equipment, group interaction, classroom meetings, and long retreats because the excessive time demands of these activities disrupt busy schedules. The essentials are healthy living habits combined with medical management at home and work.

Reversing cardiovascular disease and preventing its relentless outcomes require the following: understanding the fundamentals of the heart and health, eating easily prepared, widely available low-fat foods, enjoying moderate exercise, abstaining from smoking, taking antioxidant vitamins, and controlling weight. Incorporating cholesterol-lowering or cardiovascular drugs with these steps ensures optimal outcomes. In most people, reversal treatment produces a sense of well-being and reduces or eliminates symptoms. It dramatically lowers the risk of cardiovascular death, heart attack, chest pain, stroke, and the need for balloon dilation or bypass surgery.

Nevertheless, many physicians do not recognize, understand, or support reversal treatment. Others do not know how to do it, lack the time to implement it, and are compensated more for doing invasive procedures. The medical profession in general is heavily oriented toward surgical or catheter procedures for the definitive diagnosis and primary treatment of cardiovascular disease. This orientation is due to tradition, training, available technology, patient expectations, the satisfaction of immediately "fixing" the problem, and reimbursement incentives. But regardless of whether your own physician is a specialist or general practitioner with limited time, expertise, or interest, this book shows how to use the physician as a "consultant" in the self-directed management of your health. It indicates what questions to ask medical staff and how to manage your reversal program and doctor. Since physicians are usually willing to prescribe and monitor appropriate cholesterol-lowering or cardiovascular drugs, you should be able to complete the program and prevent or reverse coronary heart disease by following the recommendations in this book.

Reversal treatment can replace surgical or catheter procedures as the principal or definitive approach for treating cardiovascular disease in most patients. In some specific circumstances, however, an individual may need balloon dilation or bypass surgery in addition to reversal treatment. This book provides criteria and guidelines for these mechanical procedures to identify the minority of patients who need them.

Although most people with vascular or coronary heart disease have success with the approach used in this book, no treatment has a guaranteed outcome; some risk of heart attack or complications of vascular disease may remain for any individual, as is the case with bypass or vascular surgery and balloon dilation. In some people, the application of these principles is difficult and complex due to advanced atherosclerosis, incomplete adherence to lifestyle guidelines, adverse reactions to medications, individual differences in responses to treatment and aggressiveness of the vascular disease, lack of knowledge or communication between physician and patient, unrealistic expectations of success, and many other factors affecting clinical outcomes. Neither the publisher nor I can be responsible for the health care of any reader or for the results of any reader's treatment of vascular disease using these guidelines.

PART 1

Understanding the Heart and the Dangers of Coronary Heart Disease

✓ The Heartbeat of Life

✓ The Pumping Heart

✓ The Coronary Arteries

✓ Blood Pressure and the Heartbeat

✓ Cholesterol and Coronary Heart Disease

✓ The Damaged Heart

✓ Heart Failure

✓ The Electrocardiogram and the Heartbeat

✓ Sudden Death

✓ Dysfunctional Coronary Arteries—A Time Bomb

✓ The Silver Lining

✓ Blood Clots in Coronary Arteries

✓ Narrowed Arteries and Swirling Flow

✓ The Give-and-Take of the Heartbeat

✓ Narrowed Arteries and the Pumping Heart

✓ Growing New Blood Vessels—Collaterals

✓ Blue Clues to Finding the Silent Killer

✓ Rainbow Clues

✓ Early Clues

✓ Progression—The Killer Stalks

✓ Regression—You Win

The first step toward taking charge of your heart's health is to learn how the heart functions normally and what happens in coronary heart disease. This section describes how the heart and vascular system work, using pictorial representations of the heart and its coronary arteries. The illustrations and text answer the basic questions: How does the heart pump? Why are coronary arteries important? What is vascular disease? What are the causes and outcomes of coronary heart disease? How does it affect blood flow to heart muscle? How do we detect and measure it? What happens with progression? Does regression, or reversal, of coronary heart disease occur?

The Heartbeat of Life

Even before humans understood how it worked, the heart symbolized life, love, courage, generosity, loyalty, strength, endurance, and purity. All of these essential qualities of our being—physical, emotional, social, and spiritual—have been attributed to the heart. Indeed, this point of view makes good sense based on the near magical physical performance of the heart under a wide range of conditions.

During an eighty-year life span the heart beats approximately 3.4 billion times and pumps 61.1 million gallons of blood. The pump that produces this remarkable output of work is a cone-shaped sack of specialized muscle about three to four inches in diameter, four to six inches long, with walls one-half to three-quarters inch thick. It weighs only one-half to one pound depending on body size and physical conditioning.

The heart is a muscular organ in the chest with four chambers. The two thin-walled upper chambers, called the left and right atria, direct blood flow into and assist in filling the two lower, stronger pumping chambers, called the left and right ventricles. The veins carry blood flow from the body into the atria. The arteries carry the blood pumped from the ventricles out to the body. (See figure 1.1.)

The right side of the heart (the right atrium and right ventricle) pumps blood from the body through the lungs, where the blood becomes saturated with oxygen from the lungs. This oxygen-carrying blood is bright red, as compared with a darker purple red after the oxygen is extracted from the blood by the body to maintain its oxygen metabolism.

The bright red oxygenated blood flows from the lungs back to the left side of the heart (the left atrium and left ventricle), which then pumps the oxygen-carrying blood out to the body through the main large artery called the aorta and to arteries of the body. This oxygen-carrying blood is necessary for the function of all organs and sustains life.

The heart muscle itself requires oxygen-carrying blood in order to continue working. The coronary arteries carry blood flow from the aorta back to the heart muscle. Thus, the heart pumps life-sustaining, oxygen-carrying blood to the body and to its own muscle. Without oxygen-carrying blood

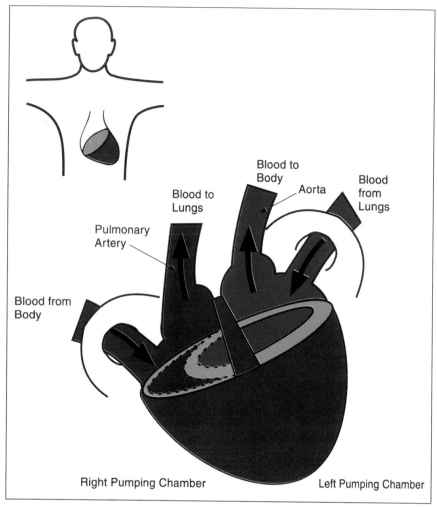

Figure 1.1. Normal Anatomy and Function of the Heart Pumping Chambers

flow, the heart muscle and brain stop functioning within a few minutes, causing death. Therefore, the heart has to pump adequate blood flow continuously at all times, particularly during hard physical exertion. Consequently, the left ventricle, which pumps the blood out to the body, has the thickest, strongest muscle of the four heart chambers. It performs the greatest amount of pumping work and needs for its own heart muscle the greatest amount of oxygen-carrying blood. The left ventricle is therefore the most important of the heart chambers.

This section focuses on the left ventricular pumping chamber, its pumping function, and its coronary arteries. To assist the reader, I have simplified the heart illustrations so that only this central pumping chamber is depicted.

The Pumping Heart

When the sack of heart muscle around this central left ventricular chamber contracts, the blood in the central chamber is squeezed or pumped out to the body. This contraction phase is called systole (pronounced *sis-toe-lee*). During systolic contraction, the heart muscle squeezes the inner pumping chamber to a smaller size like a fist squeezing water out of a rubber balloon. This squeeze generates high pressure in the heart chamber that squirts the blood into the aorta. During this systolic squeeze, the heart wall thickens as the muscle fibers shorten, much like the bulging of muscles during weight lifting. If you touched the heart muscle during contraction, you would find it to be very hard, like dense rubber.

After contraction, the heart muscle relaxes momentarily so that the pumping chamber can fill with blood in preparation for the next contraction. This relaxation phase is called diastole (pronounced dye-*ass*-toe-lee). Each sequential systole and diastole constitute a heart cycle. The heartbeat is systole, and the pause between heartbeats is diastole. A heart cycle of systole and diastole occurs at heart rates ranging normally from 45 to 100 beats per minute at rest. One second for each heart cycle is a heart rate of 60 beats per minute. With exercise, excitement, stress, or other stimuli, this rate may increase normally up to 250 beats per minute. (Figure 1.2 illustrates the normal pumping cycle.)

Heart muscle is adapted to contract rhythmically about once per second without ceasing throughout one's life. In contrast, all other muscles of the body have prolonged periods of rest such as during sleep. Heart muscle must be able to achieve a ten- to twentyfold increase in its work output from resting levels to meet the demands of the body during intense exercise.

In order to respond to such prolonged or intense workloads, heart muscle is enmeshed in a dense network of small blood vessels providing the heart muscle with a rich vascular supply. The larger coronary arteries, which course over the surface of the heart, send branches into the heart muscle, where they connect with the dense network of small blood vessels enmeshing the heart muscle. This coronary arterial system has the highest blood flow capacity of the body. It ensures that the heart muscle receives enough oxygen-carrying blood during maximum physical exertion.

The Coronary Arteries

There are three major coronary arteries. They all arise at the root of the biggest artery of the body, the aorta, which feeds blood to all other arteries. The right coronary artery courses around the right side of the heart to its back, or posterior, surface. There it turns down along the length of the back, or bottom, surface of the heart to its tip. Since it descends down the length of the back, or posterior, surface of the heart, this segment is also called the

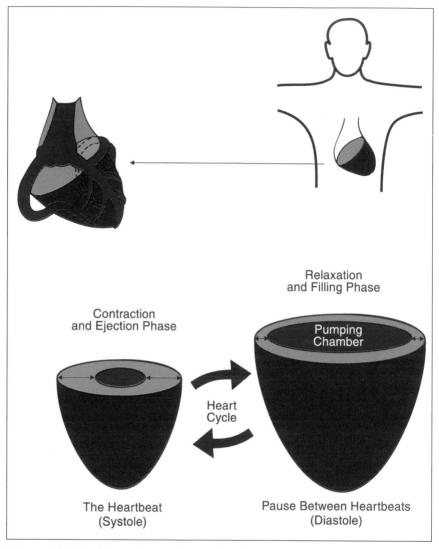

Figure 1.2. The Normal Pumping Cycle of Heart Contraction (Systole) and Relaxation (Diastole)

posterior descending coronary artery. The left main coronary artery immediately branches into the two other major coronary arteries, the left anterior descending and left circumflex coronary arteries. The left anterior descending artery is so named because it descends down the front, or anterior, surface of the heart to the tip. It is sometimes referred to as the widow-maker artery since it is the largest of the coronary arteries and blockage commonly causes death. The left circumflex gets its name from the fact that it flexes around (circum) the left side of the heart. The left circumflex and right coronary arteries form a crude ring around the base of the heart, like the base of an upside-down crown. The cage, or crest, of this crown is formed by the left anterior descending in front and the posterior descending segment of the right coronary artery in back. This crownlike structure of the coronary arteries gives rise to the name *coronary*, as in *coronation* or *setting of the crown*. (See figure 1.3 for the orientation of the heart and coronary arteries.)

The English term *cardiac*, the French word *coeur*, and the Spanish word *corazon*, all meaning heart, are derived from the Latin *corona*, meaning crown. Thus, the root of the term *coronary arteries* reflects the esteem held for royalty, the center of sociobiological organization. The words *heart* in English and *Herz* in German are metaphors for strength and vitality.

Blood Pressure and the Heartbeat

With heart contraction, blood in the pumping chamber is ejected from the heart under high pressure. The blood squirts into the aorta through a one-way flap valve called the aortic valve. The pressure surge and blood ejected into the aorta with each heart squeeze expand it somewhat, like the inflation of a long, narrow balloon. This surge of blood and pressure with each heartbeat is transmitted through the aorta to all the arteries of the body and causes the throbbing of the pulse, which is easily felt in the wrist arteries and neck. During the relaxation phase of the heart, diastole, the aortic valve closes. The closed valve prevents blood in the aorta from leaking backward into the emptied pumping chamber. During diastole, blood flowing forward from the lungs then fills the pumping chamber in preparation for the next heart contraction. During this diastolic relaxation phase, the blood pressure in the aorta is maintained by the elastic recoil of the aorta. The pressure in the aorta during diastole associated with its elastic recoil serves to maintain some pressure between heartbeats. This pressure during diastole maintains blood flow to the body between heart contractions.

The highest pressure generated in the aorta during heart contraction is called systolic pressure. The lowest pressure in the aorta between heartbeats is called diastolic pressure. The measurement of blood pressure is usually given as two numbers. The first and higher number is systolic pressure during heart contraction. It is written above or before the second and lower number, which is the diastolic pressure present between heartbeats. (See figure 1.4.) A blood pressure measurement gives the pressure at which blood circulates in the body. It does not describe the volume or adequacy of blood flow. Blood pressure is therefore analogous to oil pressure in a car, which shows the pressure at which the oil circulates but not the volume or flow of oil in the engine.

The units of blood pressure are expressed as millimeters of mercury based on medical custom. The unit millimeters of mercury refers to that pressure at the bottom of a column of mercury in a glass tube attached to a

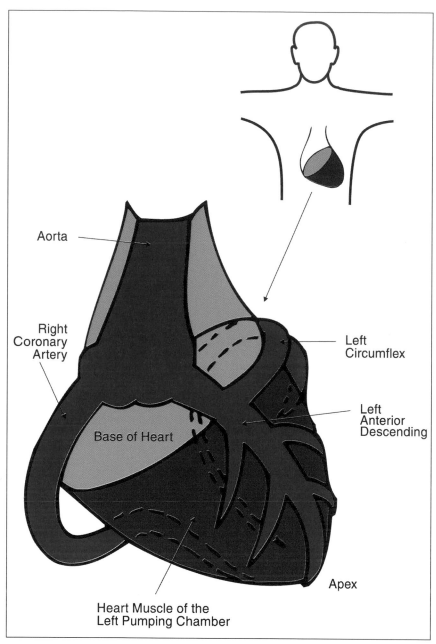

Figure 1.3. Orientation of the Heart and Coronary Arteries

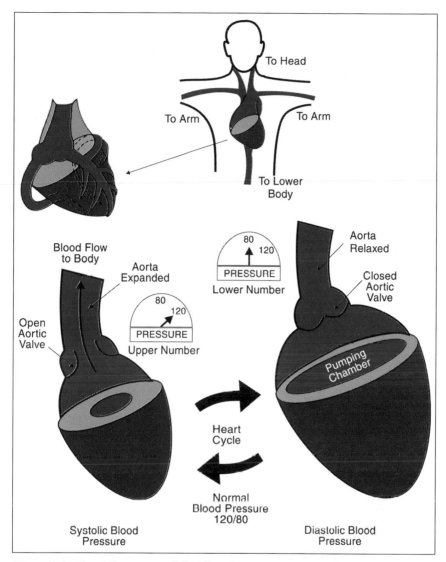

Figure 1.4. Blood Pressure and the Heartbeat

blood pressure cuff around the arm. The systolic blood pressure is normally approximately 120 millimeters of mercury, which is equivalent to approximately 0.3 pounds per square inch (psi) if expressed like the pressure in an automobile tire. A tire pressure of 25 psi is equivalent to 1,200 millimeters of mercury, or ten times the normal blood pressure.

Blood pressure is measured by inflating an air cuff around the arm until the artery in the arm is compressed shut with no blood flow through it.

The air cuff is then deflated slowly until the first squirt of blood into the collapsed artery is heard with a stethoscope placed over the artery. The pressure in the cuff at the first sound heard as the blood begins to squirt through the partially compressed artery is systolic pressure. The pressure in the cuff when there is no more squirting noise (because the artery is no longer compressed) is the diastolic pressure.

Cholesterol and Coronary Heart Disease

Cardiovascular disease is principally due to cholesterol deposited from the blood into the walls of arteries throughout the body. This cholesterol deposition causes scarring and calcification of the artery, giving rise to the term *hardening of the arteries*, or *atherosclerosis*. Atherosclerosis leads to partial or complete blockages of the arteries and inadequate blood flow to various parts of the body. Coronary heart disease is caused by atherosclerosis of the coronary arteries, which restricts the blood supply to the heart muscle; hence the synonym, *coronary artery disease*.

The buildup of cholesterol in the walls of the arteries is slow, accumulating over many years, commonly starting when a person is twenty to thirty years old. This cholesterol accumulation is increased by smoking, high blood cholesterol levels, high blood pressure, fatty food, genetic tendencies, inactivity, and other risk factors reviewed later.

The cholesterol deposit is covered by the inner lining of the artery, which forms a fibrous cap on the cholesterol in the arterial wall. The cholesterol causes inflammation, which weakens the shoulder of this fibrous cap where it joins the wall of the artery. A *cholesterol plaque* is the term applied to the combination of the cholesterol deposition, the fibrous cap, inflammation, scarring, and calcium deposition. A cholesterol plaque grows slowly over many years, merging with many other cholesterol plaques along the artery so that the wall of the artery is infiltrated with cholesterol diffusely but irregularly throughout its length. The cholesterol buildup is greater in some segments, causing localized, more severe narrowings called stenoses.

There are substantial mechanical stresses at the shoulder of the fibrous cap. The pulsing pressure of each heartbeat exacerbates these stresses and further weakens the fibrous tissue at the shoulder. If the mechanical stresses and inflammation weaken the shoulder attachment enough, the fibrous cap may break or rupture at one of its corners.

When this plaque ruptures at the shoulder, the blood pressure forces blood under the ruptured cap, lifts it up into and partially blocks the artery. The cholesterol and tissues under the fibrous cap come in contact with blood, causing the blood to clot. This clot, or thrombosis, then causes more blood clotting, which extends into the inside, or lumen, of the artery and further blocks it, either completely or partially. The blood clot in the coronary artery is called a coronary thrombosis. It may partially or completely block blood

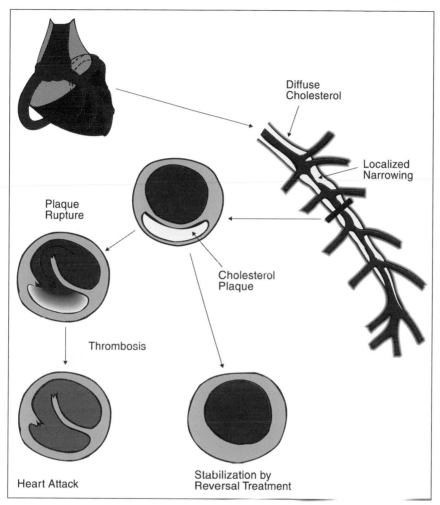

Figure 1.5. Cholesterol, Heart Attack, and Reversal Treatment

flow to the heart muscle. Partial blockage of blood flow in the coronary artery causes chest pain. Complete blockage of blood flow causes a heart attack. (See figure 1.5.) The medical term for a heart attack is *myocardial infarction*. It indicates death of the heart muscle supplied by the blocked artery.

Plaque rupture typically occurs at sites in the coronary artery where the cholesterol buildup is relatively new, without severe narrowing of the artery and without extensive scarring or calcification. With this early atherosclerosis, the fibrous cap of the soft, mushy, young plaque is thin and easily ruptured. Therefore, a person with coronary atherosclerosis without a significant narrowing of the artery may feel well and do strenuous exercise without limitations or symptoms since there is adequate blood flow through the coronary artery. However, minutes later the plaque may rupture, thereby causing thrombosis and a heart attack.

Like coronary heart disease, cardiovascular disease throughout the body is caused primarily by cholesterol deposition in the walls of the arteries. It is associated with several factors that increase the risk, such as smoking, high blood pressure, high cholesterol levels in blood, and a family history of cardiovascular disease. The cholesterol stimulates inflammation, scarring, and calcification, which narrow the artery and limit its blood flow. This process of atherosclerosis usually affects arteries in some parts of the body more than others. As noted, coronary heart disease involves the coronary arteries to the heart muscle. Blockage of the coronary arteries causes chest pain, heart attack, sudden death, or heart failure. Atherosclerosis of arteries to the brain (cerebrum) is called cerebrovascular disease. Blockage of cerebral arteries causes a stroke, associated with paralysis, speech difficulty, loss of consciousness or sensation, and perhaps death. Peripheral vascular disease involves the arteries to the limbs, particularly the legs, where blockage may result in leg pain during exercise, loss of toes, foot, or lower leg. The terms *coronary artery disease, coronary heart disease, coronary atherosclerosis* are used interchangeably. The term *cardiovascular* is somewhat more general, referring to the heart and other arteries throughout the body.

Someone with atherosclerosis of the arteries to the brain (cerebrovascular disease) or in the legs (peripheral vascular disease) is more likely to have coronary atherosclerosis as well. However, having one of these types of cardiovascular diseases does not necessarily mean that the other types are present. Most commonly these types of cardiovascular disease occur independently, but they do appear often enough together to have some association. Why similar risk factors produce one form of cardiovascular disease in an individual without the other types of disease is not known. For example, stroke is somewhat more associated with high blood pressure than is coronary artery disease, even though high blood pressure is a risk factor for both problems.

Reversal treatment markedly lowers levels of cholesterol in the blood and stops its deposition in the arterial wall. In addition, previously deposited cholesterol is absorbed out of the arterial wall. With removal of cholesterol from the wall of artery, the fibrous cap adheres to the arterial wall; it cannot rupture, and the plaque stabilizes. The risk of plaque rupture, thrombosis, and therefore of a heart attack markedly decreases. The artery becomes somewhat bigger, and areas of localized narrowing in the artery become somewhat less severe. Although cholesterol and inflammation are removed in this process of partial regression, the scarring and calcification remain unchanged, so the artery does not return to normal. However, the narrowing becomes less severe, and coronary blood flow improves.

When cholesterol is removed from the arterial wall, the risk of plaque rupture is markedly reduced, even though the severity of the narrowing decreases only modestly. There is a corresponding marked reduction in heart attacks, death, unstable chest pain, strokes, and need for bypass surgery or balloon dilation. Cholesterol removal from the arterial wall occurs optimally at the lowest blood levels of LDL cholesterol (the low-density, or "low down lipid," or bad cholesterol) and at the highest levels of HDL cholesterol (the high-density, or "highly defensive," good cholesterol). The HDL cholesterol serves as a transporter to remove the LDL cholesterol from the arterial wall. Therefore, HDL cholesterol should be increased as much as possible and LDL cholesterol reduced as much as possible.

More vigorous cholesterol lowering than has been conventionally employed is necessary to achieve stabilization or reversal of coronary heart disease. In recent studies, people with coronary heart disease following standard dietary guidelines of the American Heart Association for 20 to 30 percent of calories as fat showed progression of coronary heart disease. Those who were treated more vigorously with lower-fat food and/or cholesterol-lowering drugs showed regression or stopped progression of coronary heart disease.

The Damaged Heart

Sudden blockage of a coronary artery usually occurs during plaque rupture and thrombosis, which stop blood flow to the heart muscle. Blockage of flow in the coronary artery for more than thirty to sixty minutes causes a heart attack, or myocardial infarction, in which a segment of the heart muscle dies. (See figure 1.6.) The contraction of this heart segment then stops. The damaged heart wall thins and later forms a scar. If the interruption of blood flow to the heart muscle is only temporary, lasting five to ten minutes, the heart muscle may be only temporarily stunned. During this stunning period the heart muscle fails to contract. However, it may recover its function over a period of weeks without scarring.

Normally with each heart contraction, 50 percent or more of blood in the pumping chamber at the end of diastole is ejected into the aorta. This fraction, or percentage, of blood in the pumping chamber that is ejected with each heartbeat is called the ejection fraction. It is normally 50 percent or greater. When approximately 23 percent of heart muscle is damaged and stops contracting, the ejection fraction falls below 50 percent. With progressive heart damage, the ejection fraction may fall further, to only 8 percent or 10 percent. This level of pumping impairment causes fatigue, limited exercise capacity, difficulty breathing, ankle swelling, and shortened life span.

Heart Failure

After a heart attack that damages part of the heart, the surrounding normal parts of the pumping chamber contract more vigorously than normal to compensate for the damaged nonfunctioning segments. This compensatory

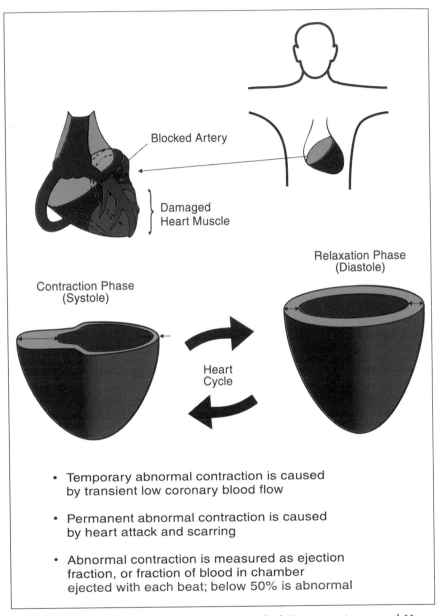

Blocked Artery

Damaged
Heart Muscle

Relaxation Phase
(Diastole)

Contraction Phase
(Systole)

Heart
Cycle

- Temporary abnormal contraction is caused
  by transient low coronary blood flow

- Permanent abnormal contraction is caused
  by heart attack and scarring

- Abnormal contraction is measured as ejection
  fraction, or fraction of blood in chamber
  ejected with each beat; below 50% is abnormal

Figure 1.6. The Damaged Heart Due to a Blocked Coronary Artery and Heart Attack

overcontraction maintains a normal amount of blood ejected with each heartbeat until approximately 23 percent of the pumping chamber is permanently damaged or scarred. With a large heart attack or several heart attacks that cause cumulative damage of greater than 23 percent of the pumping chamber, the ejection fraction falls below the normal 50 percent.

Over a period of months to years, the overworked normal segments of the pumping chamber become fatigued with less efficient pumping function. The heart enlarges, which makes its contractile force weaker and pumping action less effective. The ejection fraction falls progressively lower. The heart then fails to pump enough blood to the body organs, causing a condition called heart failure. (See figure 1.7.) In heart failure, inadequate blood flow to the kidneys causes retention of fluid, which collects in the lungs. This fluid in the lungs makes breathing very difficult with a sense of suffocation. Normal breathing sounds heard with a stethoscope change to bubbling sounds—a sign of fluid in the lungs. In addition, fluid may collect in the ankles, causing them to swell. The low blood flow to the body causes fatigue and reduced exercise capacity. The symptoms of heart failure are therefore short-windedness, fatigue, ankle swelling, and inability to do physical activity.

Development of heart failure may be sudden, over a few hours, as a consequence of a large heart attack. It may also develop slowly over a period of months to years as the heart slowly enlarges from progressive damage or weakening. Heart failure is treated by diuretics (which rid the body of excess fluid), drugs that strengthen heart contraction, and other drugs that reduce the workload on the heart, allowing it to function more effectively. The latter drugs also minimize the progressive heart enlargement that signifies progressive heart failure and shortened survival.

The Electrocardiogram and the Heartbeat

The rate at which the heart beats and the regularity of the heartbeat are controlled by specialized tissues of the heart called the pacemaker and conduction system. The pacemaker fires off electrical impulses at regular intervals like a biological electric clock. These electrical impulses are conducted throughout the heart muscle by a network of fine biological electrical "wires." The distribution of the pacemaker impulses throughout this circuitry is coordinated in order to stimulate the heart muscle to contract simultaneously everywhere around the pumping chamber. With this coordinated contraction, the pumping chamber squeezes efficiently and uniformly during systole. Consequently, with each heartbeat a blood pressure is generated and blood is squirted into the aorta, where it is fed to the rest of the body.

This electrical activity of the heart is recorded as an electrocardiogram (ECG) by an ECG machine. (See figure 1.8.) The ECG machine is essentially

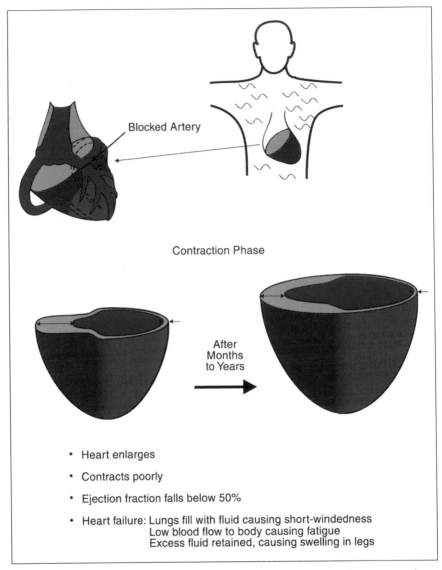

Contraction Phase

Blocked Artery

After
Months
to Years

- Heart enlarges
- Contracts poorly
- Ejection fraction falls below 50%
- Heart failure: Lungs fill with fluid causing short-windedness
  Low blood flow to body causing fatigue
  Excess fluid retained, causing swelling in legs

Figure 1.7. Heart Failure Due to Heart Enlargement over Months to Years after a Heart Attack

a sensitive voltmeter that measures the electrical activity of the heart in millivolts, or one-thousandth of a volt. Each electrical impulse spreading throughout the heart is recorded as a voltage spike on the ECG. Each of these voltage spikes triggers a mechanical contraction, or systole. Systole is followed by the relaxation phase of diastole, during which the electrical conducting system and heart muscle recover or recharge in preparation for the next heartbeat.

Sudden Death

Sudden blockage of a coronary artery may alter the heart's electrical be-havior. At the borders of damaged areas of the pumping chamber, abnormal electrical pacemaking activity may develop, called an arrhythmia. These ab-normal pacemakers may fire off electrical signals that override the normal pacemaker function. Abnormal pacemaker sites usually drive the heart at very fast rates of up to 250 beats per minute. They also cause an abnormal

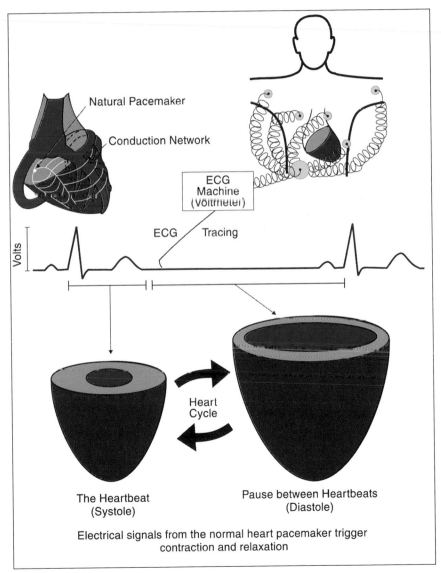

Figure 1.8. The Electrocardiogram and the Heartbeat

ECG. The abnormal ECG signals are typically wide and slurred, whereas normal ECG signals are sharp and narrow.

When the heart is driven by these fast, abnormal pacemakers, the pumping function is impaired because the relaxation phase of the heart cycle is not long enough to allow adequate filling of the pumping chamber for the following contraction. Since the heart does not pump enough blood to the body, the blood pressure falls. This fall in blood pressure may reduce blood flow to the brain, causing fainting or brain damage. Blood flow in the coronary arteries is also reduced, leading to further heart damage, which impairs pumping still more and causes further fall in blood pressure. This vicious cycle may cause death within a few minutes. (See figure 1.9.) Because of this risk, some patients with potentially dangerous arrhythmias are monitored in an intensive coronary care unit where the arrhythmia may be immediately treated if it occurs.

Disruption of the normal electrical behavior of the heart may become so extreme that the electrical signals are completely disorganized. When the electrical signals become completely disorganized or chaotic, the pumping chamber does not contract rhythmically. It simply quivers without any pumping action. In this case, the ECG shows wavy irregular lines without the rhythmic electrical signals normally seen. In the absence of heart pumping, there is no blood pressure and death also quickly follows. With appropriate equipment and experienced personnel immediately available, as in a coronary care unit, an electrical shock may be applied across the chest wall with two electrical paddles in order to restore coordinated electrical activity and pumping function. Unfortunately, this benefit may be only temporary. The usual outcomes of progressive coronary heart disease are heart attacks leading to heart failure or sudden death. However, reversal treatment as described in this book can stop progression or partially reverse coronary atherosclerosis and prevent heart attacks that cause heart failure and sudden death.

Dysfunctional Coronary Arteries—A Time Bomb

Plaque rupture and heart attack cause structural damage to the heart muscle that is fixed and irreversible. However, before this structural damage occurs, coronary atherosclerosis alters the functioning of the coronary arteries. Functional abnormalities are dynamic and may change over a period of minutes to months. They may cause transient reduction in blood flow in the coronary arteries. This reduction in blood flow to the heart muscle may cause chest pain; sometimes it may be clinically silent and not cause any symptoms.

Coronary arteries normally become larger, or dilate (vasodilate), under conditions of exercise or stress. However, as explained in more detail later, smoking, hypertension, high cholesterol levels in blood, or cholesterol deposition in the arterial wall interferes with this normal vasodilation. Under

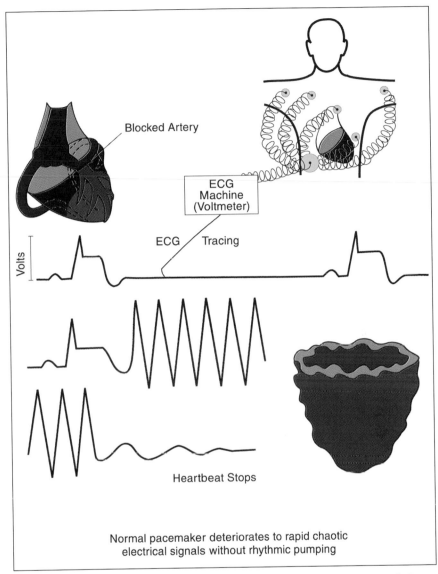

Blocked Artery

ECG
Machine
(Voltmeter)

ECG   Tracing

Volts

Heartbeat Stops

Normal pacemaker deteriorates to rapid chaotic
electrical signals without rhythmic pumping

Figure 1.9. Sudden Death Due to Coronary Heart Disease or Heart Attack Causing Abnormal Heart Rhythm

these conditions, the coronary artery may go into spasm or constrict (vasoconstriction) during stress, exercise, or even at resting conditions. The coronary artery may vasoconstrict diffusely along its entire length or at local sites of cholesterol plaque. This vasoconstriction may transiently reduce coronary blood flow, cause partial thrombosis, or contribute to partial plaque rupture, which narrows but does not completely block the artery. (See figure 1.10.)

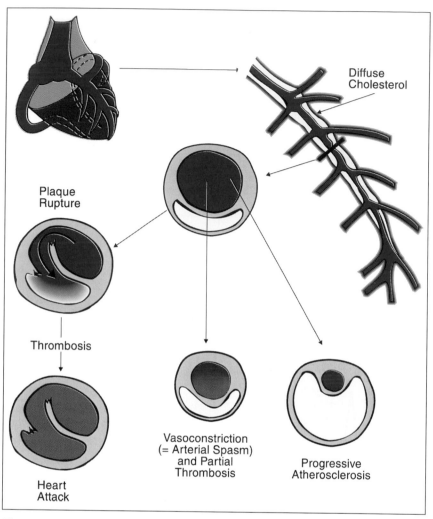

Figure 1.10. Dysfunctional Coronary Arteries—A Time Bomb Leading to Chest Pain or Heart Attack

Atherosclerosis may also progressively narrow the coronary artery slowly by accumulating cholesterol, scarring, and calcium in the wall of the coronary artery. The buildup of these deposits is usually greatest on one side of the artery, making it appear lopsided or eccentric when viewed in cross section. However, even such severe narrowing of the coronary arteries is not completely fixed. Sites of severe narrowing may retain the capacity for dynamic changes, including transient worsening (vasoconstriction) or improvement (vasodilation). These dynamic changes occur principally in the segment of the arterial wall that is not yet calcified and scarred.

Chest pain may be a sign of any of several different heart problems, such as heart attack, coronary artery spasm, or progressive accumulation of cholesterol in the arterial wall causing a localized narrowing. All of these abnormal processes restrict blood flow in the coronary arteries, which causes the chest pain.

The Silver Lining

The dynamic functional changes in the coronary arteries of vasoconstriction and vasodilation are largely controlled by a thin layer of vascular cells that line the inner surface of the artery. This thin lining is called the endothelium (pronounced end-o-*thee*-lee-um). Normal endothelial function causes the coronary artery to enlarge, or vasodilate, with increasing blood flow to heart muscle in response to exercise or stress. Smoking, hypertension, high levels of cholesterol in blood, or cholesterol deposited in the wall of the artery impairs the normal function of the endothelium. The loss of normal endothelial function may cause vasoconstriction, or further transient narrowing, of the artery at sites of cholesterol plaque or previously narrowed areas due to cholesterol buildup. This vasoconstriction may in turn reduce blood flow to the heart muscle during resting conditions or in response to exercise or stress. (See figure 1.11.)

Blood Clots in Coronary Arteries

Other functional changes in the coronary arteries involve interaction between the endothelial lining and small particles in the blood responsible for clotting, or thrombosis. These small particles are called platelets. Normally, platelets circulate in the blood in a quiescent state without sticking to the endothelium or inside walls of the coronary artery. Normal endothelium secretes two substances that prevent platelet clumping, or clot formation. They also cause vasodilation of the coronary artery with improved blood flow. These beneficial substances are called prostacyclin and nitric oxide.

Smoking, high blood pressure, high levels of cholesterol in the blood, or cholesterol deposited in the arterial wall impairs normal endothelial function and inhibits the secretion of the beneficial substances. Worse, the injured endothelial lining secretes an excess of a substance called thromboxane, which promotes clotting and vasoconstriction. The platelets circulating in the blood are activated by contact with the damaged endothelium and by the thromboxane. The activated platelets form sticky clumps, which adhere to the damaged arterial wall; they also activate other platelets, which then form several layers of platelets. These layers of clumped platelets progress to a blood clot, or thrombosis, in the artery. (See figure 1.12.)

Commonly, endothelial injury due to smoking, high blood pressure, elevated cholesterol, or other noxious stimuli may cause only partial thrombosis and spasm of the artery that are transient. However, the spasm and

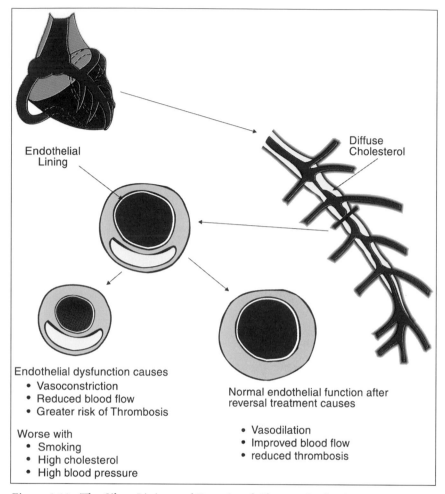

Figure 1.11. The Silver Lining and Functional Changes in the Coronary Arteries

thrombosis may partially or completely block blood flow in the artery like a plaque rupture. Over several days to weeks, the clots that adhere to the arterial wall may become incorporated into the scarring process. The result is progressive, permanent, structural narrowing of the artery.

The endothelium secretes thirty or more substances similar to prostacyclin or thromboxane that may also have opposing effects on the function of the coronary artery and platelets. The normal balance of their combined effects are to vasodilate the coronary artery and inhibit clumping of the platelets. However, with injury to the endothelial cells, which inhibit their function, the balance of these various substances is shifted toward causing arterial spasm, platelet clumping, thrombosis, and low coronary blood flow. The commonest causes of injury to the endothelium are smoking, elevated cholesterol levels in blood, cholesterol deposition in the arterial wall, and high blood pressure.

All arteries throughout the body demonstrate this delicate balance between substances that inhibit blood clotting platelets (vasodilate the arteries) and those that clump platelets (vasoconstrict the arteries). This balance serves to protect the individual from bleeding to death after external trauma. For example, after a finger is cut, the cut may bleed profusely. However, this injury to the endothelium of the blood vessels causes secretion of substances that produce platelet clumping, thrombosis, vasoconstriction, and blockage of the damaged arteries. The bleeding therefore stops, and healing occurs.

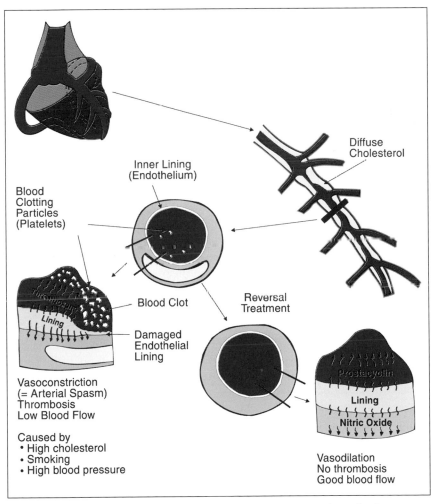

Figure 1.12. Blood Clots in Coronary Arteries—Coronary Thrombosis

Thus, these processes serve a protective function after external injury. However, after internal injury of the endothelium caused by smoking, high blood pressure, or elevated cholesterol, the same reaction may have deleterious effects. These harmful effects include vasoconstriction of the artery, thrombosis, and low blood flow resulting in chest pain or heart attack.

Reversal treatment of coronary heart disease by lowering cholesterol, controlling blood pressure, and stopping smoking heals the damaged endothelium and restores the balance of these substances to normal. The arteries then vasodilate, platelet clumping is inhibited, and blood flow improves. Consequently, the accompanying chest pain that occurs with these transient imbalances also improves. With reversal treatment, the person with coronary heart disease therefore feels better, has markedly reduced risk of heart attack and improved longevity.

Narrowed Arteries and Swirling Flow

In the absence of reversal treatment, coronary artery disease progresses in two ways. Cholesterol continues to accumulate in the walls of the coronary arteries with associated scarring, calcification, and progressive diffuse narrowing. Localized narrowings may also develop and worsen due to partial plaque rupture and partial thrombosis without complete blockage of the artery. After partial thrombosis, the clot on the wall of the artery is incorporated into the wall as a scar that thickens it and narrows the artery. Characteristically, these localized narrowings are scattered throughout the coronary arteries in addition to the diffuse narrowing.

The localized, more severe narrowings in coronary arteries cause flow eddies, or swirling flow, that dissipate the pressure wave transmitted from the aorta with each heartbeat. The pressure in the coronary artery downstream from the narrowing is therefore lower than the pressure upstream, before the narrowing. This lowered pressure is associated with lower coronary blood flow caused by the resistance of the localized, more severe narrowing. In addition to the effects of localized narrowings, blood flowing along the entire length of the diffusely narrowed arteries is subject to friction between the layers of blood flow in the artery and the arterial walls. The friction of flow increases markedly with more severe diffuse narrowing. It also is worse with greater thickness of the blood, analogous to thicker motor oil in an engine due to its higher viscosity. This viscous friction slows blood flow further and also dissipates the pressure wave normally transmitted from the aorta through the coronary artery. (See figure 1.13.)

Coronary blood flow capacity is reduced by the formation of flow eddies downstream beyond the localized narrowing and by the viscous friction along the length of the diffusely narrowed arteries. The reduction in blood flow capacity is particularly severe under conditions of stress, when higher blood flow is needed by heart muscle.

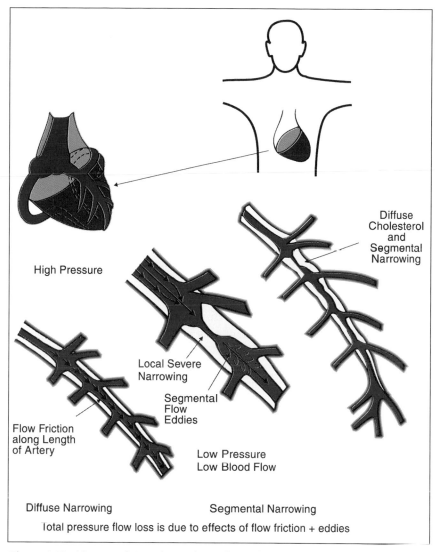

High Pressure

Local Severe
Narrowing

Segmental
Flow
Eddies

Flow Friction
along Length
of Artery

Low Pressure
Low Blood Flow

Diffuse
Cholesterol
and
Segmental
Narrowing

Diffuse Narrowing   Segmental Narrowing

Total pressure flow loss is due to effects of flow friction + eddies

Figure 1.13. Narrowed Arteries and Swirling Flow—Effects of Diffuse and Segmental Narrowing of Coronary Arteries on Blood Flow and Pressure in the Artery

The severity of narrowing is usually described in terms of percent narrowing. Since this local segmental narrowing is called a stenosis, the term *percent stenosis* is used, referring to the percent reduction in the diameter of the inside of the artery, or lumen, as seen on an X-ray picture of the artery called an angiogram or an arteriogram. However, percent stenosis is just one dimension of several measurements of the diseased coronary artery that determine its severity.

The dimensions of the localized coronary artery narrowing *and* the dimensions of the entire artery along its length determine how severely blood flow capacity is limited. The most important specific dimensions affecting blood flow capacity include:

1. The length of the arterial narrowing.
2. The absolute cross-sectional size of the artery at its narrowest point.
3. The relative percent reduction in the cross-sectional size compared with adjacent segments of the artery without localized narrowing.
4. The shape of the narrowing that determines its streamlining.

Therefore, measuring the percent narrowing alone, as is done clinically on coronary arteriograms, is an incomplete, inaccurate measure of severity of the narrowing. The single dimension of percent narrowing does not reflect how limited coronary blood flow will be. Nor does it indicate severity of flow limitation because it does not account for the absolute size of the artery, the length of the narrowing, or its shape, all of which also determine flow capacity. To correctly quantify severity of narrowing requires measurement of all these dimensions. The effect of each dimension is then integrated by computer, using fluid dynamic equations that predict the correct flow capacity.

Normally, at resting conditions, workload of the heart muscle is relatively low. Therefore, coronary blood flow is also fairly low but adequate for the low work demands at resting conditions. Under such conditions, the effects of flow eddies and viscous friction are small, even with severe narrowing, and blood flow throughout the heart is adequate and uniformly distributed. Consequently, someone with fairly severe narrowing of the coronary arteries may have enough blood flow to the heart at resting conditions and experience no chest pain or symptoms.

During intense exercise, coronary blood flow normally increases in order to meet the increased workload on the heart. In an atherosclerotic, narrowed coronary artery, the needed increase in flow is limited by flow eddies and viscous friction, which become markedly worse as flow rises in response to work demands. The worsening flow eddies and viscous friction cause a progressively greater resistance to flow as coronary blood flow tries to increase during exercise. There is inadequate blood flow to heart muscle for meeting work demands, thereby causing chest pain on exertion. Once exercise is stopped and the workload on the heart decreases, coronary blood flow falls, flow eddies and viscous friction diminish. Resistance to flow decreases, and normal resting flow is restored to levels adequate for low resting workloads.

Coronary artery narrowing therefore reduces maximum flow capacity to meet the demands of increased heart work. This capacity to increase coronary blood flow is called coronary flow reserve. Normally, coronary flow reserve in a healthy young adult is 3.5 to 4.0. In other words, coronary blood flow can increase by 3.5 to 4.0 times baseline resting levels. Factors responsible for reducing coronary flow reserve include coronary artery narrowing, cholesterol deposition in the arterial wall, elevated cholesterol levels in blood, smoking, and hypertension. People affected by one or more of these factors will have an improvement in coronary flow reserve after successful reversal treatment.

The Give-and-Take of the Heartbeat

Normally, there is adequate flow of blood through the coronary arteries and throughout the wall of the heart muscle in the relaxation phase between heartbeats (diastole). However, during systole the powerful contraction of the heart muscle squeezes down the network of small blood vessels enmeshing the heart muscle. This squeeze is so powerful that the small blood vessels collapse, stopping blood flow to the inner layers of the heart muscle where the squeezing forces are greatest. Diastole provides a momentary period of rest without heart muscle contraction. The network of small blood vessels opens up and provides good blood flow throughout the wall of the heart muscle in preparation for the next heartbeat. (See figure 1.14.)

The diastolic period between heartbeats therefore allows two crucial events. The pumping chamber fills with oxygen-carrying blood flowing forward from the lungs; coronary blood flow reaches the heart muscle delivering oxygen throughout the wall. Both of these steps are essential for the next contraction to occur. Although coronary blood flow is momentarily stopped during the systolic squeeze, coronary blood flow to the heart muscle during the relaxation phase between heartbeats is high enough to meet the needs of the heart muscle over the entire heart cycle. Thus, the heart pumps life-sustaining, blood-carrying oxygen to the rest of the body during the heartbeat. Between beats, the heart takes the blood flow it needs from the aorta through the coronary arteries to the heart muscle in order to continue pumping.

Narrowed Arteries and the Pumping Heart

As we have seen, narrowing of the coronary arteries limits the increase in blood flow required to meet the workload demanded of the heart during exercise. This limiting effect is particularly severe during diastole, when high coronary blood flow is needed to make up for the normal absence of flow during systole. When coronary blood flow and pressure are inadequate due to coronary artery narrowing, the blood flow does not penetrate the entire thickness of the heart wall during the diastolic phase. Therefore, over the entire heart cycle, blood flow is inadequate to maintain normal contraction. (See figure 1.15.)

This deficiency of blood flow to the inner layers of the heart muscle usually causes symptoms that make the individual stop whatever stressful activity is causing them. The inadequacy of blood flow and pressure to the heart muscle is called ischemia. It also causes characteristic changes on the ECG, as during an exercise stress test (discussed in part 3). Ischemia may also occur at resting conditions if the narrowing is severe enough. The symptoms caused by inadequate blood flow to heart muscle are chest pain, pallor, sweating, short-windedness, weakness, ECG abnormalities, and impaired pumping function of the heart. They are warning signs of coronary heart disease.

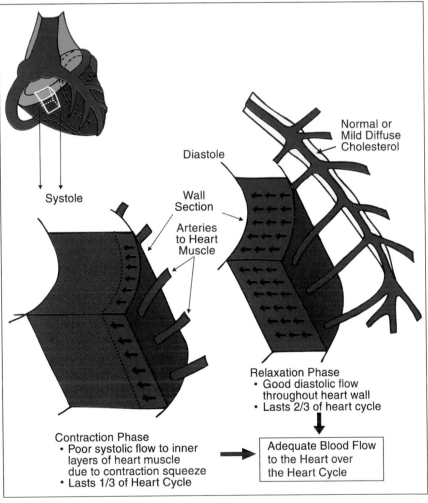

Figure 1.14. The Give-and-Take of the Heartbeat—Normal Blood Flow and Pressure to Heart Muscle during Contraction and Relaxation Phases

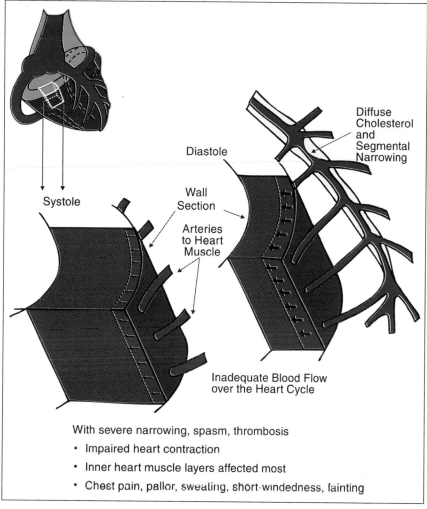

Diffuse
Cholesterol
and
Segmental
Narrowing

Diastole

Wall
Section

Systole

Arteries
to Heart
Muscle

Inadequate Blood Flow
over the Heart Cycle

With severe narrowing, spasm, thrombosis
- Impaired heart contraction
- Inner heart muscle layers affected most
- Chest pain, pallor, sweating, short-windedness, fainting

Figure 1.15. Narrowed Arteries and the Pumping Heart—Low Blood Flow and Pressure to Heart Muscle during Contraction and Relaxation Phases Due to Narrowing of the Coronary Artery

However, low coronary blood flow and ischemia may be present but cause no symptoms.

The coronary arteries may be only mildly narrowed or dysfunctional due to cholesterol deposited in the wall of the arteries. This early stage of atherosclerosis carries a significant risk of plaque rupture, thrombosis, and unexpected heart attack or sudden death. Standard stress testing does not reliably identify this silent, early stage of coronary heart disease. However, accurate quantitative pictures of blood flow in the heart muscle by positron emission tomography (PET) can be used to identify coronary atherosclerosis. Reversal treatment can then be started to heal dysfunctional arteries, reduce severity of narrowing, improve coronary blood flow, reduce or eliminate symptoms, and markedly reduce risk of heart attacks or sudden death.

Growing New Blood Vessels—Collaterals

Progression of coronary artery narrowing may occur very slowly. Complete blockage of the coronary artery may take months or even years. This slow progression allows the growth of new blood vessels from other coronary arteries into the branches of the blocked artery. These new blood vessels are called collaterals. They may grow sufficiently to form a natural bypass of the blockage, providing blood flow to the area of muscle previously supplied by the blocked artery. Well-developed collaterals may become so effective that the blood flow is as good as in the original native artery before it was blocked. Collaterals that are less well developed may provide enough blood flow to support normal heart needs and function at resting conditions but not during exercise. Consequently, chest pain may occur only during exercise when coronary blood flow is inadequate. Despite chest pain during exercise, there is little danger of a heart attack since the natural bypass through the collaterals provides enough blood flow to maintain the heart muscle. (See figure 1.16.)

Repeated controlled exercise and repetitive with mild to moderate ischemia stimulates the growth of more collaterals. Improved blood flow through this bigger network of collaterals then helps prevent ischemia during exercise and allows progressively greater intensity of exercise before ischemia occurs. The improved collaterals may eventually restore normal blood flow to heart muscle both at rest and during exercise with no symptoms or limitations of activity.

Sometimes coronary artery narrowing is so severe and hardened by calcium deposition that it cannot reverse even partially. However, reversal treatment usually stops progression or slows it enough for collaterals to grow. The collaterals then provide enough blood flow to heart muscle to prevent heart attack when the artery blocks off completely. For such severe, calcified narrowing of a coronary artery, reversal treatment "buys time" for collaterals to grow. This course of events is remarkably consistent in people with coronary heart disease who follow the reversal treatment, particularly if the pumping function of the heart is good when reversal treatment is started.

Progression of coronary artery disease may block the arteries supplying blood flow to the collaterals. Blockage of these supply arteries could then cause an even larger heart attack because the heart muscle supplied by both arteries would be affected. Reversal treatment markedly reduces the risk of progression, or blockage of the arteries supplying the collaterals. Therefore, reversal treatment is important for protecting the heart muscle even if an

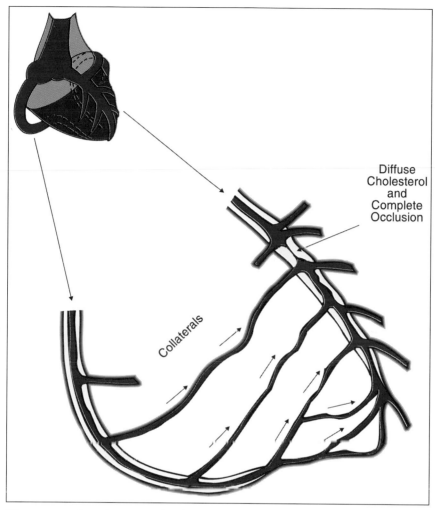

Figure 1.16. Growing New Blood Vessels (Collaterals) beyond a Blocked Coronary Artery

artery is already completely blocked and supplied by collaterals from other coronary arteries.

Blue Clues to Finding the Silent Killer

For evaluating coronary artery disease, pictures of blood flow in the heart muscle, called images, are obtained at resting conditions and during stress. In this instance, stress is pharmacologic, produced by a drug called dipyridamole. The first step is to obtain a picture of blood flow in the heart muscle at resting conditions. If there has been no previous heart attack or scarring of the heart, the image of blood flow in the heart muscle at rest is normal and uniform. If there is scarring from previous heart damage, the picture shows an abnormality, or area of low blood flow, where there is a scar. Next, dipyridamole is given intravenously, which normally increases blood flow in the heart muscle by three to four times the baseline resting levels. It is safe because the heart does not undergo an exercise workload. (While treadmill or bicycle exercise can also be used as a stress, neither of these is as reliable as dipyridamole for increasing blood flow to heart muscle.) A second blood flow image is then obtained after injecting the radiotracer during dipyridamole-induced stress when the blood flow in the heart muscle is highest. In areas of the heart not affected by atherosclerosis, the blood flow in the heart muscle is normal. In areas where there is narrowing of the coronary arteries, the maximum blood flow is reduced. This area of reduced maximum blood flow shows as an abnormal region of relatively low flow in the blood flow picture, indicating impaired coronary flow reserve. (See figure 1.17.)

Hence coronary artery disease can be detected by the picture of blood flow in the heart muscle after dipyridamole injection. The severity of this abnormality of maximum blood flow in the heart muscle indicates the severity of the narrowing in the coronary artery. Of the several technologies now available for taking pictures of blood flow in heart muscle, the most accurate one is positron emission tomography (PET). PET imaging is the only diagnostic test that can evaluate the cumulative effects of *all* the coronary artherosclerois along the length of the artery (both localized severe segmental narrowing and diffuse milder narrowing throughout the artery) and even detect the effects of risk factors on the heart. PET imaging also has the advantage of being noninvasive, requiring only an intravenous injection. The remainder of part 1 focuses on how PET images appear under various conditions of blood flow in the heart muscle. In part 3, we will take a closer look at all the tests currently used in the diagosis and treatment of coronary heart disease.

PET pictures of blood flow in heart muscle are displayed in a color scale. The warm colors (such as red, orange, and yellow) indicate good to adequate flow, respectively. The cold colors (purple, blue, and black) indicate progressively severe deficiency of blood flow in heart muscle on either resting or stress blood flow pictures.

Both diffuse atherosclerosis (see "Rainbow Clues," below) and localized severe segmental narrowing appear as abnormalities on the blood flow images. Typically, the localized segmental narrowing causes a discrete blue area with clear borders on the stress picture where the red sharply changes to blue. This sharp color change, or color gradient, shows the shift from normal blood flow to impaired blood flow in heart muscle. The location of this discrete abnormality indicates which artery is involved and where in the artery the narrowing is located.

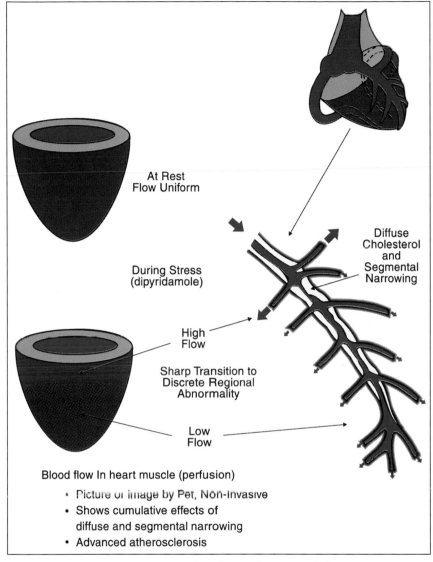

Figure 1.17. Blue Clues to Finding the Silent Killer—Blood Flow in Heart Muscle with Segmental Narrowing at Resting and Stress Conditions

Rainbow Clues

Diffuse coronary artery narrowing throughout its length causes a gradually progressive, decreased flow capacity along the length of the coronary artery. At the top of the heart (called the base of the heart), blood flow is relatively normal since the cumulative effects of diffuse narrowing are minimal within the short length of artery supplying the base of the heart. In the mid-section of the heart, coronary flow reserve is somewhat more impaired due to more cumulative effects of a greater length of diffusely narrowed artery supplying the midsection of the heart. At the tip, or apex, of the heart, the coronary flow reserve is reduced most severely due to the cumulative effects of diffuse narrowing along the entire length of the artery.

Therefore, with diffuse coronary atherosclerosis there is a gradual gradient of progressively reduced coronary flow reserve from base to apex. On three-dimensional pictures of blood flow in the heart muscle, the top (or base) of the heart is red, indicating relatively good flow; the midsection is orange to yellow, showing intermediate flow; the tip of the heart is blue to black, reflecting the lowest flow. (See figure 1.18.) This pattern of blood flow in the heart muscle with a longitudinal "rainbow" gradient of colors is different from the discrete abnormalities with sharp borders caused by more severe localized segmental narrowing of the coronary artery.

The presence of a rainbow of colors on a PET image usually indicates that the diffuse coronary narrowing is not severe enough to restrict blood flow markedly or cause chest pain. It indicates early silent coronary atherosclerosis with risk of plaque rupture and heart attack or sudden death. It may also be due to a dysfunctional coronary artery with diffuse vasoconstriction. Commonly, diffuse vasoconstriction is caused by high levels of cholesterol in the blood or by cholesterol deposited throughout the wall of the coronary artery. These "rainbow" abnormalities have been shown to disappear with reversal treatment.

Although there are several different technologies for taking pictures of blood flow in heart muscle, positron emission tomography or PET imaging is unique among all medical diagnostic tests for evaluating the cumulative effects of diffuse narrowing throughout the coronary arteries. Not even the coronary arteriogram as now used clinically is sufficiently accurate for identifying diffuse narrowing or for detecting early coronary artery disease that may cause a heart attack.

Early Clues

Early coronary atherosclerosis or risk factors such as elevated blood cholesterol, smoking, high blood pressure, and diabetes impair the function of the endothelial lining of the coronary arteries. The artery has a normal tendency to maintain a dilated or mildly enlarged state at rest, and that tendency is also impaired. Consequently, blood flow in the heart muscle at resting conditions is mildly decreased. Since the altered endothelial function is irregular and patchy along the length of the coronary arteries, a picture of blood flow in heart muscle at resting conditions is also patchy and irregular.

After dipyridamole stress is induced, the blood flow in heart muscle increases and becomes more uniform. When a new picture of blood flow is

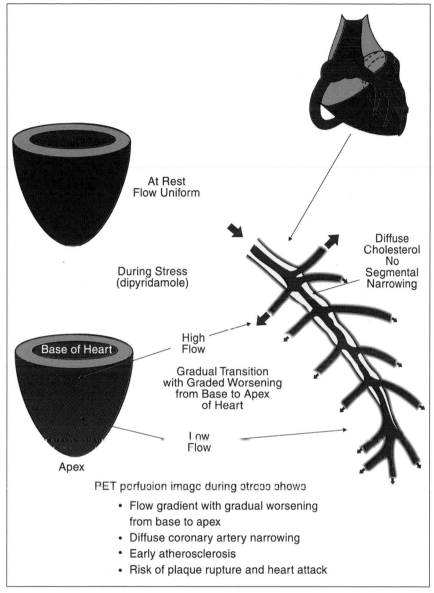

At Rest
Flow Uniform

During Stress
(dipyridamole)

Diffuse
Cholesterol
No
Segmental
Narrowing

Base of Heart

High
Flow

Gradual Transition
with Graded Worsening
from Base to Apex
of Heart

Low
Flow

Apex

PET perfusion image during stress shows

- Flow gradient with gradual worsening
  from base to apex
- Diffuse coronary artery narrowing
- Early atherosclerosis
- Risk of plaque rupture and heart attack

Figure 1.18. Rainbow Clues—Blood Flow in Heart Muscle with Diffuse Narrowing but No Segmental Narrowing at Resting and Stress Conditions

taken, the flow appears normal and evenly distributed around the heart provided there is no narrowing of the coronary artery (which limits stress flow, or maximum flow capacity).

This patchy, irregular appearance of blood flow in heart muscle at resting conditions that improves with dipyridamole stress does not cause symptoms or impair heart pumping function. It is simply a sign of abnormal function of the endothelial lining of the coronary arteries due to early coronary atherosclerosis or effects of risk factors on the heart. The abnormal picture of blood flow in the heart muscle at resting conditions is usually localized and patchy. However, it may be gradually worse toward the tip of the heart like the rainbow sign, reflecting a more uniform gradient of abnormal endothelial function toward the tip of the heart. The hallmark of these early signs is that the picture looks better and more uniform after dipyridamole stress is induced. (See figure 1.19.)

Progression—The Killer Stalks

As we have seen, narrowing of the coronary artery limits the maximum blood flow capacity in heart muscle during dipyridamole stress. On pictures of blood flow in the heart muscle, this area of limited blood flow appears as abnormal in a green, purple, or blue color, as compared with normal areas in red, orange, or yellow. Progression, or worsening of the narrowing in the coronary artery, reduces still further the maximum possible blood flow to the heart muscle. Changes in severity of the narrowing can be determined by comparing the baseline picture after dipyridamole stress is induced with a follow-up picture also taken under dipyridamole stress. If the stress picture at follow-up is worse than the stress picture at baseline, the narrowing has become more severe. (See figure 1.20.)

Worsening may also be seen on pictures of blood flow in the heart muscle obtained at resting conditions. Severe worsening on resting blood flow images, such as a red area at baseline changing to blue on the follow-up resting picture, usually indicates that a heart attack or scarring of the heart muscle has occurred. Milder worsening on resting blood flow images, such as a red area changing to orange or yellow, indicates more dysfunctional coronary arteries due to worsening function of the endothelial lining of the artery. It also suggests more cholesterol deposition in the arterial wall.

Progression of coronary atherosclerosis is associated with a high risk of heart attack, sudden death, or the need for coronary bypass surgery or balloon dilation of the narrowed arteries. Reversal treatment stops this progression, partially reverses the narrowing, and prevents these outcomes.

Regression—You Win

Reversal treatment reduces the severity of coronary artery narrowing. The abnormal endothelial lining heals, and the coronary arteries function more normally. They are more likely to enlarge (vasodilate) rather than go into spasm (vasoconstrict). Consequently, coronary blood flow to the heart muscle improves both at rest and during stress. With regression of narrowing, PET pictures during stress change—from baseline pictures in green,

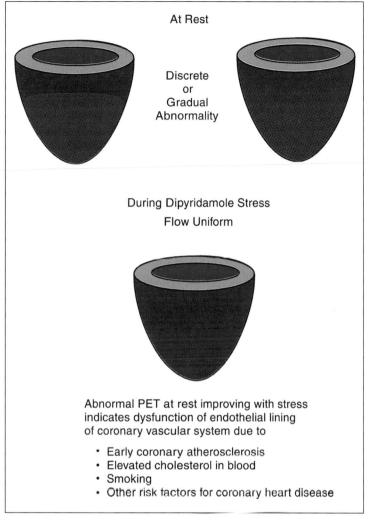

At Rest

Discrete
or
Gradual
Abnormality

During Dipyridamole Stress
Flow Uniform

Abnormal PET at rest improving with stress
indicates dysfunction of endothelial lining
of coronary vascular system due to

• Early coronary atherosclerosis
• Elevated cholesterol in blood
• Smoking
• Other risk factors for coronary heart disease

Figure 1.19. Early Clues—Blood Flow in Heart Muscle at Resting and Stress Conditions Indicating Dysfunctional Coronary Arteries Due to Bad Risk Factors or Early Coronary Atherosclerosis

purple, or blue to follow-up pictures in yellow, orange, or red. (See figure 1.21.) Similar changes are seen when baseline and follow-up pictures are obtained at resting conditions.

Regression of coronary atherosclerosis markedly reduces the risk of plaque rupture, thrombosis, vasoconstriction, heart attack, sudden death, and the need for coronary bypass surgery or balloon dilation.

Since the coronary arteriogram is commonly thought to be the most definitive test for identifying coronary atherosclerosis, it is important to compare it with PET. Blood flow in heart muscle measured by PET shows the effects of dysfunctional coronary arteries and all atherosclerosis along the *entire* length of the artery. Both localized severe segmental narrowing *and* diffuse milder narrowing throughout the artery reduce the blood flow in heart muscle. By comparison, the coronary arteriogram shows the severity of only the localized segmental narrowing. Coronary arteriograms do not show the

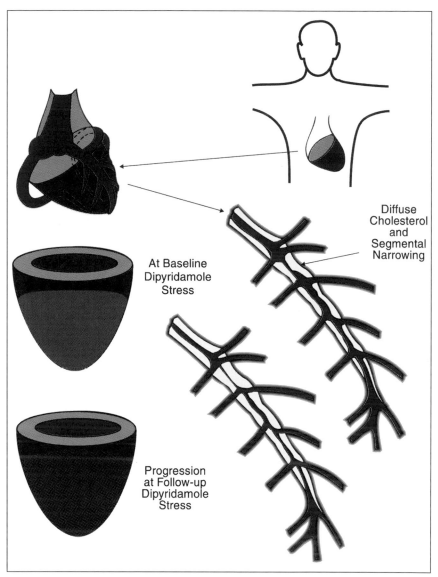

Figure 1.20. The Killer Stalks—Blood Flow in Heart Muscle with Progression of Coronary Artery Narrowing

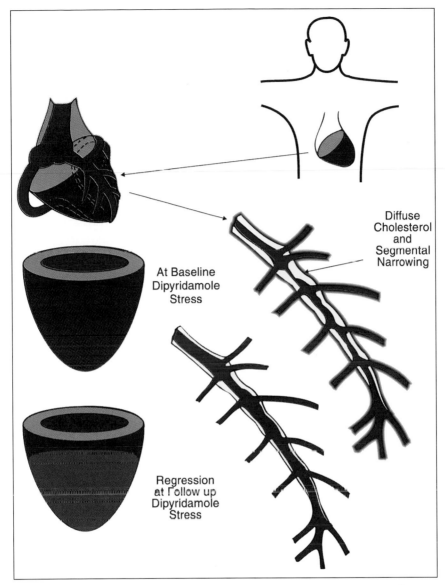

At Baseline
Dipyridamole
Stress

Regression
at Follow up
Dipyridamole
Stress

Diffuse
Cholesterol
and
Segmental
Narrowing

Figure 1.21. You Win—Blood Flow in Heart Muscle with Regression of Coronary Artery Narrowing

severity of diffuse narrowing reliably. Consequently, pictures of blood flow in heart muscle by PET show progression or regression of disease throughout the coronary arteries with an accuracy that is comparable or greater than the coronary arteriogram. Furthermore, changes in coronary blood flow occur as a function of any change in arterial diameter raised to the fourth power. In other words, a very small change in diameter of the artery that is difficult to measure accurately on an arteriogram causes a large change in blood flow that is easily seen on pictures of blood flow in the heart muscle.

The functional improvement in blood flow to heart muscle after reversal treatment (or progression in the absence of reversal treatment) can be followed best by positron emission tomography (PET). Although not widely available, PET scanners are being used more frequently and are more cost effective than in the past. The combination of PET and reversal treatment provides the basis for managing coronary artery disease without invasive and expensive procedures like arteriography, balloon dilation, or bypass surgery, thereby decreasing the costs of cardiac care.

PART 2

Who Gets Coronary Heart Disease? Why? How Can It Be Prevented or Reversed?

✓ How Prevalent Is Coronary Atherosclerosis?

✓ Risk Factors and Coronary Artery Disease

✓ Women and Heart Disease

✓ Cholesterol Lowering—Does It Work?

✓ Cholesterol-lowering Drugs Plus Very Low-Fat Food

✓ How Much Should Cholesterol Be Lowered?

✓ Can Cholesterol Levels Be Too Low?

✓ Smoking and Death

✓ Excess Body Weight and Survival

✓ Physical Fitness and Survival

T his section reviews scientific reports on the prevalence and causes of coronary heart disease; coronary heart disease in women; the role of dietary fat, cholesterol, smoking, excess weight, and physical fitness. It also reviews the extensive data indicating that cholesterol lowering improves survival and reduces the incidence of heart attacks, deaths, bypass surgery, and balloon dilation procedures.

How Prevalent Is Coronary Atherosclerosis?

Cardiovascular disease remains the leading cause of death and disability in the United States. Approximately 900,000 Americans die per year of heart disease alone, with an estimated $18 billion expended for hospital, physician, and other medical expenses. Coronary atherosclerosis is common even at relatively young ages, particularly increasing after the fourth decade in men. For women, the risk of developing coronary heart disease increases in the fifth decade of life and becomes comparable to that for men by the seventh decade.

Young trauma victims and war casualties of Korea and Vietnam have been examined for coronary atherosclerosis. Of these young men averaging between twenty-two and twenty-six years old when they died, cholesterol deposition with early coronary atherosclerosis was found in 45 to 76 percent of the hearts examined. In the community of Olmsted, Minnesota, a large number of hearts have been examined at postmortem from people of all ages who died of various causes. Early coronary atherosclerosis was also found in 41 to 72 percent of these individuals depending upon age at death. (See table 2.1.) However, not all of this early atherosclerosis progresses to clinically evident coronary artery narrowing or heart attacks.

There is a continuous healing process that counteracts the injury caused by cholesterol deposition in the wall of the arteries. Because of this healing process, significant coronary artery narrowing in these hearts is less frequent than the early changes of atherosclerosis.

As discussed previously, the common clinical measure of severity of narrowings in the coronary arteries on clinical arteriograms is percent diameter narrowing. In postmortem studies by microscopic examination, the percent narrowing of the cross-sectional lumen *area* is measured rather than percent narrowing of the lumen *diameter*. In hearts from men dying of noncardiac causes at twenty-one to twenty-six years old, 15 to 21 percent had one or more coronary arteries in which the cross-sectional size, or area, of the artery was narrowed by 50 percent or more. (See table 2.2.) A 50 percent narrowing of the cross-sectional area of the artery, called 50 percent area stenosis, corresponds to a 26 percent diameter reduction, called 26 percent diameter stenosis.

A 26 percent diameter narrowing would be considered mild coronary artery narrowing since the diameter of the artery is reduced by only one-

Table 2.1. Prevalence of Males with Coronary Atherosclerosis

Source of Heart Specimens	Prevalence of Coronary Athero- sclerosis	Average Age	No. in Sample	Reference[a]
Trauma victims	76%	26	96	J Am Coll Cardiol 1993; 22:459
Vietnam War casualties	45%	22	105	JAMA 1971; 216:1,185
Korean War casualties	77%	22	300	JAMA 1953; 152:1,090
Olmsted, Minn. postmortems	41% 72%	30–49 50–59	5,558[b]	Circulation 1984; 70:345
Heart donors	56%	54	50	Circulation 1995; 91:1,706

[a]For full names of journals, see the list of abbreviations in the bibliography.
[b]The entire data set from Olmsted included 5,558 subjects, from which the 30–49 and 50–59 age groups were selected for this table.

Table 2.2. Severity of Coronary Artery Narrowing in Males at Autopsy

Age	Percent Narrowing[a]			Reference[b]
	≥20%	≥50%	≥75%	
21	—	19%	6%	Arch Path Lab Med 1987; 111:972
22	28%	15%	11%	JAMA 1953; 152:1,090
26	—	21%	9%	J Am Coll Cardiol 1993; 22:459
30–49	—	—	41%	Circulation 1984; 70:345
50–59	—	—	72%	

[a]Of cross-sectional area of artery.
[b]For full names of journals, see the list of abbreviations in the bibliography.

quarter. More severe disease, with 50 percent diameter narrowing (corresponding to 75 percent cross-sectional area narrowing) or greater, was found in 6 to 11 percent of these young men who died of trauma or war injuries. Older men showed a greater prevalence of more severe narrowing. Approximately 56 percent of hearts transplanted from donors dying of noncardiac causes have early coronary atherosclerosis.

Coronary Artery Disease in the General Population

✓ Present in 25 to 35% of middle-aged men

✓ Present in 10 to 15% of middle-aged women

✓ Increases after menopause; women are comparable to men by seventh decade

✓ Ten times more people with the disease have no symptoms than have symptoms

✓ 60% of those suffering heart attacks or sudden death have no prior symptoms

Based on this data, 25 to 35 percent of middle-aged men have coronary atherosclerosis of potential clinical significance that began to develop in their twenties or thirties. This large population with coronary atherosclerosis without symptoms is the source of most heart attacks or sudden death, 60 percent of which occurs without prior warning symptoms. (See accompanying box.)

The prevalence of coronary heart disease at postmortem examination has not been studied in younger women as much as in younger men. This is partly due to the lower prevalence of coronary heart disease in women and to the fact that there are fewer combat casualties and violent deaths among women than among men. Therefore, the tables reflect the data published in scientific journals. Coronary heart disease in women is addressed in more detail later in part 2.

Risk Factors and Coronary Artery Disease

Coronary heart disease is caused by a complicated interplay of factors, each of which increases the risk of atherosclerosis. Some of these risk factors are:

✓ smoking

✓ abnormally high blood levels of the bad LDL cholesterol and triglycerides (a form of fat)

✓ abnormally low blood levels of the good HDL cholesterol

✓ elevated blood pressure

✓ family history of cardiovascular disease

✓ diabetes

✓ excess body weight

✓ older age

✓ male gender

✓ presence of atherosclerosis elsewhere in the body

✓ dietary fat.

Elevated blood levels of homocysteine (a by-product of amino acid metabolism) add to cardiovascular risk and may be as important as cholesterol in the basic mechanisms underlying development of atherosclerosis in some people. Elevated homocysteine may be caused by genetic abnormalities of metabolism and by kidney failure but more commonly is due to deficient dietary intake of folic acid. This risk factor is the most easily controlled of all risk factors, simply by adequate folic acid supplementation in one to two multivitamin pills each day. Most multivitamins contain 400 micrograms of folic acid, adequate for daily requirements, with two providing 800 micrograms, or 0.8 milligrams, which is therapeutic for even high levels of homocysteine. Since folic acid is found in fruits and vegetables, the recommended food plan detailed in part 4 provides adequate amounts of folic acid even without vitamin supplementation.

Stress may also be an important risk factor. It worsens the effects of other risk factors such as decreasing the good HDL cholesterol, increasing blood pressure, disrupting good dietary or exercise habits. Since stress is hard to define precisely and may vary greatly between individuals, it is difficult to quantify for scientific study. Stress involving fear, anger, or depression is associated with increased risk of heart attacks. The stress of hard work or long working hours without these emotions is not associated with cardiovascular risk if other risk factors are controlled.

There are two major forms of cholesterol in blood that have opposite effects on the risk of coronary heart disease. The low-density lipoprotein cholesterol, or LDL ("low down lipid"), causes a major risk of coronary heart disease regardless of other types of cholesterol. The high-density lipoprotein cholesterol, or HDL ("highly defensive lipid"), is a protective cholesterol that reduces the risk of atherosclerosis. When the HDL is abnormally low, this beneficial protective effect is lost. Therefore, a low HDL cholesterol in the blood is a major risk factor for developing coronary heart disease even with normal levels of LDL cholesterol.

Triglycerides are a form of fat in blood. At high levels, they are associated with coronary heart disease, particularly in some individuals where the triglycerides interact with low HDL. High levels of triglycerides in the blood in association with low HDL cholesterol levels and a family history of coronary heart disease are strongly associated with a very high risk of coronary heart disease. Such individuals have a 40 to 60 percent risk of developing coronary heart disease over their lifetime. Dietary fat separate from serum cholesterol is also an important risk factor for progression of coronary heart disease.

In different individuals, the importance of one or more risk factors may be highly variable. Some people with many risk factors for coronary atherosclerosis never develop coronary heart disease. Others with few or no risk factors and "normal" cholesterol levels in blood develop severe coronary heart disease. Therefore, development of coronary heart disease cannot always be explained by these risk factors.

Let us take a closer look at those people who are susceptible to modest or even normal risk factors and therefore have a low risk factor threshold. Maintaining cholesterol in normal ranges for these susceptible individuals is usually associated with progression of disease. Such individuals stop progressing or partially reverse their disease only with more vigorous cholesterol lowering and dietary fat restriction than is normally recommended. Their cholesterol levels and dietary fat have to be reduced below some risk threshold in order to prevent, reverse, or stabilize their disease.

Therefore, for individuals with coronary artery disease, reversal treatment does not aim for normal cholesterol levels. Treatment should reduce total cholesterol, the LDL fraction of cholesterol, and dietary fat as much as possible to well below the normal ranges. The protective HDL cholesterol should be increased as much as possible. Since dietary fat is a major risk factor for progression of coronary atherosclerosis independent of cholesterol levels (measured in blood under fasting conditions), dietary fat should be reduced as much as possible in addition to lowering cholesterol levels in blood.

It is important to differentiate public health measures for reducing risk factors for cardiovascular disease in the general population from specific treatment to reverse cardiovascular disease in an individual. Public health measures for the general public as recommended by the American Heart Association and the National Cholesterol Education Program emphasize smoking cessation, blood pressure control, mild exercise, and modest reduction in dietary fat and cholesterol. The purpose of those guidelines is to reduce the prevalence of cardiovascular disease in the general population. In individuals, such public health measures typically reduce blood cholesterol only modestly, for example, by 5 to 10 percent. For individuals with established cardiovascular disease or at high risk for developing it, these modest steps are not adequate for reliably reversing or stopping the progression of the disease. More vigorous fat reduction in food and cholesterol-lowering drugs are required in order to optimize outcomes in people with coronary heart disease.

Since many people with risk factors do not have or will not develop coronary heart disease, not all of these people should be treated by the same vigorous measures necessary for those with known or diagnosed cardiovascular disease. On the other hand, many other people known to have coronary heart disease would not receive essential reversal treatment if abnormal risk factors were the only criteria for instituting treatment. They do not have the recognized risk factors yet have developed vascular disease.

There are two principal reasons for undertaking a vigorous, lifelong reversal program. The first is multiple or severe risk factors for developing coronary heart disease. For example, a person with elevated levels of LDL cholesterol and triglycerides, a low HDL, a strong family history of coronary heart disease at young ages, high blood pressure, a smoking habit, and excess weight has a very high risk of developing coronary heart disease. This person needs reversal treatment. The second reason is a firm diagnosis of cardiovascular disease or any form of atherosclerosis based on definitive clinical evidence or by diagnostic testing regardless of what risk factors are present. For example, a heart attack is definite clinical grounds for starting lifelong reversal treatment; if cholesterol levels are "normal" in someone with a heart attack, they should be reduced to well below "normal" levels and other risk factors modified, such as breaking the smoking habit.

This second reason for reversal treatment of risk factors, a clinical diagnosis of coronary artery disease, needs to be definitive as the basis for lifelong treatment. Just as a single modestly abnormal risk factor may not be sufficient grounds for intense reversal treatment with cholesterol-lowering medications, common symptoms or tests may not be adequate for establishing the diagnosis. For example, chest pain or a positive exercise stress test suggests the presence of coronary heart disease. Someone with chest pain or a positive exercise test is more likely to have coronary heart disease than people without these findings. However, neither chest pain nor conventional exercise testing is reliable enough for definitively diagnosing coronary heart disease with sufficient accuracy to be the basis of lifelong reversal treatment. Chest pain may be due to many causes other than coronary heart disease. Many abnormal exercise tests are erroneously positive even though coronary heart disease is not present.

In contrast, a coronary arteriogram showing even mild segmental coronary artery narrowing provides a firm diagnosis for the basis of lifelong reversal treatment. However, in some instances even coronary arteriograms may appear normal in the presence of diffuse coronary atherosclerosis without significant localized segmental narrowing. This unidentified diffuse disease may result in plaque rupture and heart attack despite the normal-appearing coronary arteriograms. The coronary arteriogram is also an invasive procedure in which a catheter is inserted into the arteries of the body; it therefore has some risk of harmful side effects as well as being very costly.

Although these clinical diagnostic tests are discussed in detail later in the book, it is important here to relate them to risk factors as the basis for lifelong reversal treatment. The standard technology of exercise testing and coronary arteriography is not optimal for the accurate, efficient diagnosis and management of coronary atherosclerosis. Exercise testing is not accurate enough, and coronary arteriography is invasive and costly. However, positron emission tomography (PET) of the heart is a noninvasive, highly accurate method for identifying coronary artery disease, even very early, before symptoms develop. It is also optimal for assessing severity of more advanced disease since it shows the cumulative effects of diffuse atherosclerosis throughout the length of coronary arteries, which arteriograms often fail to show. PET is also optimal for following progression or regression of coronary atherosclerosis, with accuracy comparable to or greater than that of the arteriogram. Intensive lifelong reversal treatment by cholesterol-lowering medications and vigorous risk factor control requires a definitive diagnosis of cardiovascular disease such as a heart attack, stroke, an arteriogram, a PET scan, or combination of high risk factors.

With the need for lifelong reversal treatment established on the basis of risk factors or firm diagnosis of coronary atherosclerosis, the intensity of treatment for an individual needs to be greater than the general public health guidelines for reducing risk factors in the general population. In medical studies of low-fat diets and cholesterol-lowering drugs that were reported before 1990, cholesterol was lowered only modestly, comparable to outcomes obtained by following public health measures for modifying risk factors. This modest cholesterol lowering had only equivocal or no significant benefits for the group of subjects being treated, with no predictable benefit in specific individuals. In part as a result of these older studies, some people still question the effectiveness of cholesterol lowering for reversing or stopping the progression of cardiovascular disease.

However, current more vigorous treatment with greater cholesterol lowering and more stringent dietary fat restriction has dramatically changed the approach to cardiovascular diseases, as detailed in this book. Dietary and pharmacologic treatment to lower cholesterol markedly, together with control of other risk factors, substantially reduces the frequency of death, heart attack, chest pain, or other symptoms and the need for balloon dilation or bypass surgery. As shown subsequently, reversal treatment by vigorous cholesterol lowering, dietary fat restriction, and elimination of other risk factors is so effective that it is now a valid alternative to current widespread coronary bypass surgery or balloon dilation in individuals with coronary heart disease.

Women and Heart Disease

There are important gender differences in the symptoms, diagnosis, outcomes, and management of coronary heart disease. Death and disability in women due to coronary heart disease lag ten years behind males, rising in the fifth decade and equal to or exceeding males by the seventh to eighth decade of life.

Acute heart attack with an abnormal ECG is the most common first manifestation of the disease in men. In contrast, chest pain with a normal ECG is the most common presenting symptom in women. Women are more subject than men to other causes of chest pain that mimic but are unrelated to coronary artery disease. Of women with chest pain during exercise that is characteristic of coronary heart disease, only 60 to 70 percent have significant coronary arterial narrowing by arteriography, compared with 80 to 90 percent of men. Of women with nontypical chest pain occurring at resting conditions, only 30 to 40 percent have significant coronary artery narrowing. Of those women with still more nonspecific chest pain that is unlike heart pain, only 2 to 4 percent have significant disease identified by arteriography. On the other hand, standard coronary arteriography fails to detect or quantify diffuse coronary atherosclerosis, which is more prevalent in women than men.

The diagnostic accuracy of exercise testing for identifying coronary heart disease is particularly limited in women compared with men. Normal results of stress testing are more common in women with coronary artery disease due to their tendency to achieve lower exercise workloads and their inability to reach target heart rates. Women also have more diffuse coronary atherosclerosis that is not seen on the arteriogram or does not cause abnormalities on standard exercise testing. The diagnosis is therefore missed, and chest pain is ascribed to some other cause.

False positive stress tests are more common in women in the absence of coronary artery disease due to the higher prevalence of artifactual ECG changes. Women also commonly have artifactual abnormalities on pictures of blood flow in the heart using standard radionuclide technology due to absorption of X-ray signals by breast tissue. PET imaging does not have these false positive results and is therefore more accurate than standard heart imaging technology used with stress tests. In addition, PET more accurately shows the effects of diffuse coronary artery narrowing along the length of the coronary arteries that do not show on an arteriogram. Therefore, PET is particularly suitable for evaluating women with chest pain or risk factors.

Coronary arteriography is less frequently carried out in women than in men. Only 4 percent of women with a positive stress test using standard radionuclide pictures of blood flow in the heart subsequently undergo arteriography. The reason is that false positive results on standard stress tests are so common that a positive test is often ignored. By comparison, 40 percent of men with a positive stress test are referred for arteriography, a 10:1 ratio that is not dependent on age. Women hospitalized with chest pain appearing to be heart related are also less likely than men to undergo coronary arteriography. This is because women commonly have chest pain unrelated to coronary heart disease and because, as just mentioned, a positive stress test is frequently ignored. These differences in diagnostic testing may reflect the fact that it is harder to make a clinical diagnosis of coronary artery disease in women than in men on the basis of symptoms. They may also reflect the lower accuracy of exercise testing as the grounds for proceeding to coronary arteriography. Using PET imaging in women, with its greater accuracy, eliminates these concerns.

Of patients having chest pain due to coronary heart disease, a single diseased coronary artery is found more commonly in women than in men, who typically have multiple coronary arteries involved. Women having a heart attack as the first evidence of coronary heart disease demonstrate the same extent of coronary atherosclerosis by arteriography as do men presenting with a heart attack. Within four years after the first heart attack, more women (36 percent) than men (21 percent) will die. Although women experience the onset of coronary disease later than men, the risk of cardiac deaths in women escalates after menopause to equal that of men.

On the other hand, women have some potential advantages over men for reducing their risks of cardiovascular disease. The use of estrogens after menopause reduces the risk of cardiovascular disease. Moreover, women undergoing reversal treatment for coronary heart disease show better regression than men. In women, complications of balloon dilation and bypass surgery are higher, and short-term outcomes are less satisfactory than in men. For this reason, reversal treatment is a particularly good option for women.

Cholesterol Lowering—Does It Work?

In recent clinical studies, vigorous cholesterol lowering caused partial reversal or stopped the progression of coronary heart disease in up to 80 percent of treated subjects. Cholesterol levels in the blood were lowered by either moderate low-fat foods and cholesterol-lowering drugs or by intensive lifestyle change, with a stricter diet of very low-fat foods. The regression in severity of arterial narrowing was only modest. The percent narrowing decreased by 10 to 15 percent over one to two years. However, it was consistently observed and significant in these studies. More important, there was a much larger, major decrease in the clinical events of heart attack, death, bypass surgery, or balloon dilation in those undergoing vigorous cholesterol lowering compared with groups receiving standard treatment.

This marked clinical benefit was due to stabilization or regression of the cholesterol deposits in the coronary arteries (known as cholesterol plaques). As we saw in part 1, breakdown of the plaque or a plaque rupture leads to blood clots, or thrombosis, in the coronary artery. This clot causes sudden blockage of blood flow and severe chest pain, heart attack, or sudden death. Plaque rupture, thrombosis, and blockage of the artery characteristically occur at sites of previously mild narrowing. These sites are diffusely infiltrated with cholesterol, which causes little impairment of blood flow and no symptoms prior to plaque rupture. Therefore, an individual may feel well and be active without limitations or symptoms. However, sudden death or heart attack may occur within minutes to hours due to rupture of the plaque and thrombosis of the artery. Lowering the cholesterol level in blood causes resorption of cholesterol out of the plaques in the wall of the artery. Reduction of the cholesterol in the arterial wall by reversal treatment markedly reduces the risk of plaque rupture, thereby reducing heart attacks and deaths.

Twenty-six of twenty-seven recent medical studies showed significant benefit from reducing cholesterol levels in the blood. (See table 2.3.) The benefits were partial regression, the stopping of progression, or the prevention of cardiovascular events, such as death, heart attack, bypass surgery,

Table 2.3. Major Cholesterol-lowering Trials

Study	Outcome	Reference[a]
NHLBI	Less progression	Circulation 1984; 69:313
CLAS I	Regression, less progression	JAMA 1987; 257:3,233
CLAS II	Regression, less progression	JAMA 1990; 264:3,013
POSCH	Events reduced[b], regression, less progression	New Engl J Med 1990; 323:946 Circulation 1994; 90:1−532 J Am Coll Cardiol 1995; 26:351
Lifestyle	Regression, less progression	Lancet 1990; 336:129 Am J Cardiol 1992; 69:845 JAMA 1995; 274:894
FATS	Events reduced, regression, less progression	New Engl J Med 1990; 323:12,899 Circulation 1993; 88:2,744 J Am Coll Cardiol 1994; 23:899
UC-SCORE	Regression, less progression	JAMA 1990; 264:3,007
SCRIP	Events reduced, less progression	Circulation 1994; 89:975 J Am Coll Cardiol 1994; 24:900
Heidelberg	Regression, less progression	Circulation 1992; 86:1
CCAIT	Less progression, reduced new lesions	Circulation 1994; 89:959 Circulation 1995; 92:2,404
MARS	Regression, less progression	Ann Int Med. 1993; 119:969
PLAC I and II	Events reduced	Am J Cardiol 1995: 76:60C J Am Coll Cardiol 1995; 26:1,133
HARP	No benefit	Lancet 1994: 344:633
MAAS	Less progression	Lancet 1994; 344:633
ACAPS	Events reduced, regression	Circulation 1994; 90:1,679
SINGH	Events reduced	Br Med J 1992; 304:1,015
STARS	Events reduced	Lancet 1992; 339:563
Mediterra-nean diet	Events reduced	Lancet 1994; 343:1,454
REGRESS	Events reduced	Circulation 1995; 91:2,528
Pooled	Events reduced	Circulation 1995; 92:2,419
Meta-analysis	Events reduced	Circulation 1996; 93:1,774

Table 2.3. (continued)

Study	Outcome	Reference[a]
CARE	Events reduced	New Engl J Med 1996; 335:1,001
SSSS	Events and mortality reduced	Lancet 1994; 344:1,383 Lancet 1995; 345:1,274 Circulation 1996; 93:1,796
WOSCOPS	Events and mortality reduced	New Engl J Med 1995; 333:1,301
KAPS	Less progression	Circulation 1995; 92:1,758–1,764
LCAS	Less progression	Am J Cardiol 1997; 80:278–286
CARS	Less progression	Am J Cardiol 1997; 79:893–896
Ultrasound	Less progression	Am J Cardiol 1997; 79:1,673–1,676

[a]For full names of journals, see the list of abbreviations in the bibliography.
[b]Events are heart attack, stroke, or death or some combination of these events.

or balloon dilation. Although each study reports the details and data differently, the overall conclusions are similar. For example, the Familial Atherosclerosis Treatment Study (FATS) showed significant improvement in the arteriographic severity of coronary artery narrowing in those subjects undergoing treatment with two cholesterol-lowering medications and moderately low-fat foods compared with a control group that did not receive this treatment. In addition, the coronary events of death, heart attack, bypass surgery, and balloon dilation occurred in 21.2 percent of those without vigorous cholesterol lowering but in only 5.3 percent of those treated by this means. (See figure 2.1.) Therefore, vigorous cholesterol lowering caused a marked 75 percent reduction in coronary events. After the first six months in the FATS trial, the group treated with two cholesterol-lowering drugs had an 85 percent reduction in coronary events compared with the control group.

An example of a larger, more recent investigation was the Scandinavian Simvastatin Survival Study (4S). It evaluated the effects on survival of a common cholesterol-lowering drug called simvastatin in 4,444 individuals with coronary heart disease. Half of the subjects received simvastatin, and the other half, the control group, received placebo treatment without simvastatin. The group treated with simvastatin had a reduced incidence of death,

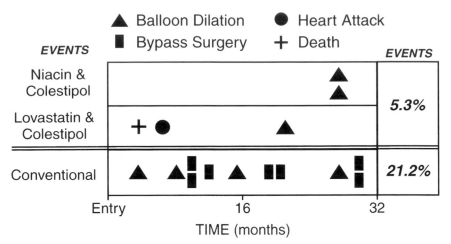

Figure 2.1. Clinical Events of Balloon Dilation, Bypass Surgery, Heart Attacks, or Death in the Familial Atherosclerosis Treatment Study (FATS). Adapted from Brown, New England Journal of Medicine 1990; 323:1,289–1,298.

heart attack, and other clinical events when compared with the control group, as summarized in table 2.4. Cholesterol lowering did not result in any increase in deaths from noncardiovascular causes, such as cancer, trauma, suicide, but rather a 5 percent decrease, a small change that reflects random variation and is not significant.

The benefit of cholesterol lowering was seen in men, women, and in older as well as younger people. Within each of these subgroups, the occurrence of coronary events, such as heart attacks, was reduced for those on the drug as compared with those not on it. (See table 2.5.) The small difference in percentages for older and younger subjects (29 percent versus 39 percent) is due to random variation; it is not a "real" or statistically significant difference in response of the older and younger subjects to simvastatin. The notion that cholesterol lowering does not benefit older people with coronary heart disease is incorrect. As shown in the 4S study, older people had significantly better survival after lowering blood cholesterol than those of comparable age without cholesterol lowering. This class of cholesterol-lowering drug is called a statin. It includes lovastatin, pravastatin, simvastatin, fluvastatin, and atorvastatin.

Another study evaluated the effect of a different cholesterol-lowering medication, pravastatin. Of 1,891 subjects with coronary heart disease, half received the drug and the other half received conventional treatment and a placebo. In subjects treated with pravastatin compared with those without it, there was a significant reduction in cardiovascular events, as shown in table 2.6. There was no increase in noncardiovascular deaths, such as cancer,

Table 2.4. Effects of Simvastatin on Clinical Events in the
Scandinavian Simvastatin Survival Study (4S)

Clinical Event	Percent Reduction[a]
Coronary death	42%
Coronary events	34%
Death from any cause	30%
Balloon dilation or bypass surgery	37%
Cerebrovascular event	37%
LDL cholesterol	35%
Noncardiovascular deaths	5%

SOURCE: Lancet 1994; 344:1,383.
NOTE: A total of 4,444 subjects with coronary heart disease were studied.
Half of them received the cholesterol-lowering drug simvastatin, and half
received conventional treatment and a placebo.
[a]In patients who took simvastatin as compared with the control group.

Table 2.5. Effects of Simvastatin on Coronary Events in the
Scandinavian Simvastatin Survival Study (4S), by Age and Gender

Subgroup	Percent Reduction in Coronary Events[a]
Men	34%
Women	35%
Age < 60 years	39%
Age ≥ 60 years	29%

SOURCE: Lancet 1994; 344:1,383.
NOTE: A total of 4,414 subjects with coronary heart disease were studied.
Half of them received the cholesterol-lowering drug simvastatin, and half
received conventional treatment and a placebo.
[a]In patients who took simvastatin as compared with the control group.

suicide, trauma, caused by the drug, indicated by the nonsignificant differences between those treated and those not treated with pravastatin.

The final example shown here is a study carried out in western Scotland on 6,595 men with elevated cholesterol but no known cardiovascular disease. Half of the subjects were treated with pravastatin, and half were not. Compared with the untreated group, the treated group had a reduced incidence of heart attacks and other clinical events, as summarized in table 2.7. There was no increase in noncardiovascular deaths caused by the drug. This study is

Table 2.6. Effects of Pravastatin on Clinical Events in the Pooled Pravastatin Trials

Clinical Event	Percent Reduction[a]
Heart attack	62%
Heart attack or death from cardiovascular disease	51%
Heart attack or death from all other causes	53%
Stroke	62%
All death, heart attack, stroke, balloon dilation, and bypass surgery	53%
Noncardiovascular death	0.2%[b]

SOURCE: Byington, Circulation 1995; 92:2,419.
NOTE: The Pooled Pravastatin Trials included PLAC I, PLAC II, REGRESS, and KAPS. A total of 1,891 subjects with coronary heart disease were studied. Half of them received the cholesterol-lowering drug pravastatin, and half received conventional treatment and a placebo.
[a]In patients who took pravastatin as compared with the control group.
[b]Deaths due to noncardiovascular causes were not increased.

Table 2.7. Effects of Pravastatin on Clinical Events in the West of Scotland Coronary Prevention Study Group (WOSCOPS)

Clinical Event	Percent Reduction[a]
Coronary event	31%
Cardiovascular death	32%
Coronary arteriography	31%
Balloon dilation or bypass surgery	37%
LDL cholesterol	26%
Noncardiovascular death	11%

SOURCE: Shepard, New England Journal of Medicine 1995; 333:1,301.
NOTE: A total of 6,595 men from western Scotland were studied. All had elevated cholesterol but no known cardiovascular disease. Half of the subjects received the cholesterol-lowering drug pravastatin, and half received a placebo.
[a]In subjects who took pravastatin as compared with the control group.

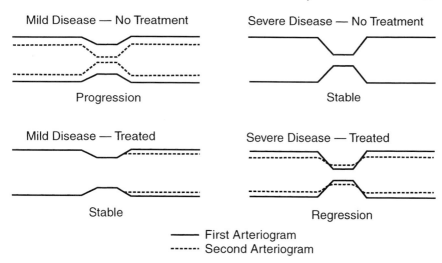

Figure 2.2. Changes in Severity of Coronary Artery Narrowing with and without Treatment by Lifestyle Changes. Adapted from Gould, American Journal of Cardiology 1992; 69:845–853.

important in demonstrating that cholesterol lowering can prevent vascular disease in people at some risk for developing it due to elevated cholesterol but who had no symptoms or diagnosis of the condition when treatment was started.

As shown in these examples, vigorous reversal treatment by cholesterol-lowering medications and moderate or very low-fat foods stops the progression of or partially reverses coronary artery disease and reduces deaths, heart attacks, strokes, balloon dilation, and bypass surgery by 40 to 73 percent or 85 percent after the first six months of treatment, compared with control groups that do not receive such treatment. In addition, there is a major decrease in symptoms, so people with coronary heart disease have less chest pain and feel better.

Coronary atherosclerosis is a diffuse process. Cholesterol is deposited throughout the wall of the artery along its entire length with a highly variable effect on the size of the artery. In some areas of the artery, plaque growth or partial rupture causes localized narrowing without complete occlusion. In other areas, the coronary arteries may be uniformly, diffusely narrowed without localized, more severe narrowing. In this case, the arteriogram may appear completely normal. In other areas, the coronary artery may remold or enlarge structurally so that the size is not narrowed despite substantial atherosclerosis in the wall. Therefore, the shape or geometry of narrowing in a coronary artery due to atherosclerosis is highly variable.

With regression in the severity of narrowing, many different dimensions of the narrowing may improve. This structural improvement may be reduction in percent narrowing (see figure 2.2.), reduction in the absolute dimensions of the narrowest segment, improved shape with smoother edges, and better streamlining of the narrowest segment. Therefore, percent narrowing alone does not adequately reflect the extent of changes in this complex geometry that affects coronary blood flow. Our study has shown that regression is characterized by improvement in percent narrowing, in the absolute size of the narrowest segment of the artery, and in the streamlining characteristics of the narrowing. Changes in the maximum flow capacity, or coronary flow reserve, expected from the integrated effects of the overall geometric changes are larger than the change in percent narrowing alone during progression or regression.

Cholesterol-lowering Drugs Plus Very Low-Fat Food

There are two ways of lowering cholesterol in order to stop progression or cause regression of atherosclerosis and prevent cardiovascular events. The first emphasizes optimal living habits, including very low-fat food with less than 10 percent of calories as fat, ideal body weight, no smoking, and regular exercise. My guidelines for this component of reversal treatment are detailed in part 4. The second way of reducing cholesterol relies on cholesterol-lowering drugs.

Most medical studies have utilized cholesterol-lowering drugs and a moderate low-fat diet. Such diets typically have 20 to 30 percent of calories as fat, following the recommendations of the American Heart Association and the National Cholesterol Education Program. These guidelines, developed as a public health initiative, are well established and widely recognized. However, this recommended percentage range of fat in the diet is too high for patients with coronary heart disease; in recent medical studies, subjects with this disease who were on diets of 20 to 30 percent fat experienced progression of their condition. On the other hand, medical studies of lower-fat diets show substantial regression.

Low-fat foods have benefits independent of and in addition to effects of cholesterol-lowering drugs. For medical purposes, levels of cholesterol and fats in blood, collectively called lipids, are typically measured after fasting for twelve hours. The reason is that eating fatty food causes a certain component of these lipids to increase during the eight hours after a meal. This surge in lipids after eating a fatty meal involves the fat called triglycerides and a cholesterol-protein complex called very low-density lipoprotein (VLDL). These levels of triglycerides and VLDL cholesterol in blood after eating may be highly variable depending upon the fat content of the food, its volume, and the time that has elapsed since eating. In order to standardize conditions, blood is always obtained under fasting conditions when measuring cholesterol levels (known as fasting cholesterol levels). (See figure 2.3.) Most scientific studies of cholesterol have measured fasting cholesterol levels in order to follow the effects of the cholesterol-lowering drugs.

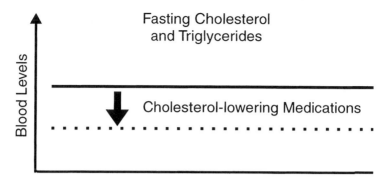

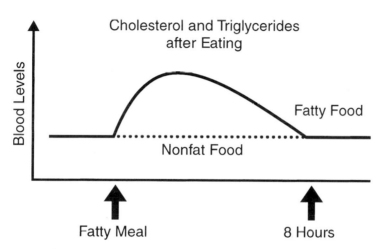

Figure 2.3. Blood Levels of Cholesterol and Triglycerides Measured after Fasting Do Not Reflect Abnormal Elevations of Very Low-Density Lipids (VLDL) and Triglycerides after Eating a Fatty Meal. Adapted from Patsch, Arteriosclerosis and Thrombosis 1992; 12:1,336–1,345.

The low-density components of the cholesterol and the triglycerides that increase after a meal are particularly prone to cause atherosclerosis (hence the term *atherogenic*). The amount of increase in these blood lipids after a fatty meal is greater in people who have coronary heart disease than in those who do not. Because the lipid increase in the blood after eating a fatty meal may persist for six to eight hours, and because most people eat three meals per day, the arterial wall is exposed to atherogenic material for a substantial part of each twenty-four-hour period.

Progression of coronary heart disease is closely associated with the size and extent of the increase in blood lipids after eating. (See figure 2.4.) The

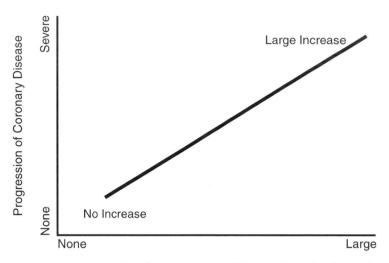

Figure 2.4. Progression of Coronary Artery Narrowing on Arteriograms Related to Extent of the Surge in Blood of the Very Low-Density Lipoprotein (VLDL) Cholesterol Fraction and Triglycerides after Eating a Fatty Meal. Adapted from Karpe, Atherosclerosis 1994; 106:83–97.

size of this increase in lipids after eating is more closely associated with progression of coronary atherosclerosis than are the fasting cholesterol levels.

Even if fasting cholesterol levels are lowered by drugs, the lipid response after eating a fatty meal may remain abnormally high and prolonged for eight hours. Lowering fasting cholesterol levels in blood by drug treatment is beneficial; however, lowering fasting cholesterol levels by the statin class of drugs does not alter the lipid surge in blood after eating fatty food. Very low-fat food eliminates the after-eating increase in lipid components in blood that accelerates atherosclerosis. Although cholesterol-lowering drugs without a very low-fat diet reduce cardiovascular deaths by 40 to 60 percent, a significant risk of cardiovascular events remains due in part to the lipid surge following a fatty meal, even with a diet containing 20 to 30 percent fat. In the absence of cholesterol-lowering drugs, low-fat food also reduces cardiovascular deaths by 40 to 50 percent but with remaining cardiovascular risk since cholesterol levels are not reduced as much as with cholesterol-lowering drugs. Very low-fat food *combined* with cholesterol-lowering drugs reduces both fasting cholesterol levels and the after-eating lipid surge. Therefore, the twenty-four-hour exposure of the arterial wall to atherogenic lipids in the blood is minimized by the combination of very low-fat food and cholesterol-lowering drugs, particularly by treatment with two or more cholesterol-lowering drugs. My clinical experience also indicates that the risk

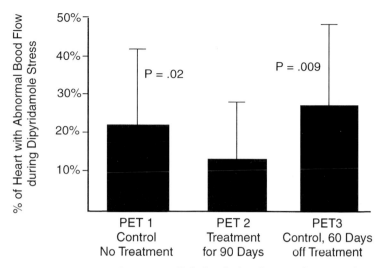

Figure 2.5. Improvement in Myocardial Blood Flow by PET from Baseline Control (PET 1) Compared with Ninety Days of Cholesterol-lowering Treatment (PET 2) Compared with Sixty Days after Stopping Treatment as a Follow-up Control (PET 3). Adapted from Gould, Circulation 1995; 89:1,530–1,538.

of cardiovascular events is maximally reduced by combining cholesterol-lowering drugs and very low-fat food.

The program presented in this book utilizes a combination of cholesterol-lowering drugs and very low-fat food designed to maximize cholesterol lowering over the twenty-four-hour day as quickly as possible. The program accelerates early plaque stabilization and early protection against coronary events. The beneficial effect of vigorous cholesterol lowering on the lining of the artery is seen in a short period of time, even days to weeks. In people with coronary heart disease, there is decreased chest pain, increased exercise capacity, and heightened sense of well-being, usually beginning within two weeks. Within three months after undertaking a reversal program, there is improved blood flow to heart muscle, as shown by PET imaging. (See figure 2.5; a probability, or p value, of less than 0.05 indicates that the changes observed are significant statistically and not due to random chance.) The combination of cholesterol-lowering drugs and very low-fat foods also reinforces adherence since the marked, rapid drop in cholesterol levels is a motivating factor.

Most people are willing to make major changes in their diet and lifestyle if the outcomes are definite, occur quickly, and make them feel better. Consequently, this program utilizes a very low-fat food plan with specific recommendations tailored to each individual. In my experience of treating people with coronary atherosclerosis by a combined regimen of very low-fat foods and cholesterol-lowering drugs, 90 percent or greater stop progressing, stabilize, or partially reverse their disease with a corresponding decrease in symptoms, heart attacks, strokes, and death. Moreover, people who adhere to the program usually do not need to have balloon dilation or bypass surgery, since the response to this treatment regimen is so consistent and effective.

The abnormal function of the blood vessel lining due to elevated cholesterol or coronary heart disease starts to heal within weeks to months after undertaking vigorous cholesterol lowering. More recent studies indicate that improved function of the endothelial lining of arteries and blood flow begin within hours after lowering cholesterol levels. Correspondingly, impaired function of the endothelial lining and decreased blood flow may occur within hours after a fatty meal. With this improved function of the endothelium by vigorous cholesterol lowering, symptoms of chest pain usually decrease and exercise capacity increases, with a sense of well-being over a period of days to weeks. With prolonged endothelial healing and stabilization of plaque, there is also a marked decrease in the risk of coronary events, such as death, heart attacks, strokes, bypass surgery, and balloon dilation. The protection against these cardiovascular events is observed to begin at approximately six months of treatment and improves to maximal reduction in risk at two to five years.

How Much Should Cholesterol Be Lowered?

How much should cholesterol be lowered for optimal reversal? In a large population followed for medical studies, cholesterol levels in blood were directly related to death rates due to coronary heart disease. Higher cholesterol levels were associated with higher death rates; lower cholesterol levels, lower death rates. (See figure 2.6.) There was a continuous decline in death rates with decreasing cholesterol levels down to 140 mg/dl. In countries where the population has very low cholesterol levels—for example, in China, where cholesterol levels average 120 to 140 mg/dl—coronary heart disease is uncommon.

In the 4S study, discussed earlier, people with normal or only modestly elevated LDL cholesterol levels showed a reduction in death rates after treatment that was comparable to the reduction for people with higher LDL cholesterol levels undergoing the same treatment. The treated subjects with either normal or high cholesterol levels had fewer deaths than those without cholesterol lowering.

In the FATS study, also discussed earlier, people with coronary heart disease and LDL cholesterol that was normal or only moderately elevated showed regression of coronary artery narrowing after further cholesterol lowering. The improvement in narrowing was as much as or more than in patients with higher LDL cholesterol levels undergoing comparable treatment. Therefore, people with coronary heart disease and "normal" cholesterol levels benefit from further cholesterol lowering.

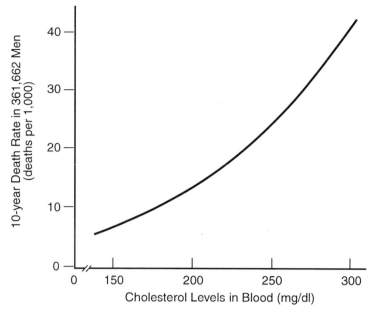

Figure 2.6. Relation of Blood Cholesterol Levels to Deaths Caused by Heart Disease in 361,622 Subjects Screened for the MRFIT Trial. Adapted from Circulation 1994; 89:1,329–1,445.

An analysis of two recent studies shows that people with coronary heart disease who had normal or only modestly elevated cholesterol levels also had fewer coronary events after cholesterol-lowering treatment than those without cholesterol lowering. (Figure 2.7 shows the correlation between cholesterol level and frequency of coronary events.) The coronary events were reduced in parallel with progressive lowering of cholesterol levels down to much lower than the "normal" value of 200 mg/dl. These cholesterol-lowering studies, population data, and the progressively decreasing risk of cardiovascular deaths with decreasing blood cholesterol levels down to 140 mg/dl all indicate that achieving cholesterol levels well below the normal of 200 mg/dl improves outcomes in coronary heart disease. For this reason, one of the goals of my program for stabilizing or reversing cardiovascular disease is a total cholesterol of 140 mg/dl, as discussed in part 4.

A low level of HDL cholesterol, particularly associated with elevated triglycerides, is commonly associated with coronary heart disease. When followed over a period of thirteen years, people with coronary heart disease and low HDL levels do not survive as well as those with normal HDL levels. (See figure 2.8.)

Increasing HDL reduces the cardiovascular risk. In the 4S trial study, subjects with low HDL cholesterol had markedly improved survival after treatment with simvastatin compared with subjects not receiving this treat-

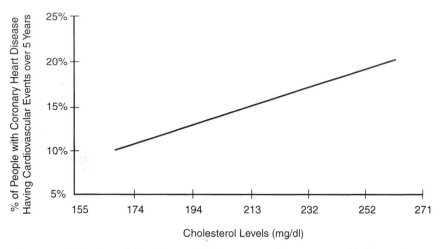

Figure 2.7. Relation of Cardiovascular Events over Five Years to Cholesterol Levels in Treated and Untreated Control Subjects. Adapted from Yusuf, Circulation 1996; 93:1,774–1,776.

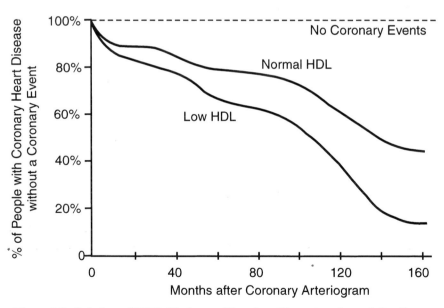

Figure 2.8. Relation of HDL Cholesterol Levels to Heart Attacks and Cardiovascular Deaths. Adapted from Miller, Circulation 1992; 86:1,165–1,170.

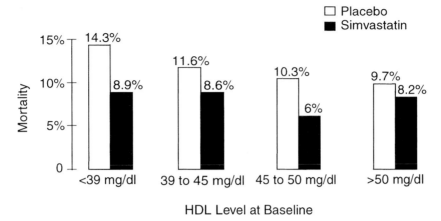

Figure 2.9. Baseline HDL and Deaths in the Scandinavian Simvastatin Survival Study (4S). Adapted from Lancet 1995; 345:1,274–1,275.

ment. (See figure 2.9.) Consequently, people with coronary heart disease who have low HDL levels and even normal LDL levels undergo reversal treatment in my program; LDL levels are lowered further by very low fat food and the statin class of drugs; the HDL levels are raised by specific medications, weight loss, adequate dietary protein, exercise, and smoking cessation. All of these steps are necessary to raise the HDL optimally.

These studies indicate that *everyone* with coronary heart disease should be treated by cholesterol lowering as much as possible below the level of cholesterol at which their disease developed. In addition, people at high risk for developing coronary heart disease will also profit from cholesterol lowering. If the HDL cholesterol is low, it should be increased toward normal as much as possible. In order to maximize stabilization or partial reversal of atherosclerosis and protection against death, heart attacks, strokes, bypass surgery, or balloon dilations, this treatment program recommends a total cholesterol below 140 mg/dl, an LDL cholesterol below 90 mg/dl, and an HDL cholesterol over 45 mg/dl, very low-fat foods, lean body mass, stress control, and moderate physical activity.

As noted earlier, lowering cholesterol in the blood to normal levels is not always adequate to cause regression of coronary heart disease. However, lowering cholesterol to well below normal levels is beneficial, as demonstrated by the following clinical example: A sixty-five-year-old man had no symptoms when I first saw him for blood pressure management. He had a total cholesterol level in his blood of 253 mg/dl, LDL 201 mg/dl, HDL 51 mg/dl, and triglycerides of 224 mg/dl, ate high-fat food, and had hypertension. These risk factors were present for many years prior to his being seen by me. At medical evaluation he had a PET study of his heart (a diagnostic test

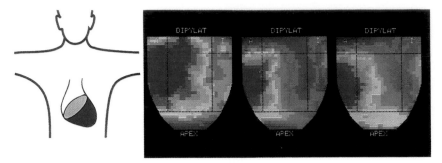

Figure 2.10. Progression of Coronary Artery Disease with Inadequate Reversal Treatment and Subsequent Regression with More Vigorous Treatment. Adapted from Gould, Lancet 1995; 346:750–753.

discussed in detail in part 3). PET images during dipyridamole stress initially showed a mild abnormality in the blood flow to the bottom, or inferior, part of the heart muscle (see left panel of figure 2.10). In PET pictures of blood flow in the heart muscle, warm colors (red, yellow) indicate good blood flow and cold colors (green, blue, black) indicate poor blood flow. These results indicated mild coronary heart disease causing mild reduction in blood flow to heart muscle during stress. However, he had no symptoms such as chest pain or short-windedness.

He was treated with moderate doses of a cholesterol-lowering drug and instructed in detail about the very low-fat food regimen. Although he faithfully took his cholesterol-lowering medication, he did not adhere to a low-fat diet during the first year of treatment. His total cholesterol was reduced to 175 mg/dl, LDL 95 mg/dl, HDL 53 mg/dl, and triglycerides 136 mg/dl average values over the first year, a substantial improvement over baseline values. After one year of these "normal" cholesterol levels and poor control of dietary fat, a repeat PET scan showed marked worsening indicated by dark blue areas (see middle panel of figure 2.10). He had also developed mild chest pain on exertion for the first time just prior to the PET scan. On reviewing the worsening in his PET pictures, this patient decided to adhere to a strict low-fat diet over the next year. He was also switched to a more effective dose of another cholesterol-lowering medication. The combination of very low-fat foods and optimal doses of a cholesterol-lowering drug reduced his total cholesterol to an average of 110, LDL 49, HDL 51, and triglycerides 94 mg/dl over the following year. A repeat scan after a year of this more vigorous treatment showed improvement (see right panel of figure 2.10). Although green areas remain, the abnormality of blood flow is less severe than in the blue areas of the middle picture. This improvement indicated partial reversal and stabilization of his coronary heart disease. His chest pain on exertion also disappeared. The patient has remained well and pain free for the past five years. This clinical example illustrates the importance of vigorous reversal treatment to achieve optimal results.

Can Cholesterol Levels Be Too Low?

Although there clearly are benefits resulting from vigorous cholesterol lowering in patients with coronary heart disease, there has been some concern that very low cholesterol levels may be associated with increased deaths due to other noncardiovascular causes (such as cancer, trauma, or suicides). This concern arose after several studies found such an association in their general, unselected population of subjects.

In these large population studies, there is a small percentage of people who have preexisting medical conditions, such as cancer, depression, alcoholism, gastrointestinal diseases, or addictive behavior such as drug addiction or smoking, all of which reduce appetite and may impair nutrition in association with very low cholesterol levels. These preexisting conditions not only lower cholesterol levels but may also cause death unrelated to cardiovascular disease. Therefore, in such studies, there may be an association between death caused by the preexisting nonvascular disease and low cholesterol levels.

However, if the people with these preexisting nonvascular medical conditions are screened out and removed from the analysis, there is no increase in deaths associated with low cholesterol levels. These observations are documented by the relative risk ratio, which is the ratio of deaths per 1,000 people with low cholesterol to deaths per 1,000 people with normal cholesterol. When people with preexisting medical conditions are excluded from the analysis, the relative risk ratio is close to one, indicating that deaths are not increased in subjects with low cholesterol. (See table 2.8.) Three large scientific studies support this conclusion.

Table 2.8. Risk of Violent or Noncardiovascular Deaths in Subjects with Low Cholesterol Who Have No Preexisting Confounding Conditions

No. of Subjects	Risk Ratio[a]	Reference[b]
10,898	0.97	Vartiainen Br Med J 1994; 309:445
7,049	1.10	Iribarren JAMA 1995; 273:1,926
4,444	0.95	4S Lancet 1994; 344:1,383

[a]Risk ratio is the mortality with low cholesterol divided by the mortality with normal cholesterol.
[b]For full names of journals, see the list of abbreviations in the bibliography.

Table 2.9. Risk of Violent Deaths in Finnish Subjects with Low Cholesterol

Risk Factor	Risk Ratio[a]
Smoking	2.28
Alcohol	1.11
Systolic blood pressure	1.09
Low cholesterol level	1.02
Years of education	.97

SOURCE: Vartiainen, British Medical Journal 1994; 309:445.
NOTE: A total of 10,898 Finnish men with specific risk factors for coronary heart disease were studied.
[a]Risk ratio is the mortality with a given risk factor divided by the mortality without the risk factor.

In a general population that includes people with preexisting, nonvascular medical problems or addictive behavior, the association between low cholesterol and increased noncardiovascular deaths can be identified as due to the preexisting condition or addictive behavior. For example, in a Finnish study, increased deaths with a relative risk ratio of greater than one were associated with smoking, excess alcohol, and high blood pressure. (See table 2.9.) However, other characteristics of the population such as low cholesterol levels and years of education were *not* associated with an increase in deaths.

In the 4S trial, reviewed previously, there was no increase in death rates due to cancer, trauma, suicides, or other noncardiovascular causes in those individuals treated with cholesterol-lowering drugs. In other words, these deaths were not caused by any adverse effects of the cholesterol-lowering drugs. The percentage of patients in whom drugs were discontinued because of side effects of the drugs was comparable to the percentage of people stopping the inert placebo without active ingredients given to the control group on a random basis. (See table 2.10.) Therefore, neither the active ingredients of the cholesterol-lowering drugs nor lowered cholesterol itself had significant side effects.

This section on cholesterol lowering and the benefits of vigorous reversal treatment of coronary heart disease can be summarized as follows: There is decreased chest pain due to coronary heart disease, increased blood flow to heart muscle, decreased heart attacks, decreased deaths, decreased strokes, decreased balloon dilation, decreased coronary bypass surgery, decreased days of hospitalization, decreased costs of medical care, and few adverse reactions to cholesterol lowering, especially when compared with the risks of balloon dilation and coronary bypass surgery. (See table 2.11.) This body of scientific information is the basis for the principally noninvasive

Table 2.10. Side Effects and Noncardiovascular Deaths in the Scandinavian Simvastatin Survival Study (4S)

Group[a]	Side Effects[b]	Noncardiovascular Deaths
Simvastatin	10%	2.1%
Placebo	13%	2.2%

SOURCE: Lancet 1994; 334:1,383.
[a]Of 4,444 subjects, half were given the cholesterol-lowering drug simvastatin, and half were given a placebo.
[b]Includes only those side effects leading to discontinuance of treatment.

Table 2.11. Summary of Outcomes after Reversal Treatment and after Balloon Dilation or Bypass Surgery

Outcome	After Reversal Treatment	After Bypass Surgery or Balloon Dilation
Chest pain	Reduced	Reduced
Blood flow to heart muscle	Improved	Improved
Heart attacks, strokes	Reduced	Little benefit
Deaths	Reduced	Little benefit
Bypass surgery, balloon dilation	Reduced	Repeated often
Cost of medical care	Lower	Higher

management of coronary heart disease by reversal treatment combined with noninvasive PET imaging to identify or follow changes.

Smoking and Death

Smoking kills. It kills both the smoker and those in the environment exposed passively to cigarette smoke. Smoking is responsible for more deaths in the United States than alcohol, motor vehicle accidents, or any other dangers. (See table 2.12.) As an addictive, lethal drug, tobacco kills twenty times as many people as all other addictive drugs together, such as heroin, cocaine, and amphetamines. It is astonishing that such an addictive, lethal drug, tobacco or nicotine, is not regulated as a drug. It is accepted as a routine business at enormous profits to the tobacco industry, although now there are numerous antismoking lawsuits pending that may change this attitude somewhat. However, it causes an enormous burden of death, disability, and costs

Table 2.12. The Leading Causes of Death in the United States
in 1990

Cause of Death	No. of Deaths
Tobacco	400,000
Diet and activity	300,000
Alcohol	100,000
Infection	90,000
Toxins	60,000
Firearms	35,000
Sexual behavior	30,000
Motor vehicles	25,000
Illicit drugs	20,000

SOURCE: McGinnis, Journal of the American Medication Association 1993;
270:2,207–2,212.

for health care. People get upset and excited about "hard drugs," especially
for younger people, but tolerate a far more insidious, addictive drug that kills
and disables on a much greater scale: indeed smoking kills and cripples more
people in the United States than any other threat to life.

Diseases directly caused by smoking, leading to death or disability, include coronary heart disease, cerebrovascular disease, cancer, and chronic
lung disease. Both smoking and passive smoke exposure:

✓ Damage the endothelial lining of the arteries.
✓ Activate blood clotting, leading to increased thrombosis.
✓ Cause constriction of arteries that slows blood flow.
✓ Accelerate atherosclerosis and plaque rupture.
✓ Reduce HDL, thereby accelerating atherosclerosis.
✓ Increase the number of heart attacks and strokes.
✓ Damage genes of cells, resulting in cancer.
✓ Destroy lung tissue.
✓ Reduce the oxygen-carrying capacity of blood.
✓ Cause addiction to nicotine.

The toxins in cigarette smoke include nicotine, carbon monoxide,
polycyclic aromatic hydrocarbons, and many other compounds less well
defined than these poisons. The effects of cigarette smoke are immediate,
within minutes of exposure, prolonged after exposure, and cumulative. Exposure of nonsmokers for twenty minutes to environmental tobacco smoke

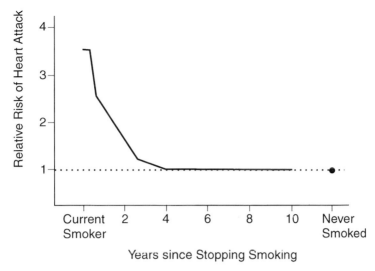

Figure 2.11. Decreased Risk of Heart Attack in Women Who Have Stopped Smoking. Adapted from Rosenberg, New England Journal of Medicine 1990; 322:213–217.

in an elevator lobby of a hospital increased the sensitivity for forming blood clots up to 60 percent of the level of active smokers. Some of the scientific publications documenting these conclusions are listed in the references at the end of the book.

Stopping smoking is an essential step in this reversal regimen. For those addicted to cigarettes, nicotine patches are a useful aid, to be used under medical supervision. For nonsmokers, eliminating passive exposure to tobacco smoke in the environment is essential. Anyone who does not recognize these facts and tolerates exposure to tobacco smoke has a significant health problem with a high risk of premature death and disability. Failure to recognize or accept these facts regarding active or passive smoke exposure simply reflects disregard for health. This disregard is perhaps due to advertising and financial interests of tobacco companies, true self-destructive addiction to the drug nicotine, lack of good sense, peer pressure, or other self-destructive tendencies. Smoking is equivalent in outcome to violent crime, hard drug addiction, and suicide, but results in far more widespread death and disability because it has been socially acceptable, although attitudes are recently changing.

Breaking the smoking habit eliminates this major cause of death and risk from cardiovascular disease. As an example for women, within two to four years after stopping smoking, the relative risk of heart attack due to smoking dramatically falls and approaches the risk for someone who never smoked. (See figure 2.11.)

Excess Body Weight and Survival

Body weight reflects the balance of total calories eaten and caloric expenditure. Some people maintain lean body mass despite high calories in their food, such as 3,000 or more calories per day. They have high metabolic rates that burn the calories without gaining weight, or they may be physically very active. Other people may gain weight on low-caloric intake such as 1,200 to 1,500 calories per day, even if they are physically active. The balance between weight and calories consumed in food is highly variable and highly individualized. Normal weight ranges are also highly variable, depending on body build, self-image, how one feels at a given weight, social attitudes, and many other factors.

Excess body weight or weight gain reflects excess calories and excessive or richer food for whatever level of activity or metabolism characterizes the person. For a given individual, excess weight causes higher cholesterol levels than a lower weight does. When carefully defined in comparison with average values for age and height, excess body weight is directly related to increased risk of death and disability, particularly from coronary heart disease. In the studies that were the basis for figures 2.12 and 2.13, weight was normalized to height squared (raised to the second power). This normalization takes into account body size related to height in the weight of the person. As weight normalized for body size increases, risk of death also increases. As weight normalized for body size decreases, the risk of death decreases. This relation between excess weight or weight gain and risk of death affects both men and women but to differing degrees, for unknown reasons.

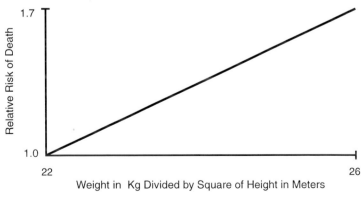

Figure 2.12. Body Weight and Risk of Death for Men. Adapted from Lee, Journal of the American Medical Association 1993; 270:2,823–2,828.

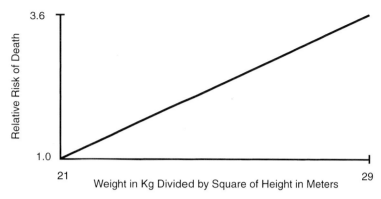

Figure 2.13. Body Weight and Risk of Death for Women. Adapted from Willett, Journal of the American Medical Association 1995; 273:461–465.

Physical Fitness and Survival

Physical activity has long been associated with healthy living. For example, in a long-term, eighteen-year study of people who were physically unfit initially but then became physically fit, survival was improved over those who remained unfit. (See figure 2.14.)

In another study, summarized in figure 2.15, death rates observed in inactive people (expressed as the relative maximal risk of 100 percent) were compared with those seen in more active people. As activity level rose, the death rate fell—up to 50 percent lower in very active people. The data in these different studies were obtained and analyzed by different methods. Consequently, they are presented in different types of graphs, but the conclusions are similar.

On the basis of studies like these, we know that regular physical exercise is an important part of this comprehensive program for preventing/ reversing coronary heart disease. The beneficial effects of exercising regularly, of being fit, or becoming fit include the following:

1. Improved survival and decreased deaths compared with those who are not physically fit.
2. Improved weight control due to burning calories, otherwise added as excess weight associated with elevated cholesterol and increased risk of death.
3. Increased levels of the good HDL cholesterol that reduce the risk of atherosclerosis.
4. Improved sense of well-being and control of one's body and life.
5. Slowed progression of narrowing in the coronary arteries due to atherosclerosis.

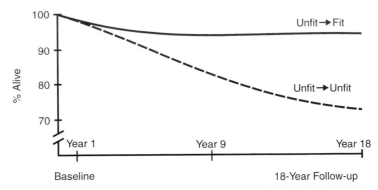

Figure 2.14. Yearly Survival and Physical Fitness through Eighteen Years of Follow-up. Adapted from Blair, Journal of the American Medical Association 1995; 273:1,093–1,098.

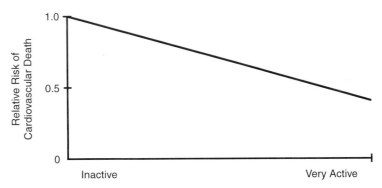

Figure 2.15. Relative Risk of Cardiovascular Death and Level of Physical Activity. Adapted from Pate, Journal of the American Medical Association 1995; 273: 402–407.

In part 2, we have reviewed the scientific basis for noninvasive reversal treatment of cardiovascular disease. In part 3, for comparative purposes, it is important for us to examine the conventional, more widespread approach to cardiovascular disease. This approach relies primarily on standard exercise stress testing, coronary arteriography, coronary bypass surgery, and balloon dilation.

PART 3

Steering through the Medical Maze

✓ The Importance of a Definitive Diagnosis

✓ Standard Exercise Stress Tests—True or False Answers?

✓ Other Noninvasive Tests for Atherosclerosis

✓ How Accurate Is the Coronary Arteriogram?

✓ Percent Narrowing—An Inaccurate Measurement of Severity

✓ High Tech for the Heart

✓ Accuracy of Positron Emission Tomography (PET)

✓ Blood Flow in Heart Muscle after Reversal Treatment

✓ Two People, Two Outcomes—Real-Life Examples

✓ Other Tests—What Do They Show?

✓ Does Coronary Bypass Surgery Prolong Your Life?

✓ PET for Determining Who Needs Bypass Surgery or Balloon Dilation

✓ Balloon Dilation of Narrowed Coronary Arteries

✓ Chest Pain: Reversal? Balloon? Bypass?

✓ Costs of Reversal Treatment, Balloon Dilation, and Bypass Surgery

✓ Economics, Ethics, and Politics of Cardiovascular Disease

✓ Managing Your Physician

P eople are commonly overwhelmed by a variety of emotions and questions on first recognizing their vascular or coronary heart disease, or their high risk of having it. Fear of death, disability, and pain makes it difficult to ask the right questions, objectively understand the options, or develop a rational plan. The urge to quickly resolve those intense emotions often interferes with acquiring enough accurate information to make good decisions. Consequently, many people passively accept tests and procedures without asking the hard questions of their physicians, without understanding what cardiovascular disease is, what and why diagnostic tests or treatment procedures are needed, and what alternatives are available. These tests and procedures may be more or less useful, but they may also be unnecessary or harmful. Other people are so frightened they don't do anything at all; more information about the problem is unwelcome, even though essential for good decision making.

Years of experience and many scientific studies have yielded new insights into the tests, procedures, and treatments used by doctors, particularly cardiovascular specialists, for vascular and coronary heart disease. Although commonly used tests and procedures may have been or are beneficial in some circumstances, accumulating evidence indicates that they may now be unnecessary for the most part, ineffective or harmful in comparison with newer diagnostic and treatment methods.

This section outlines the usefulness, the truths, and the failures of current, widely used tests and procedures for coronary artery disease. The purpose is to provide an accurate base of knowledge for the enlightened, active management of one's own health.

The Importance of a Definitive Diagnosis

Many people with cardiovascular disease have no symptoms and feel well. Many others have clear-cut symptoms indicating a problem, but the extent and severity of disease are unknown. Coronary atherosclerosis may develop without narrowing the artery or without limiting blood flow to heart muscle. Therefore, coronary artery disease may be silent, causing no symptoms or disability until a cholesterol plaque ruptures, blocks an artery, and causes chest pain, heart attack, or death. The first symptom of coronary heart disease may be a catastrophic event. For this reason, everyone with a firmly established diagnosis of coronary heart disease, even in a mild early form, or after a heart attack, should undergo reversal treatment regardless of whether symptoms or physical limitations are present.

Chest pain or other symptoms may be nonspecific and due to some other problem unrelated to the heart. However, because chest pain may also be a warning sign of coronary heart disease, it is important to make a definitive diagnosis by a reliable test administered by a physician. The diagnostic test may rule out coronary artery disease or may identify it in either early or advanced stages. If coronary artery disease is excluded, and risk factors not increased, intensive treatment may not be needed, but a healthy diet and lifestyle are recommended to prevent future problems. For undertaking intense lifelong reversal treatment involving very low-fat food and cholesterol-lowering medications, a definitive diagnosis by a reliable test is essential. The intensity of lifestyle modification, dietary change, and use of cholesterol-lowering or cardiovascular drugs are justifiable only for severe risk factors or only if cardiovascular disease is definitively diagnosed even in early form before symptoms arise. The regimen for reversing cardiovascular disease described here requires an accurate diagnosis of cardiovascular disease, since the treatment is vigorous and lasts throughout a lifetime.

There is a major difference between the diet and lifestyle modifications needed for treating firmly diagnosed coronary artery disease and those recommended as general public health measures for reducing cardiovascular disease in the population at large. The latter do not require definitive diagnostic information about everyone in the population because they are quite modest in their intensity and scope; they are not adequate to reverse or stop progression of cardiovascular disease in an individual who has coronary atherosclerosis or high risk factors for developing it. The intensity of reversal treatment necessary for an individual with coronary heart disease is not appropriate for the general population, most of whom do not have cardiovascular disease. Certainly, smoking cessation, reduction in dietary fat and cholesterol, control of hypertension, and adequate exercise are desirable public health goals. The essential difference between these public health preventive measures and reversal treatment of an individual is the degree or vigor of lowering fat in the diet and the use of cholesterol-lowering or cardiovascular drugs.

The intensity of such treatment requires a definitive diagnosis of cardiovascular disease, atherosclerosis, dysfunctional arteries, or high risk factors.

Standard Exercise Stress Tests— True or False Answers?

The standard stress test uses ECG monitoring or standard radiotracer technology to obtain relatively crude pictures of blood flow in the heart during exercise. In people with suggestive chest pain, standard exercise testing using standard radiotracer technology has an accuracy of only 50 to 75 percent. In other words, only half to three-quarters of patients tested will be accurately diagnosed (as either having coronary artery disease or not having it). In patients with no symptoms undergoing these tests, the accuracy is worse, only 30 to 50 percent, with erroneous results in 50 to 70 percent. This poor accuracy of standard exercise testing is well documented by eight scientific reports published since 1983 and involving 3,232 patients. Therefore, these standard stress tests are not reliable enough for definitively diagnosing or excluding coronary heart disease in an individual as the basis for choosing lifelong reversal treatment. Symptoms alone, such as chest pain, are also not sufficiently reliable indicators of disease to begin reversal treatment.

The terms *diagnostic sensitivity* and *diagnostic specificity* are used to describe the accuracy of exercise tests for identifying coronary heart disease proven to be present by coronary arteriography. Sensitivity indicates the percentage or number of people with a positive stress test out of 100 patients having proven coronary heart disease by coronary arteriography. A sensitivity of 87 percent means that of 100 patients with coronary heart disease, 87 percent will have a positive stress test. However, 13 out of 100 (13 percent) will have a normal stress test that misses the coronary heart disease which is present. Specificity indicates the percentage or number of individuals having a normal stress test out of 100 normal people who do not have significant coronary heart disease by coronary arteriography. A specificity of 54 percent means that of 100 normal individuals, only 54 will have a normal stress test; 46 out of 100 (46 percent) will have a false positive test result, even though these individuals have no coronary heart disease by coronary arteriography.

The accuracy of standard radionuclide technology for obtaining pictures of blood flow in heart muscle under stress conditions is also measured in terms of its diagnostic sensitivity and specificity. This standard technology usually refers to single photon emission tomography (SPECT) using standard radiotracers of either thallium or technetium sestimibi for taking the pictures of blood flow in the heart. In seven different scientific articles reporting on results in 3,232 patients studied with standard stress tests using standard radiotracer technology, the diagnostic sensitivity was, on average, 87 percent. Thirteen percent of these patients had normal exercise tests despite having coronary artery disease documented by coronary arteriography. The diagnostic specificity was 54 percent, indicating that 46 percent had false positive exercise SPECT studies with no significant coronary artery disease by coronary arteriography. In other words, 46 percent of the arteriograms were done as a consequence of erroneous or artifactual results of stress testing. (See table 3.1.) From one point of view, these coronary arteriograms were unnecessary procedures incurring substantial risk and cost as a result of suboptimal technology for stress testing. The patients in these studies were primarily clinical populations with chest pain or other symptoms. In subjects without symptoms, the diagnostic accuracy of standard stress testing is worse.

Of middle-aged men without symptoms or chest pain who have a positive exercise test, only one-third have or develop coronary heart disease while two-thirds do not. For example, in 407 symptom-free subjects with one or more risk factors for cardiovascular disease followed for four years after a standard thallium exercise stress test, the test results did not predict who had a cardiac event or who did well. In this study, 58 percent of subjects who had

Table 3.1. Accuracy of Standard Thallium Exercise Testing

Sensitivity[a]	Specificity[b]	No. of Patients	Reference[c]
83%	47%	197	Van Train J Nuc Med 1986; 27:17
85%	52%	1,096	Ranhosky Circulation 1988; 78:II 432
95%	71%	210	DePasquale Circulation 1988; 77:316
82%	62%	461	Iskandrian J Am Coll Cardiol 1989; 14:1,477
94%	52%	81	Bungo Chest 1983; 83:112
94%	44%	342	Van Train J Nuc Med 1990; 31:1,168
75%	53%	845	Schwartz Circulation 1993; 87:165
		3,232	

SOURCE: Circulation 1994; 90:1,558.
[a]The average diagnostic sensitivity was 87 percent.
[b]The average diagnostic specificity was 54 percent.
[c]For full names of journals, see the list of abbreviations in the bibliography.

a cardiac event had had a previously normal standard exercise test using the thallium radionuclide pictures of the heart. Of those patients who did have a cardiac event, only 52 percent had a positive thallium exercise test and 48 percent with a positive test did not. As illustrated in this example, standard exercise tests now commonly done do not reliably predict or exclude future cardiovascular events in symptom-free subjects with risk factors but no known coronary heart disease. This observation has been confirmed by several other studies listed in the references and also included in the section "Chest Pain: Reversal? Balloon? Bypass?" later in part 3.

In current cardiology practice, exercise testing is used as a noninvasive first step in evaluating an individual for coronary heart disease. However, due to its widely recognized inaccuracy, it is not considered a definitive test. If it is positive, a more definitive test, such as a coronary angiogram, is done. If symptoms strongly suggest coronary heart disease despite a normal exercise stress test, a coronary angiogram may be obtained anyway, in order to get a definitive answer confirming or ruling out coronary heart disease.

It is common practice that people with no symptoms commonly undergo exercise testing as part of a yearly physical. However, in such individuals, based on the above observations, the diagnostic accuracy is only 30 to 50 percent, with a 50 to 70 percent error in both men and women. Consequently, the standard stress test with standard radionuclide pictures of blood flow in the heart is not sufficiently accurate for reliably identifying coronary heart disease in individuals as the basis for lifelong reversal treatment.

Other Noninvasive Tests for Atherosclerosis

For atherosclerosis of the arteries to the brain (cerebrovascular disease) or in the legs (peripheral vascular disease), the most accurate noninvasive diagnostic tests utilize ultrasound such as Doppler-ECHO technologies. These arteries are close to the skin and accessible by ultrasound waves. Consequently, ultrasound works particularly well for cerebrovascular or peripheral vascular disease. Results of Doppler-ECHO tests indicating cerebrovascular or peripheral vascular disease are adequate grounds for undertaking lifelong reversal treatment. However, the relatively small size of coronary arteries, their location deep in the chest, their curving tortuous paths, and bouncing heart motion limit the value of ultrasound for assessing the coronary arteries.

How Accurate Is the Coronary Arteriogram?

Since symptoms and exercise testing are not sufficiently definitive for the diagnosis of coronary heart disease, the coronary angiogram has been traditionally used to rule out or confirm the presence of coronary artery disease and its severity. (See figure 3.1.) The coronary angiogram is also called the coronary arteriogram. Coronary arteriography is an invasive diagnostic test in which a small tube or catheter is inserted into the arteries of an arm or leg. The catheter is threaded backward through the artery to the base of the heart and positioned at the origin of the coronary arteries. A liquid that absorbs X rays, called contrast media, is then injected into the coronary artery while an X-ray movie of the heart is taken. This X-ray dye momentarily fills up the artery, replacing the blood during its injection. The X-ray movie then outlines the inside, or lumen, of the artery as a black-and-white movie picture that shows narrowing or irregularities in the inner edges due to cholesterol

---

Reversal treatment should be undertaken for individuals with:

1. prior heart attack or stroke
2. coronary artery disease by coronary angiogram
3. coronary artherosclerosis by PET imaging
4. high risk factors for coronary heart disease
5. cerebrovascular or peripheral vascular disease by Doppler-ECHO tests.

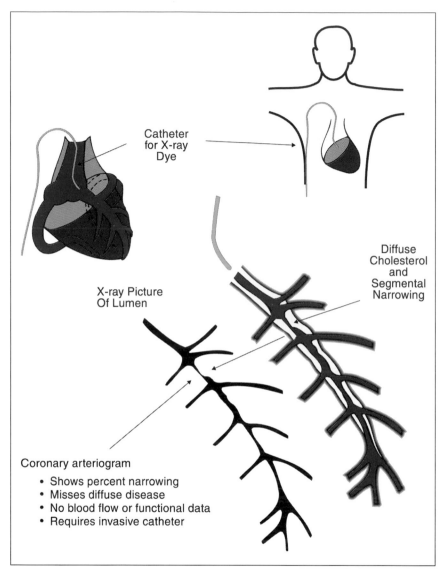

Catheter
for X-ray
Dye

Diffuse
Cholesterol
and
Segmental
Narrowing

X-ray Picture
Of Lumen

Coronary arteriogram
- Shows percent narrowing
- Misses diffuse disease
- No blood flow or functional data
- Requires invasive catheter

Figure 3.1. The Coronary Arteriogram

buildup in the arterial wall. However, the cholesterol buildup in the arterial wall itself cannot be seen in the X-ray picture; it is only implied by the narrowing of the arterial opening.

In clinical application, the coronary arteriogram is played on a small movie screen. It is visually reviewed by a cardiologist, who makes visual estimates of the severity of narrowing (called stenosis) based on the moving picture of X-ray images, as discussed in part 1. The severity of the narrowing is traditionally described in terms of percent diameter narrowing. For example, a 70 percent diameter narrowing means that the diameter of the inside of the artery is 70 percent smaller than the diameter of an adjacent normal-appearing segment of the artery on the X-ray pictures. In this instance, the size of the artery remaining open for blood flow has a diameter that is only 30 percent of the adjacent normal-appearing diameter. Traditionally, percent diameter narrowing of 0 to 50 percent is considered mild or insignificant. A severity of 50 to 75 percent diameter narrowing is considered moderate. Over 75 percent diameter narrowing is considered severe.

There are several major limitations of coronary arteriography as it is now widely used in clinical practice. First, the coronary arteriogram fails to identify or measure diffuse narrowing throughout the length of the artery. The only measurement taken, percent diameter narrowing, is determined by comparing the diameter of the narrowest point in the artery with that of an adjacent segment of the artery considered to be normal. However, in fact, this adjacent reference segment is usually also narrowed by the presence of diffuse disease. The measurement of percent diameter narrowing is therefore inaccurate because the adjacent referenced segment is also narrowed.

For patients with cholesterol diffusely deposited in the arterial wall throughout its length, there is no normal reference segment in the entire artery for purposes of determining the percent narrowing. In many instances, the coronary arteriogram appears completely normal with no segmental narrowing despite severe diffuse coronary atherosclerosis throughout the length of the coronary arteries. In a study of subjects with elevated cholesterol levels, the coronary arteriogram erroneously appeared normal in 79 percent of subjects with diffuse cholesterol deposition and atherosclerosis throughout the length of the coronary arteries; the presence of this extensive disease was proven by an invasive catheter ultrasound picture of the arterial wall obtained at the time of the arteriogram. Thus, the arteriogram misses 79 percent of the diffuse coronary atherosclerosis that can cause plaque rupture and heart attacks. This diffuse coronary atherosclerosis missed by the arteriogram may severely reduce blood flow capacity, cause chest pain, plaque rupture, heart attack, or sudden death.

There are other major deficiencies in current visual estimates of severity of coronary artery disease. Experienced, board-certified cardiologists on the average estimate severity of moderate narrowing on the coronary arteriogram as being 30 to 60 percent more severe than it actually is by objective computerized measurement. (This error in visually assessing stenosis severity is called an overestimation; see figure 3.2.) Computer techniques for measuring severity of narrowing on coronary arteriograms have been repeatedly proven accurate in experimental studies, more accurate than visual estimates by cardiologists. Cardiologists' overestimations appear to be due to such factors as training from a mentor's example rather than learning from objective

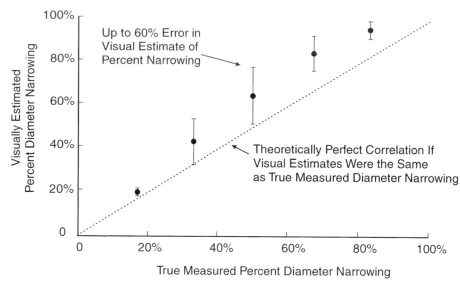

Figure 3.2. Errors in Visual Estimates of Severity of Narrowing on Coronary Arteriograms. Adapted from Fleming, Journal of the American College of Cardiology 1991; 18:945–951.

measurements or from examples of known stenosis severity, and being under pressure to overdiagnose severity as grounds for procedures that are financially rewarding.

The consequences of these erroneous visually based estimates of stenosis severity on coronary arteriograms may be serious, resulting in unnecessary bypass surgery and/or balloon dilation. In a study of patients undergoing balloon dilation of a narrowed coronary artery, the visually estimated severity by board-certified cardiologists averaged 85 percent diameter narrowing before balloon dilation. However, the actual severity measured objectively by accurate, automatic computer analysis of the same arteriograms averaged only 68 percent. The visually estimated severity after balloon dilation was 30 percent diameter narrowing. The actual severity measured by objective computer analysis following balloon dilation was 49 percent diameter narrowing. By visual estimates, the change in severity from 85 to 30 percent diameter narrowing was an improvement of 55 percent diameter narrowing units. However, the actual improvement in severity by balloon dilation was from 68 to 49 percent diameter narrowing, a change of only 19 percent diameter narrowing units. So there was a 180 percent error in the estimated benefits of balloon dilation by visual interpretation of board-certified cardiologists (calculated as 55% − 19% ÷ 19% = 180%).

Thus, by visual estimates balloon dilation appears to substantially open the artery. However, objective measurements show the benefits of balloon dilation to be considerably less. Several other scientific reports have confirmed comparable errors as widespread practice in cardiovascular medicine.

Percent Narrowing—An Inaccurate Measurement of Severity

Even if measured accurately, the percent diameter narrowing on the arteriogram does not indicate or reflect the flow capacity of a narrowed coronary artery. The maximum flow through a narrowed artery or its coronary flow reserve is determined not just by the relative percent diameter narrowing. Other dimensions have important effects on coronary blood flow. These other important dimensions include the absolute cross-sectional size of the artery, the length of the narrowing, the number of sequential other narrowings in the artery, the diffuse narrowing throughout the length of the artery, the shape of the narrowing, and the extent of functional abnormalities such as vasoconstriction or partial blood clot or thrombosis in the coronary artery which may also impede coronary blood flow.

Consequently, a graph relating maximum flow capacity or coronary flow reserve to percent diameter narrowing or stenosis on coronary arteriograms shows no consistent relation. Rather, the data are randomly located on the graph in a "scattergram." (See figure 3.3.) If there were a correlation between blood flow and percent narrowing, the dots of the scattergram would

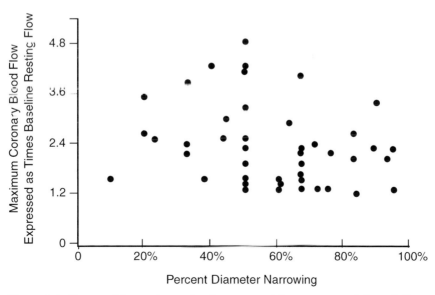

Figure 3.3. Percent Narrowing—An Inaccurate Measurement. Adapted from White, New England Journal of Medicine 1984; 310:819–824.

not be randomly located on the graph but would fall along a straight diagonal line. Thus, percent diameter narrowing, even when properly measured, is a poor, misleading, or inaccurate measurement of severity of coronary artery disease.

Despite its shortcomings, coronary arteriography continues to be widely used in clinical practice, whereas more sophisticated, advanced analysis of the entire coronary artery tree by computer methods is rarely used. The computer techniques require additional knowledge, time, and effort, retraining one's visual judgment of severity, and moderation of a common disregard for objectivity, resulting in fewer procedures and their associated financial rewards.

High Tech for the Heart

Positron emission tomography, or PET, is the most accurate high-tech medical imaging technology for measuring or taking pictures of blood flow and metabolism in heart muscle. It is different from all other technologies, such as computed tomography (CT, commonly called CAT scanning) and magnetic resonance imaging (MRI), both of which take images of the anatomical structure of the heart. Consequently, CT and MRI are not used clinically for evaluating active processes of the heart, such as its blood flow and metabolism. PET is a technology that images these dynamic processes of blood flow and metabolism in the heart muscle by using very small amounts of radiotracers which are injected intravenously. These radiotracers emit positrons, or positive electrons, which convert to paired X-ray signals that are detected or imaged by unique electronics in a scanner that looks like a large thin doughnut. It is thin enough to prevent claustrophobia. With the use of specific radiotracers, images can be obtained of blood flow in the heart muscle or its metabolic processes necessary for heart contraction. For imaging blood flow in heart muscle, the PET tracers most commonly used are rubidium-82 and nitrogen-13 ammonia. They are safe and without side effects. These PET radiotracers have very short half-lives and last only minutes to hours. Consequently, the X-ray dose is much lower than standard conventional radiotracers now used clinically for imaging the heart. (See figure 3.4.)

PET of the heart requires only an injection of the radiotracer into an arm vein. It does not require insertion of a catheter into the artery or threading the catheter back to the base of the heart, as in coronary arteriography. PET is therefore to be considered "noninvasive," with little significant risk.

PET radiotracers have the unique characteristic of emitting pairs of X-ray beams in opposite directions. These paired X rays allow a unique electronic detection method called coincidence counting. It produces the most

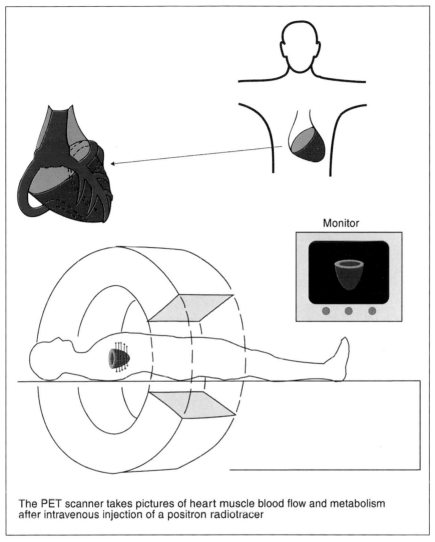

The PET scanner takes pictures of heart muscle blood flow and metabolism after intravenous injection of a positron radiotracer

Figure 3.4. Positron Emission Tomography (PET) of the Heart

accurate pictures of blood flow or metabolism in the heart. With standard radionuclide imaging, the X-ray signals from the back of the heart are absorbed by the surrounding chest wall, liver, or other organs. This absorption of the X-ray signals causes errors, or artifacts, in pictures made using standard imaging technology. In PET these artifacts are corrected so that more accurate quantitative pictures are obtained of blood flow or metabolism in the heart. PET is therefore more accurate than standard radiotracer pictures. (See figure 3.5.)

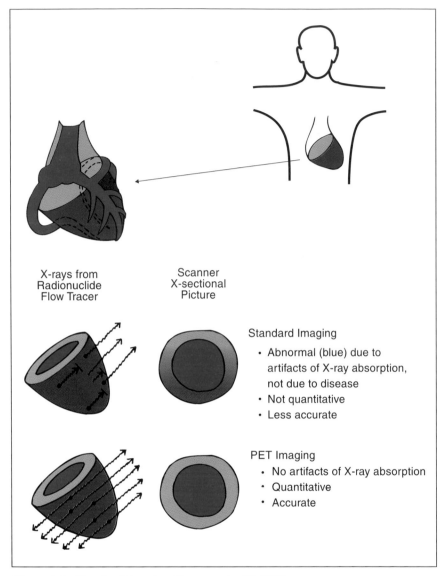

X-rays from
Radionuclide
Flow Tracer

Scanner
X-sectional
Picture

Standard Imaging

- Abnormal (blue) due to
  artifacts of X-ray absorption,
  not due to disease
- Not quantitative
- Less accurate

PET Imaging

- No artifacts of X-ray absorption
- Quantitative
- Accurate

Figure 3.5. Standard Imaging Compared with PET

Accuracy of Positron Emission Tomography (PET)

As discussed earlier, the accuracy of a diagnostic test is described by two terms, sensitivity and specificity. The sensitivity is measured as the number of people with a positive test out of 100 people with coronary artery disease. It is therefore the percentage of people with coronary heart disease who have a positive test identifying that disease. Those people having a normal test despite having coronary heart disease have a false negative result. The specificity

Table 3.2. Accuracy of Cardiac Position Emission Tomography (PET)

Sensitivity[a]	Specificity[b]	No. of Patients	Reference[c]
94%	95%	193	Demer Circulation 1989; 79:825
94%	95%	48	Gupta Am Heart J 1992: 122:293
98%	93%	208	Williams Journal of Myocardial Ischemia 1990; 2:38
95%	82%	132	Go J Nuc Med 1990; 31:1,899
95%	100%	50	Gould J Am Coll Cardiol 1986; 7:775
84%	88%	81	Stewart Am J Cardiol 1991; 67:1,303
98%	100%	51	Tamaki J Nuc Med 1988; 29:1,181
97%	100%	32	Schelbert Am J Cardiol 1982; 49:1,197
97%	100%	60	Yonekura 1987; 113:645
		855	

SOURCE: Circulation 1994; 90:1,558.
[a]The average diagnostic sensitivity was 95 percent.
[b]The average diagnostic specificity was 95 percent.
[c]For full names of journals, see the list of abbreviations in the bibliography.

is measured as the number of people with a negative, or normal, test out of 100 people who are normal (that is, without coronary heart disease). It is therefore the percentage of normal people without heart disease who also have a normal test result indicating that disease has been excluded. Those normal people who have positive test results despite being normal have a false positive test.

Positron emission tomography (PET) detects coronary artery disease with a diagnostic accuracy of 95 percent or greater. In 855 patients reported in nine scientific publications, the diagnostic sensitivity was 95 percent and the specificity was also 95 percent. (See table 3.2.) A specificity of 95 percent indicates that 95 percent of individuals with normal arteriograms also had prior normal PET scans. A sensitivity of 95 percent indicates that 95 percent of individuals with coronary atherosclerosis by coronary arteriography are correctly identified by PET imaging.

On the other hand, the standard arteriogram fails to show diffuse coronary atherosclerosis, is frequently misinterpreted, and does not provide functional information on blood flow capacity or the status of the lining of the artery. Since all of these factors affect coronary blood flow, PET is often more sensitive and accurate than both arteriography and standard exercise testing for evaluating coronary atherosclerosis. PET eliminates the frequent false positive tests and reduces unnecessary coronary arteriograms. Individuals definitively identified as having coronary atherosclerosis by PET may undergo vigorous reversal treatment without an arteriogram. Progression or regression of coronary artery disease can also be followed by PET with an accuracy that is comparable or greater than the quantitative changes in severity as measured by coronary arteriography.

Blood Flow in Heart Muscle after Reversal Treatment

Coronary artery narrowing due to cholesterol buildup in the walls of the coronary artery limits or reduces the maximum blood flow through the artery during stress. Reversal treatment decreases severity of this narrowing and increases blood flow through the artery to the heart muscle of people with coronary heart disease. To determine the extent of this narrowing, and consequently the blood flow capacity, PET takes pictures of blood flow in heart muscle during induced stress. Stress for this purpose is produced by using a drug called dipyridamole which makes blood flow in the heart muscle increase by three to four times baseline resting blood flow if the coronary arteries are normal. This normal increase in coronary blood flow produced by dipyridamole is much more than occurs after exercise stress. If the arteries are narrowed by cholesterol buildup, the flow induced by dipyridamole is restricted or limited to a lesser increase, for example, to 1.5 to 2 times baseline flow.

PET is accurate not only for diagnosing coronary heart disease but also for following its progression or regression. Reversal treatment reduces the size and severity of blood flow abnormalities seen on a PET picture of the heart. With PET, the progression or regression in the severity of the narrowed coronary arteries can be accurately followed without using invasive catheters.

The orientation of three-dimensional PET images of blood flow in heart muscle is shown, in figure 3.6, in right (septal), front (anterior), left (lateral), and back (inferior) views, illustrated in relation to the coronary arteries. The colors in each view show relative blood flow in heart muscle. The color scale is graded, ranging from maximum flow in the heart muscle in red (100 percent) downward in 5 percent increments corresponding to the stepped color scale through red, yellow, green, blue, to black representing the lowest blood flow in the heart muscle. Warm colors of red, yellow, orange indicate relatively good flow; yellow indicates intermediate blood flow; and green, blue, black indicate relatively low blood flow.

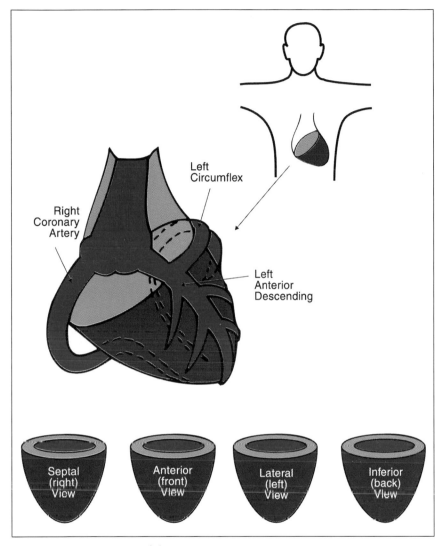

Figure 3.6. Orientation of the Heart on PET Images

Two People, Two Outcomes—Real-Life Examples
Regression

Figure 3.7 shows PET images during stress before (upper row) and during stress after intense cholesterol lowering for five years (lower row). After the treatment period, the area of abnormal blood flow under stress, as seen on the upper baseline by PET (green and blue), becomes markedly smaller. This change indicates better, more uniform blood flow throughout the heart

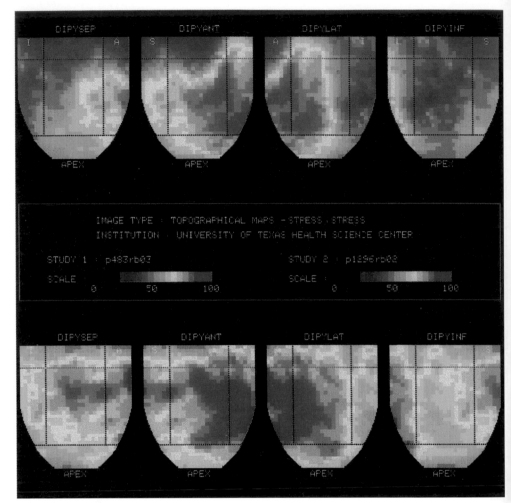

Figure 3.7. Example of Regression of Coronary Artery Disease by PET. Adapted from Gould, Journal of the American Medical Association 1995; 274:894–901.

muscle (more yellow, red, and white colors) as a result of reversal treatment. Such regression on reversal treatment reduces markedly the risk of heart attack or sudden death, and the need for coronary bypass surgery or balloon dilation.

Progression

Figure 3.8 shows PET images during stress at baseline before (upper row) and during stress after five years of conventional medical treatment without a low-fat diet or cholesterol-lowering drugs (lower row). There is worsening (areas of green and blue) on the follow-up PET image character-

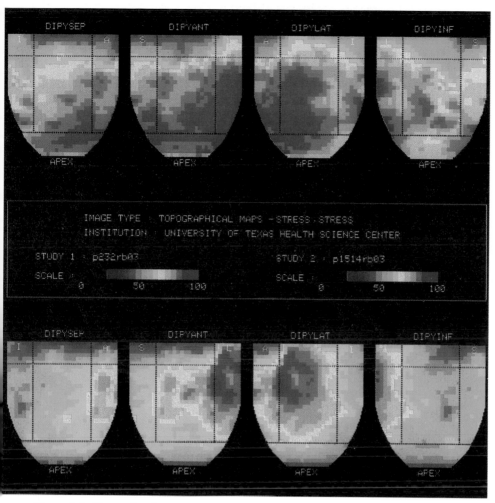

Figure 3.8. Example of Progression of Coronary Artery Disease by PET. Adapted from Gould, Journal of the American Medical Association 1995; 274:894–901.

istically seen in people with coronary atherosclerosis who are not on reversal treatment. Such progression is associated with a high risk of heart attack or sudden death, and the need for coronary bypass surgery and balloon dilation.

Thus, the components for the principally noninvasive management of coronary heart disease are as follows:

✓ Cardiac PET with dipyridamole stress is used as the primary definitive diagnostic test.

✓ Vigorous reversal treatment is provided by very low-fat foods, cholesterol-lowering medications, and lifestyle changes.

✓ Progression or regression is monitored by PET.

✓ For reversal failure (the rare cases where coronary artery disease progresses despite good treatment, or where patients do not adhere to a good program or cannot tolerate medications), standard invasive procedures of coronary arteriography, balloon dilation, or bypass surgery are appropriate.

Other Tests—What Do They Show?

A number of diagnostic tests are used for evaluating the heart. Each test has advantages and disadvantages. Each has its proponents who vigorously support their use. The approach here focuses on noninvasive diagnosis and management of coronary heart disease based on reversal treatment. Because reversal treatment is beneficial for those who have been diagnosed with coronary artery disease, an accurate, specific diagnosis of coronary artery disease is a key component of the complete comprehensive program. From this perspective, any diagnostic test should meet the following criteria:

1. Noninvasive, except for an intravenous injection.
2. High diagnostic accuracy comparable to or better than that of coronary arteriography in order to decide whether or not lifelong reversal treatment is advisable; there must be accuracy both in identifying atherosclerosis present (sensitivity) and in identifying normals (specificity) by ruling out coronary artery narrowing.
3. Reliable detection of early atherosclerosis or dysfunctional coronary arteries due to abnormal endothelial lining of the artery or due to mild early atherosclerosis.
4. Assessment of coronary artery function, such as endothelial function and maximum blood flow capacity in the heart muscle.
5. Proven accuracy for showing progression or regression of coronary artery disease as well as or better than coronary arteriography.

The different kinds of noninvasive diagnostic tests can be classified by several conceptually simple characteristics. The first major characteristic is the type of stress testing. All types of stress testing have a common purpose: to stimulate increased coronary blood flow to the heart muscle in order to assess the maximum work of the heart or flow capacity of the coronary arteries. This stress can be treadmill exercise or bicycle exercise, either upright or lying on one's back. Or the stress can be pharmacologic, induced by special drugs that substitute for exercise stress, a technique I first developed in the seventies using the drug dipyridamole.

The stress drug dipyridamole and a similar one, adenosine, stimulate increased coronary blood flow to the heart muscle by directly dilating the coronary arteries. They increase coronary blood flow by three to four times baseline values, much greater than during exercise, and therefore are more useful for detecting early mild narrowings of the coronary arteries that limit only the maximum levels of highest coronary blood flow. The effect of these drugs does not depend on the ability or willingness to exercise hard. Heart work is increased only minimally compared with the heavy workload on the heart with exercise. Since the increase in blood flow is greater with these drugs than with exercise, abnormally restricted flow capacity due to narrowing in the coronary arteries is more readily identified on pictures of blood flow in the heart muscle. Both drugs have been used safely in millions of tests. However, dipyridamole has fewer side effects than adenosine.

For each of these stress drugs or for exercise stress, PET technology for taking diagnostic pictures of the blood flow in the heart muscle is better than current commonly used standard imaging technology.

A third drug used for stress is called dobutamine. It mimics exercise by increasing the heart rate and heart pumping work. It does not increase coronary flow as much as dipyridamole or adenosine. Either dobutamine or exercise stress is optimal for testing pumping function, or work capacity, of the heart. Heart pumping function may be reduced by several health problems unrelated to coronary atherosclerosis, including high blood pressure, excess alcohol consumption, primary heart muscle deterioration, diabetes, abnormal valvular function, severe viral infections of the heart, and several other systemic diseases. In these conditions, stress tests using dobutamine or exercise may show abnormally reduced work capacity of the heart, even when the coronary arteries and blood flow to the heart are normal.

Therefore, these tests do not specifically indicate whether coronary artery blood flow is affected by atherosclerosis. In contrast, dipyridamole and adenosine test the actual blood flow capacity of the coronary arteries. They are therefore more useful for identifying coronary atherosclerosis. However, they do not provide information about the pumping function or work capacity of the heart.

The second major characteristic of noninvasive diagnostic heart tests is the type of data obtained about heart function. One category of data involves measuring heart pumping function. The second type of data, obtained during exercise, is recorded on the electrocardiogram. The third, and final, type appears as pictures of the blood flow in heart muscle. All of these approaches are briefly reviewed below.

Heart Pumping Function

Data on the pumping function of the heart are acquired by taking pictures by ultrasound, by radionuclide methods, by magnetic resonance imaging (MRI), or by fast CT scanning (called CAT scanning). The most widely used of these four technologies for assessing pump function are ultrasound (called ECHO) and radionuclide methods (called MUGA, or multiple gated acquisition). Although there are technical differences, both ECHO and MUGA give comparable information on the pumping function of the heart. This pumping function is usually measured as the ejection fraction, or the fraction of blood in the pumping chamber ejected with each heartbeat. The contraction of heart muscle in each localized region of the heart is also measured in order to detect localized segments of damaged heart muscle. (For background on the pumping function and detection of localized damage, see part 1.) Regional abnormalities in the heart contraction are typically associated with damage caused by a heart attack. Reduction of overall heart pumping function and ejection fraction is associated with either heart attacks or a variety of other causes unrelated to atherosclerosis.

ECHO or MUGA tests are carried out at rest and/or during exercise or dobutamine stress. Abnormal pumping function of the heart shown by these tests done under resting conditions indicates significant heart damage from some cause. Severity of the reduction in heart pumping function indicates severity of damage to the heart muscle.

If the pumping function of the heart is normal at resting conditions, stress is often used to test the maximum work capacity of the heart. The purpose is to reveal milder or transient pumping abnormalities that are not apparent under the resting conditions. The stress used is typically supine bicycle exercise or dobutamine. Under the workload on the heart produced by these stresses, pumping function normally increases. With stress, the ejection fraction normally increases to meet the workload of delivering more blood to the body. If the pumping function deteriorates and ejection fraction falls during stress, the heart muscle is impaired by some cause that has to be identified by further testing.

The cause may be narrowing of the coronary arteries, which limits blood flow to the heart muscle and thereby prevents the heart muscle from contracting harder to meet the workload demanded during stress. This limited blood flow is what makes the ejection fraction fall. However, as we have seen, there are many causes other than coronary atherosclerosis that make the pumping function deteriorate with stress. In these other conditions, the coronary arteries may be normal, but the work capacity of the heart is impaired, causing an abnormal ECHO or MUGA test.

On the other hand, coronary atherosclerosis and narrowing of the coronary arteries may be present, but the pump-function test may be normal.

Therefore, all tests that measure heart pumping function, either at resting conditions or under stress, are not specific for identifying or ruling out coronary atherosclerosis. Neither do they adequately indicate the severity or changes in severity with progression or regression of coronary heart disease. While these tests are valuable in clinical management, they are not reliable or specific enough for deciding either on lifelong reversal treatment for coronary atherosclerosis or on the procedures of bypass surgery or balloon dilation.

ECG Stress Testing

The standard ECG stress test on a bicycle or treadmill records the electrical behavior of the heart by ECG during exercise stress. An abnormal ECG response to stress may be due to inadequate blood flow to heart muscle caused by narrowing of the coronary arteries. However, abnormal ECG responses are frequently observed in individuals with normal heart function and no coronary atherosclerosis. Abnormal ECG responses during exercise typically also occur in the presence of high blood pressure or cardiac enlargement due to any cause other than coronary atherosclerosis. Therefore, the ECG stress test is also an indirect test for coronary heart disease. It is not accurate or reliable enough to be the basis for deciding on lifelong reversal treatment of coronary atherosclerosis.

Blood Flow Capacity in the Heart Muscle

The final major type of data from noninvasive heart tests is that which directly measures or takes pictures of coronary blood flow in the heart muscle. Pictures of blood flow in heart muscle may be obtained by several technologies. These include positron emission tomography (PET), standard radionuclide methods (called SPECT), magnetic resonance imaging (MRI), and fast CT (CAT scanning). The diagnostic accuracy of PET is 95 percent or higher, as previously noted. The diagnostic accuracy of standard radionuclide technology is 50 to 70 percent due to errors or artifacts caused by absorption of X-ray signals by the chest and tissues surrounding the heart. (See figure 3.5.) Neither MRI nor fast CT provides pictures of blood flow in the heart muscle of clinical value. Both have been studied experimentally but have not been shown to be suitable for routine clinical application.

Fast CT has been used to take pictures of calcium deposited in atherosclerotic coronary arteries in response to cholesterol injury. Since calcium deposition commonly occurs in the arterial wall as well as cholesterol deposition, identifying calcium indicates the presence of atherosclerosis. This test has been used to screen for coronary heart disease by detecting the calcium associated with atherosclerosis. However, most men over forty-five years old have identifiable calcium in their coronary arteries without significant narrowing of the coronary arteries. For women, the same is true at a somewhat older age. The presence of calcium in the coronary arteries, identified by fast CT, does not indicate impaired blood flow capacity in the coronary arteries. More recently, extensive severe coronary artery disease causing heart attack has been demonstrated in younger people with normal fast CT pictures demonstrating no calcium in the coronary arteries. Furthermore, fast CT has not been shown to indicate progression or regression of coronary atherosclerosis.

From the perspective of noninvasive management of coronary heart disease based on intensive, lifelong reversal treatment, the only technology

Table 3.3. Comparative Accuracy of Current Diagnostic Tests for Coronary Heart Disease

Diagnostic Test	Sensitivity	Specificity
ECG exercise stress test	66%	77%
Exercise radionuclide angiogram	90%	58%
Dobutamine stress ECHO	78%	93%
Thallium or sestimibi stress test[a]	87%	54%
Dipyridamole or adenosine PET	95%	95%

SOURCE: Circulation 1989; 80:87; Circulation 1981; 64:586; Journal of the American College of Cardiology 1992; 19:1,203; Circulation 1994; 90:1,558.
[a]Thallium and sestimibi are standard radionuclides used for stress testing with standard technology (see text for details).

that fulfills the criteria for a noninvasive test to definitively identify or rule out coronary artery disease is positron emission tomography (PET). It is accurate and reliable enough for diagnosing and following progression or regression of coronary artery disease. For a comparison of the accuracy of these various tests in terms of their sensitivity and specificity, see table 3.3.

Does Coronary Bypass Surgery Prolong Your Life?

Historically, the basis for deciding on coronary bypass surgery was typical chest pain caused by coronary heart disease that could not be relieved by medical treatment. However, now bypass surgery is commonly done principally because of visually apparent narrowing on the coronary arteriogram. This justification given for doing bypass surgery based on the appearance of the arteriogram is that it will prevent heart attack or death.

During coronary bypass surgery, a vein is removed from the leg and one end is sewn into the base of the aorta. The other end is sewn into the coronary artery beyond any segmental narrowing, thereby bypassing the blockage in the coronary artery. (See figure 3.9.) Alternatively, there is an artery normally present on the inside surface of the front chest wall, called the internal mammary artery. It can be moved from its usual location and sewn into the coronary artery beyond a segmental narrowing. This bypass is then called an internal mammary artery graft. Multiple bypass grafts may be placed beyond multiple narrowings of the coronary arteries. Either leg veins or internal mammary arteries can be used in men or women.

In scientifically well-designed medical studies of coronary bypass surgery for stable, chronic chest pain due to coronary heart disease, overall survival for patients undergoing bypass surgery is not significantly better than

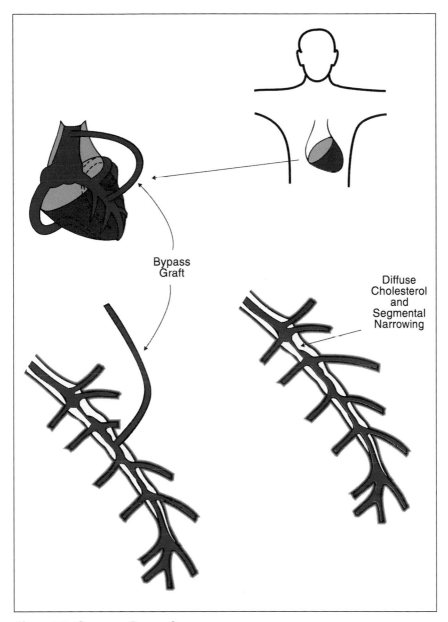

Figure 3.9. Coronary Bypass Surgery

it is for those who do not have surgery. In the same studies, the incidence of heart attacks is not significantly lower in patients who have had bypass surgery than in those without surgery. For example, in the study by the Veterans Administration, the survival rate after initial bypass surgery was not significantly higher (only 9 percent) than that after initial medical treatment.

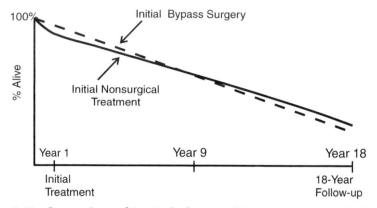

Figure 3.10. Comparison of Survival after Initial Bypass Surgery and after Initial Nonsurgical Treatment in All Patients with Stable Coronary Heart Disease. Adapted from Circulation 1992; 86:121–130.

The 9 percent difference between the surgical and medical outcomes was within the statistical noise, or random biological variability, expected from the number of patients studied and was therefore not significant. Even at eighteen-year follow-up in this Veterans Administration study, bypass surgery did not significantly improve overall survival. (See figure 3.10.)

Patients can be classified as being at high risk of dying from coronary heart disease based on the appearance of the arteriogram and pumping function of the heart. More specifically, there is *both* severe narrowing of all three major coronary arteries in the heart *and* reduced pumping function due to previous heart attack. In the Veterans Administration study, patients classified as being at high risk by the presence of both these findings did have significantly higher survival rates after initial bypass surgery than did those without surgery. However, this benefit of improved survival disappeared at twelve to fifteen years of follow-up. By eighteen years of follow-up, there was no difference between those patients with and those without bypass surgery. (See figure 3.11.)

For those patients with normal heart pumping function (normal ejection fraction), survival was worse in the group undergoing bypass surgery at the beginning of the study than in the group that did not have surgery. However, this worsened survival was not significant since the difference was within the range of random variability in the data. The important point here is that patients with normal heart pumping function do not show better survival after bypass surgery than those patients treated without surgery. (See figure 3.12.)

The effects of coronary bypass surgery on survival can also be analyzed by combining several of the larger studies. This type of analysis is called meta-analysis. In the best-known meta-analysis of coronary bypass surgery,

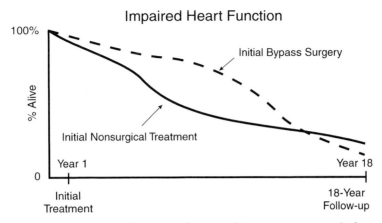

Figure 3.11. Comparison of Survival after Initial Bypass Surgery and after Initial Nonsurgical Treatment in Patients with Impaired Heart Pumping Function and Stable Coronary Heart Disease. Adapted from Circulation 1992; 86:121–130.

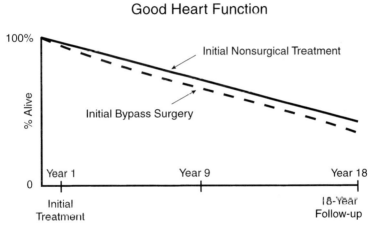

Figure 3.12. Comparison of Survival after Initial Bypass Surgery and after Initial Nonsurgical Treatment in Patients with Normal Heart Pumping Function and Stable Coronary Heart Disease. Adapted from Circulation 1992; 86:121–130.

the overall survival of patients was improved by 17 percent after initial bypass surgery compared with patients treated without initial surgery. This difference was greater than statistical variability, or noise, and was therefore considered significant. Medical treatment in these studies did not include vigorous cholesterol-lowering efforts such as effective reversal treatment with low-fat foods and cholesterol-lowering drugs.

Compared with this 17 percent improvement in survival after coronary bypass surgery, the improvement or reduction in overall deaths after

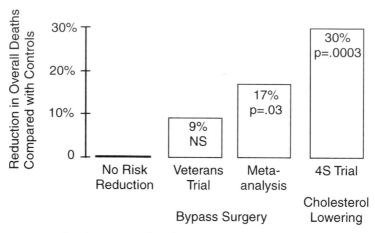

Figure 3.13. Reduction in Deaths after Bypass Surgery and after Cholesterol-lowering Treatment Compared with Untreated Controls in Separate Trials. Adapted from Circulation 1992; 86:121–130; Lancet 1994; 344:563–570; Lancet 1994; 344:1,383–1,389.

cholesterol lowering is 30 to 60 percent (in the largest of the cholesterol-lowering studies comparable to the surgical studies). In these separate scientific trials, cholesterol lowering improved overall survival substantially more than did bypass surgery. (See figure 3.13; for explanation of p values see figure 2.5; NS means not significant statistically.) Since both diet and drugs have been shown to significantly improve survival, one might anticipate even less potential benefit from bypass surgery when directly compared with cholesterol lowering.

Coronary bypass surgery is often used for patients with severe, progressive chest pain present even at resting conditions. This medical problem is called unstable angina. In a scientifically well-designed study of patients with unstable angina, coronary bypass surgery improved survival compared with patients initially treated without surgery *only* if heart pumping function was impaired by previous heart attack. Importantly, in the patients with unstable angina who had *normal* pumping function, bypass surgery was associated with a *higher death rate* than in similar patients treated without initial surgery. (See figure 3.14.) These results suggest that coronary bypass surgery may be beneficial in patients with severe chest pain only if all three coronary arteries are involved *and* the pumping function of the heart is impaired. In patients with unstable angina and *normal* pumping function, bypass surgery may be potentially harmful since it results in significantly lower survival rates than does nonsurgical reversal treatment.

In a more recent study called the Asymptomatic Cardiac Ischemia Pilot (ACIP), 558 middle-aged people with severe coronary narrowing on their arteriogram and an abnormal stress test were divided into three groups. One

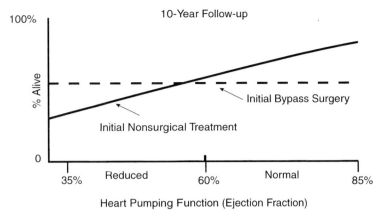

Figure 3.14. Comparison of Survival after Initial Bypass Surgery and after Initial Nonsurgical Treatment in Patients with Unstable, Progressive Chest Pain Due to Coronary Heart Disease. Adapted from Scott, Circulation 1994; 90 (Supplement 2): II20–II23.

group received only drugs used for chest pain and no treatment that systematically lowered cholesterol; the second group underwent balloon dilation; and the third group had bypass surgery. After two years, the death rates were 6.6 percent in the first group treated with standard drugs for chest pain, 4.4 percent in the group undergoing balloon dilation, and 1.1 percent in the group undergoing bypass surgery. These results appear to support the use of bypass surgery for patients with an abnormal stress test and severe coronary artery narrowing on the arteriogram. The data also suggest that survival after bypass surgery is better than after balloon dilation.

However, there are several problems with the study which raise major challenges to these conclusions. The primary problem is that the group treated exclusively with medications did not undergo systematic cholesterol lowering or reversal treatment using cholesterol-lowering drugs or low-fat diet, steps previously shown to improve survival more than any earlier reports on bypass surgery or balloon dilation. A second problem is that two-year follow-up is too short a time for making definitive conclusions on long-term survival in the three treatment groups. Finally, balloon dilation, the commonest treatment procedure for coronary heart disease, was not much better than the poor medical treatment provided to the control group by receiving no cholesterol-lowering drugs.

Why the ACIP study did not utilize cholesterol-lowering reversal treatment in the group taking only medications is a mystery to me. Why would anyone withhold treatment that has been proven to prolong life more than any other treatment for coronary heart disease in more studies and longer studies than all the combined studies of bypass surgery and balloon dilation ever done? This exclusion of proven beneficial treatment is unethical and invalid science, in my opinion. I can only conclude that the planners of this study were ignorant of the cholesterol-lowering trials, did not believe them, or were anxious to have the outcomes favor balloon dilation and bypass surgery by withholding treatment known to benefit the group taking medications only. At best, no conclusions can be drawn from this study about the relative merits of balloon dilation and bypass surgery compared with reversal treatment.

In a more recent, larger, better-designed scientific study called the RITA-2 (the second randomized intervention treatment of angina) Trial, the number of deaths and heart attacks in people undergoing balloon dilation was much higher than in those treated without balloon dilation, even without systematic cholesterol lowering.

PET for Determining Who Needs
Bypass Surgery or Balloon Dilation

People with impaired pumping function of the heart due to coronary heart disease benefit more from coronary bypass surgery in terms of improved survival than do people with normal heart pumping function. However, within this group of patients with impaired heart pumping function, there are two different populations with different prognoses; one group does not improve after bypass surgery, while the other does. The first group comprises people with permanent, fixed scarring of the heart due to previous heart attack; this group does *not* improve pumping function of the heart after bypass surgery. In the second group are patients who have areas of the heart that are injured and contract poorly, but whose heart muscle is still alive or viable. This injured-but-viable heart muscle recovers its function after bypass surgery. Bypass surgery on these patients with impaired pumping function but viable heart muscle also improves their survival. Failure to do bypass surgery in these patients is associated with a high risk of death. Thus, the accurate identification of such patients who are optimal candidates for bypass surgery is an important clinical decision; similarly, exclusion of those patients with only scars from undergoing unnecessary bypass surgery is an equally crucial clinical decision that requires informed, objective judgments by a cardiovascular specialist not influenced by economic incentive.

There are four essential questions that a person considering coronary bypass surgery or balloon dilation should ask the cardiovascular specialist.

1. What is the pumping function of my heart? It is measured as the percentage of blood in the pumping chamber ejected out of the heart into the aorta and body with each heartbeat. This fraction of blood pumped out by the heart is called the ejection fraction and should normally be over 50 percent. Neither balloon dilation nor coronary bypass surgery has been shown to improve survival, prevent heart attacks or deaths in people with normal pumping function of the heart. In a very small minority of people with normal ejection fraction who have blockages of the main trunk of the left coronary artery at its origin from the aorta, coronary bypass surgery improves survival—but only if this left main diameter narrowing is greater than 60 percent. These types of patients constitute less than 1 percent of those undergoing bypass surgery.

If the ejection fraction is less than 50 percent, the person considering balloon dilation or bypass surgery has a reasonable probability of improved survival but no guarantee. If the ejection fraction is over 50 percent, balloon dilation or bypass surgery will not likely improve survival or prevent future heart attack; on average in large studies, the only benefit derived from either procedure was relief of chest pain that had failed to improve by medical treatment. In large trials involving patients who did not have chest pain or whose chest pain was effectively treated by medicines, and whose heart pumping function was normal, only vigorous cholesterol lowering was demonstrated to improve survival and prevent heart attacks.

2. *Does my heart have damaged, poorly pumping heart muscle that is still alive or viable but has inadequate blood flow?* If this is the case, the impaired blood flow can be improved by balloon dilation or bypass surgery.

There are several diagnostic tests for identifying patients with impaired pumping function of the heart that is still viable and suitable for coronary bypass surgery. The most accurate of these tests is PET imaging of the metabolic activity of the heart muscle.

In four major university cardiovascular centers, the clinical decision for or against coronary bypass surgery using other traditional tests was incorrect in one-third (31 to 39 percent) of cases based on PET imaging of viable heart muscle. (See table 3.4.) In these university-based studies, the risk of cardiac events was very high, 24 to 50 percent, for patients in whom the decision for or against bypass surgery was incompatible with PET results. (See table 3.5.) For patients in whom the decision for or against bypass surgery was compatible with PET, the risk of death was markedly lower; the risk was still significant due to the advanced stages of coronary disease in the patients in all of these studies. Nevertheless, survival was markedly improved when decisions for or against bypass surgery were made on the basis of PET imaging of the heart muscle for viability (which bypass surgery benefited) or for the presence of scarred, permanently damaged heart tissue (which did not benefit from the surgery).

When it comes to determining whether or not impaired pumping function of the heart will improve after bypass surgery:

- ✓ PET is the best method of all the diagnostic technologies.
- ✓ PET offers accuracy that is 25 percent better than the other technologies.
- ✓ Total PET costs per study are comparable to costs of conventional tests.

Table 3.4. Potential Errors in Current Decisions for or against Balloon Dilation or Bypass Surgery in Patients with Impaired Heart Pumping Function

| No. of Patients in Study | Patients with Unsupported Decisions[a] | | Reference[b] |
	No.	%	
35	13	37%	Yoshida J Am Coll Cardiol 1993; 22:948
82	32	39%	Eitzman J Am Coll Cardiol 1992; 20:559
129	40	31%	Lee Circulation 1994; 90:2,687
93	34	37%	Di Carli Am J Cardiol 1994; 73:527

[a]Number of patients with decisions for or against balloon dilation or bypass surgery that were incompatible with viability by PET.
[b]For full names of journals, see the list of abbreviations in the bibliography.

Table 3.5. Frequency of Cardiac Events in Patients with Impaired Heart Pumping Function Who Decided for or against Balloon Dilation or Bypass Surgery

No. of Patients in Study	Cardiac Events after Decision Compatible with PET	Cardiac Events after Decision Incompatible with PET	Reference[a]
35	10%	50%	Yoshida J Am Coll Cardiol 1993; 22:948
82	12%	32%	Eitzman J Am Coll Cardiol 1992; 20:559
129	17%	35%	Lee Circulation 1994; 90:2,687
93	10%	24%	Di Carli Am J Cardiol 1944; 73:527

[a]For full names of journals, see the list of abbreviations in the bibliography.

Other tests based on current standard technology, discussed earlier in this part of the book, provide only an approximate measure of viability but are more widely available than PET. However, for advanced severe disease where a wrong decision carries a very high risk of death, PET imaging provides the best data for clinical decisions.

3. What is my risk of dying, having a heart attack or stroke as a complication of the procedure? As reported in large studies, the average overall risk of dying as a complication of balloon dilation or bypass surgery is 1 out of every 200 to 1 out of every 100 people undergoing these procedures. For more complicated or advanced heart or vascular disease or if other illnesses are present such as lung disease, this risk may increase to 1 death out of every 20 patients undergoing these procedures. The risk of adverse effects such as nonfatal heart attacks or strokes is also significant, ranging from 1 out of every 100 to 1 out of 20 people undergoing these procedures. More experienced medical centers doing greater than 250 such procedures per year have better average outcomes than centers doing fewer procedures. The person contemplating balloon dilation or bypass surgery should know the risk of undergoing either procedure and the experience of the doctor who will carry it out.

4. Can I first undergo reversal treatment with cholesterol-lowering drugs, low-fat foods, and medications to reduce my chest pain, and then see if such treatment obviates the need for balloon dilation or heart surgery? Since reversal treatment has been shown to improve survival and prevent heart attacks more than any other treatment for coronary heart disease, it makes sense to undergo balloon dilation or bypass surgery only if one's condition fails to improve after four to six months of reversal treatment. Since no large scientific studies have shown that balloon dilation or bypass surgery prevents heart attacks or death, there is no hurry to undergo these procedures without at least trying reversal treatment first.

The above remarks do not apply to all patients, however, since these conclusions are based on groups of patients studied for averaged or overall outcome. Some individuals may not be willing to undertake or adhere to a strict effective reversal treatment, or it may be ineffective in unusual circumstances. Although uncommon, some individuals may have continuing or progressive chest pain due to coronary heart disease, despite cardiovascular drugs and several months of vigorous cholesterol lowering and low-fat food. In such instances, the atherosclerotic process may be so active that coronary bypass surgery or balloon dilation may be indicated as a short-term, immediate measure to provide relief of pain. These procedures do not prevent continuing progression of atherosclerosis with its substantial risk of graft closure, recurrence of narrowing, or plaque rupture resulting in heart attack or death. Therefore, reversal treatment should be undertaken after bypass surgery or balloon dilation in such cases in order to optimize the overall outcome.

The reason for bypass surgery failing to improve survival in large groups of patients with coronary heart disease and normal pumping function is that bypass surgery by itself does not alter the progression of the basic disease process. It may buy the patient temporary relief of pain, but plaque rupture and coronary events will continue in the absence of a vigorous reversal program. Therefore, the argument frequently given for bypass surgery or balloon dilation, to "prevent a heart attack or dying," is fundamentally incorrect. These procedures do not reduce the risk of heart attack or death in groups of patients with normal ventricular function, since the atherosclerotic process continues unless a vigorous reversal program is instituted. The scientific literature indicates that the best treatment for preventing heart attack and death due to coronary artery disease is reversal treatment with vigorous cholesterol lowering and control of other risk factors.

Balloon Dilation of Narrowed Coronary Arteries

Balloon dilation of a coronary artery narrowing is also called balloon angioplasty. In this procedure, a small balloon on the end of a small, long tube called a catheter is threaded through a narrowing in the coronary artery which is visualized by coronary arteriography. The balloon is then inflated briefly under high pressure, thereby expanding the narrow segment. The balloon is then deflated and withdrawn, leaving an enlarged artery at the site of previous narrowing. Balloon dilation of one or several narrowings can be done during one cardiac catheterization procedure. (See figure 3.15.)

Balloon dilation is now commonly used instead of coronary bypass surgery in many instances, with over 400,000 patients undergoing balloon dilation per year in the United States. It is now commonly done as the primary treatment for coronary heart disease in patients who have no symptoms or have symptoms of chest pain. It is commonly used for patients having a heart attack due to acute sudden coronary blockage or patients experiencing severe, new chest pain caused by sudden partial blockage of a coronary artery. Balloon dilation is also commonly used in patients with long-term, stable chest pain due to coronary heart disease and in patients with modestly narrowed arteries on an arteriogram in the absence of any symptoms.

Although balloon dilation is currently the most common first therapeutic procedure for coronary artery narrowing, there are many problems and limitations with its use. Current standardized guidelines require that a patient who is being considered for balloon dilation have objective evidence that the coronary artery narrowing on the arteriogram is severe enough to warrant the procedure. The narrowing should be at least severe enough to cause an abnormal stress test of some kind or chest pain that is not controlled by medical treatment. However, only 29 percent of Medicare patients have an exercise test before this procedure is done in the United States. This fact suggests that cardiologists simply don't believe whatever results the stress test might show and proceed directly to balloon dilation without it. Of those patients with a previously known heart attack undergoing balloon dilation, only 9 percent have an exercise test before the procedure. Thus, 71 to 91 percent of Medicare patients undergo balloon dilation based on visual estimates of

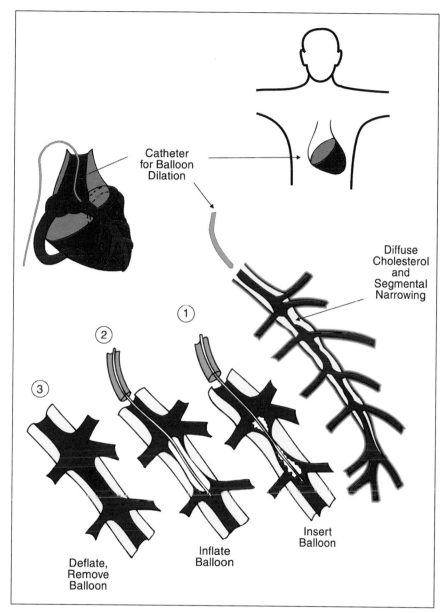

Figure 3.15. Balloon Dilation of a Narrowed Coronary Artery

of the severity of narrowing on the diagnostic arteriogram, despite the widely recognized, well-documented errors of visually estimating severity.

Visually estimated severity of narrowing on coronary arteriograms is often the primary reason for doing balloon dilation, despite errors ranging from 30 to 60 percent in estimating percent diameter narrowing. Although

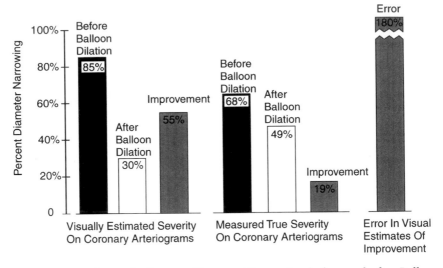

Figure 3.16. Change in Percent Diameter Narrowing before and after Balloon Dilation as Estimated Visually Compared with Objective Measurements by Computerized Analysis of Coronary Arteriograms. Adapted from Fleming, Journal of the American College of Cardiology 1991; 18:945–951.

these errors were discussed earlier, it is important to bring them up again since many procedures done on the basis of erroneous estimates of severity do not benefit the patient and incur some risk of adverse complications. Furthermore, there are errors of up to 180 percent in estimating the benefits of balloon dilation.

For example, according to visual estimates by board-certified cardiologists, the percent diameter narrowing before balloon dilation is 85 percent. By visual estimates, this severity improves to 30 percent diameter narrowing after balloon dilation, an apparent visual improvement of 55 percent diameter narrowing units. However, objective accurate measurements by proven computer analysis have shown in the same patients that the true narrowing was only 68 percent diameter narrowing before balloon dilation and improved to only 49 percent diameter narrowing after balloon dilation. This improvement is actually only 19 percent diameter narrowing units by objective measurements. (See figure 3.16.) The absolute size, or diameter, of narrowing on coronary arteriograms in this study was 0.4 mm before the balloon dilation, increasing to only 0.6 mm at six months after balloon dilation. This improvement is only 0.2 mm in the diameter of the narrowest segment. Such a small change cannot be seen or accurately measured visually on an arteriogram. The improvement in blood flow in the coronary arteries as a result of balloon dilation may be very limited due to diffuse disease present or reoccurrence of narrowing. These minimal changes and errors in the estimated benefit have been confirmed in several medical studies.

Balloon dilation widens the narrowest part of the artery principally by stretching and breaking the arterial wall. There is some compression of the softer cholesterol material in the arterial wall. This stretching and breaking of the arterial wall results in injury to the arterial wall that usually heals with scar formation on the inside of the arterial wall. There is also elastic rebound of the artery to a smaller diameter after the balloon is deflated. This elastic rebound and internal scarring cause recurrence of the coronary narrowing to the same or greater severity as the original narrowing in 40 percent of arteries undergoing balloon dilation. Of patients having balloon dilation, 39 to 40 percent subsequently have a heart attack, undergo repeat balloon dilation, or require bypass surgery.

Recently, the balloon dilation procedure has benefited from the use of an insertable tube made of expandable steel mesh, called a stent. In the pre-insertion, unexpanded state, this small wire mesh tube is mounted on the deflated balloon and inserted through the catheter into the narrowed segment of the coronary artery. When the balloon is inflated, the stent expands, opens up the narrowed segment, and locks into place so that the artery is held open temporarily. However, scar tissue grows through the mesh of the stent and causes reoccurrence of narrowing in 25 to 30 percent of cases. Therefore, use of stents inside the artery has not significantly reduced the recurrence of narrowing. High-speed burrs have also been used to ream out the narrowed coronary artery like a Roto-Rooter. But such techniques do not reduce the recurrence of narrowing either. By reasonable criteria, balloon dilation and Roto-Rooter procedures with or without stents fail to keep the artery open in 25 to 40 percent of patients.

Since balloon dilation does not require anesthesia, a heart-lung bypass machine, or cutting open the chest, it is considered safer than coronary bypass surgery. However, in the largest database reported, from California, the mortality figures were not insignificant. (See table 3.6.) Overall deaths associated with balloon dilation were 1.4 percent, or between 1 and 2 persons in every 100, comparable to mortality with coronary bypass surgery. For elective balloon dilations in patients without an immediate heart attack, deaths occurred in 0.8 percent. When balloon dilation was done in patients for an active heart attack, death occurred in 4.2 percent. Emergency coronary bypass surgery may be necessary when attempted balloon dilation fails, and causes complete blockage of the artery. Rapid emergency surgery for complications of balloon dilation was required in 4.5 percent of elective balloon dilations and in 7.1 percent of patients undergoing balloon dilation for a heart attack. The mortality at emergency surgery for complications of balloon dilation in these patients was high at 7.3 percent. Therefore, the risk of carrying out balloon dilation is higher than generally realized and comparable to that for bypass surgery.

Although more than twenty-seven well-designed scientific studies have been done on the effects of cholesterol lowering, there are *no* well-designed

Table 3.6. Complications of Balloon Dilation in California Patients

Clinical Event	All Procedures	Elective Procedures	Emergency Procedures
Death at balloon dilation	1.4%	0.8%	4.2%
Emergency bypass for balloon complications	5.0%	4.5%	7.1%
Death at emergency bypass	7.3%	5.5%	12.0%

Source: Ritchie, Circulation 1993; 88:2,735.
Note: A total of 24,833 balloon dilations were done as elective (81%) or emergency (19%) procedures.

scientific studies comparing the outcomes of balloon dilation with those of reversal treatment without balloon dilation or bypass surgery. Until recently, the only data on long-term outcome after balloon dilation have been obtained by following the medical course of large numbers of patients who have had balloon dilation or alternative treatment of chest pain without balloon dilation, bypass surgery, or reversal treatment. Such clinical follow-up studies are subject to the biases of each patient's physician in deciding whether or not to carry out balloon dilation. Therefore, in such clinical follow-up studies, it is uncertain that the group of patients undergoing balloon dilation is comparable to the group of patients who do not have balloon dilation.

In such follow-up studies, the long-term outcome of balloon dilation has been assessed by determining the hazard ratio. This hazard ratio is calculated as the percentage of patients with heart attacks or deaths after balloon dilation divided by the percentage of patients with heart attacks or death during the same period of time without having undergone balloon dilation. A hazard ratio of less than one would indicate that balloon dilation reduced heart attacks and death compared with patients on medical treatment without balloon dilation. (See figure 3.17.) Confidence intervals—the vertical bars on the hazard-ratio graph—show the statistical variability, or limits of random variability (or noise), in the data. At five-year follow-up after balloon dilation, the hazard ratio was not significantly lower than the limits of statistical noise. In other words, balloon dilation did not significantly prevent heart attacks or deaths compared with medical treatment without balloon dilation. Even in patients with severe, advanced coronary atherosclerosis of all three coronary arteries and very tight narrowing of the big artery in front of the heart (the left anterior descending coronary artery), balloon dilation did no more good in preventing death or heart attack than treatment without balloon dilation. It is important to emphasize that medical treatment in this study did not include reversal treatment, which has been shown to improve survival in other studies.

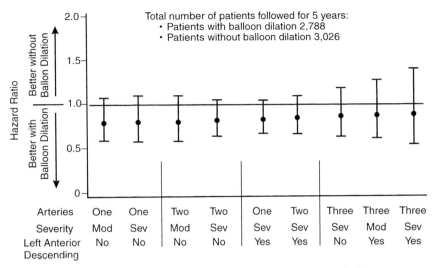

Figure 3.17. Comparison of Survival after Balloon Dilation and after Treatment without Balloon Dilation. Adapted from Mark, Circulation 1994; 89:2,015–2,025.

A more recent, scientifically superior study tested the effects of balloon dilation on heart attacks and deaths. It was called the RITA-2 (the second randomized intervention treatment of angina) Trial. The results showed that people undergoing balloon dilation for stable chest pain due to coronary heart disease suffered more deaths and more heart attacks than those who did not undergo balloon dilation. (See figure 3.18.)

These data suggest three fundamental problems with the current application of balloon dilation:

1. The basic clinical decision for selecting most patients for balloon dilation is fundamentally flawed since it relies on visually estimated severity of coronary artery narrowing that is known to be inaccurate.
2. Functional measurements of severity by exercise testing or imaging blood flow during stress are not done in most patients or are inaccurate or misleading.
3. There is no scientifically documented evidence that balloon dilation reduces the incidence of death or heart attacks any more than reversal treatment does, regardless of the severity of narrowing.

(For a summary of the various limitations of balloon dilation, see table 3.7.)

Even more remarkably, of people who have undergone coronary bypass surgery or balloon dilation, fewer than 25 to 30 percent are treated with cholesterol-lowering medications after the procedure. Despite the existence

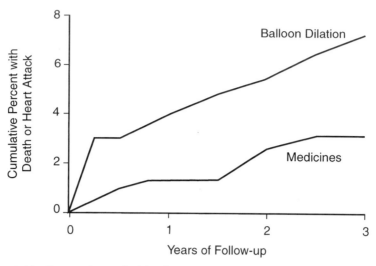

Figure 3.18. Comparison of Risk of Heart Attack and Death after Balloon Dilation and after Medical Treatment in the RITA-2 Trial (Randomized Intervention Treatment of Angina). Adapted from Lancet 1997; 350:461–468.

of over twenty-six major studies showing benefits of cholesterol-lowering treatment, most people do not undergo reversal treatment after bypass surgery or balloon dilation. Consequently, the disease progresses in these untreated people, who then commonly have additional bypass surgery or balloon dilation.

Why is balloon dilation so widely used with such little scientific basis for its application or outcome in patients who have no symptoms or stable chest pain due to coronary heart disease? Some of the reasons are strong economic incentives, reimbursement policies, training, traditional approaches to cardiovascular disease, demands by patients for a "quick fix," traditional economically driven standards of practice set by professional organizations, and the inherent intuitive urge to make a narrowed opening larger or bypass it using a mechanical procedure. For whatever reasons, there is excessive use of these expensive and potentially risky procedures as opposed to cheaper, safer, and more effective reversal treatment.

Because of such observations, major changes in reimbursement policies for cardiovascular care are presently in the works. The role and freedom of individual choice by physicians, professional societies, and patients are rapidly diminishing as third-party payers recognize the limited benefits and excessive costs of balloon dilation and coronary bypass surgery. However, the benefits of reversal treatment are generally not recognized. Even structured, effective reversal programs are not reimbursed. It is therefore essential that the consumers, namely, people with coronary heart disease, as well as health

Table 3.7. Limitations of Balloon Dilation

Patients undergoing balloon dilation without prior stress test	71–91%
Error in visual estimates of narrowing on arteriograms	30–60%
Change in percent diameter narrowing after balloon dilation[a]	
Visually estimated improvement	55%[b]
Measured true improvement (in same subjects)	19%[c]
Error in visually estimated improvement	180%
Patients with reoccurrence of narrowing	40%
Failures due to repeat dilation, heart attack, or bypass surgery	39%
Poor performance in reducing the frequency of heart attacks and death	
Failure to address diffuse disease	

SOURCE: Circulation 1993; 87:1,489; and Journal of the American College of Cardiology 1991; 18:945.

[a]The actual increase in size of the artery six months after balloon dilation was one half millimeter (0.5).

[b]Visually estimated percent diameter narrowing before balloon dilation was 85 percent; after balloon dilation, 30 percent. Subtracting the second figure from the first resulted in the 55 percent visually estimated improvement.

[c]Measured true percent diameter narrowing before balloon dilation was 68 percent; after balloon dilation, 49 percent. Subtracting the second figure from the first resulted in the 19 percent measured true improvement.

care managers and physicians, understand these issues in order to recognize the effectiveness of new technologies and reversal treatment that optimize cardiovascular care with better outcomes at lower cost than current invasive procedures.

There are two circumstances where balloon dilation or bypass surgery may be medically essential, although the supporting scientific data are quite limited. If chest pain due to coronary heart disease progresses after three to four months of reversal treatment, including cardiovascular drugs, vigorous cholesterol lowering, and low-fat food, balloon dilation or bypass surgery should be considered. The disease may be too advanced or aggressive for reversal treatment alone to abolish chest pain in a short time. However, vigorous reversal treatment should be continued after the procedure in order to control aggressive ongoing atherosclerotic processes over the longer-term future. In these circumstances, the balloon dilation or bypass surgery may "buy time" for the reversal treatment to work. Recurrence of narrowing after balloon dilation may require a repeat procedure in 30 to 40 percent of cases. However, this type of recurrence is due to a slow scarring process, not to cholesterol buildup. Moreover, its onset is commonly slow enough to allow collateral development, which often makes repeat balloon dilation unnecessary (provided angina can be controlled by medication).

The second circumstance where balloon dilation may be essential is for the treatment of a heart attack within hours of onset. Severe or sudden chest pain that does not improve with aggressive medical treatment may suggest an impending heart attack. Under such circumstances, balloon dilation may be indicated as an immediate short-term fix to the problem. In contrast, coronary bypass surgery in such patients, as discussed earlier, improves survival only if heart pumping function is impaired. Bypass surgery in such patients with normal pumping function may actually reduce survival. In such patients, surgery should be considered only if the unstable, severe chest pain cannot be managed medically and balloon dilation is not appropriate for technical reasons.

Chest Pain: Reversal? Balloon? Bypass?

Chest pain due to narrowing of the coronary arteries often leads to coronary arteriography and balloon dilation or bypass surgery as the primary initial treatment. This approach is justified on the grounds of preventing a heart attack or death. There are several fundamental flaws in this argument, however. As shown previously, scientific studies have demonstrated that on the average in large groups of subjects, bypass surgery or balloon dilation does not prevent heart attacks or death. These procedures do not reduce the incidence of heart attacks or deaths any more than other medical treatments do. Plaque rupture and thrombosis of the coronary arteries continue with progressive atherosclerosis, despite such procedures. Patients with stable chest pain or an abnormal ECG during daily activities or during exercise testing do not have a higher risk of future heart attacks or higher mortality rates than patients with coronary heart disease without chest pain and with normal ECG. (See figure 3.19.)

People with coronary heart disease have a higher risk of heart attacks and deaths than people without coronary heart disease. Stable chest pain or an abnormal ECG during daily activities or during a stress test may identify people with coronary heart disease and increased risk of heart attack or death by virtue of having coronary heart disease. However, for people with known coronary heart disease, stable chest pain or ECG changes during daily activities or stress testing are not associated with higher risk than that seen in people with coronary heart disease without stable chest pain or ECG changes during daily activities or exercise testing.

For patients who have recently had a heart attack, an abnormal stress test has some predictive value if the stress testing is done within one to two months after the heart attack. Progressive refractory chest pain that does not respond to vigorous antianginal and cholesterol-lowering treatment is also a

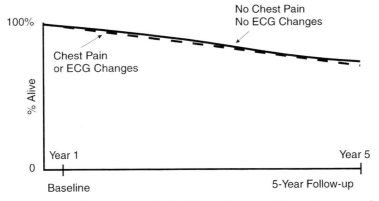

Figure 3.19. Survival in Patients Who Have Coronary Heart Disease with and without Chest Pain or ECG Changes Indicating Inadequate Blood Flow Due to Narrowed Arteries. Adapted from Gandhi, Journal of the American College of Cardiology 1994; 23:74–81, and Miller, Journal of the American College of Cardiology 1994; 23:219–224.

reason for balloon dilation or bypass surgery. However, in the general non-hospitalized population of people with stable coronary heart disease, those who have an abnormal exercise test or ECG abnormalities during daily activities are not at higher risk for future heart attacks or death than people with coronary heart disease without these symptoms or signs. Therefore, an abnormal exercise test or ECG abnormalities during daily activities should not be the only basis for carrying out bypass surgery or balloon dilation.

Severe coronary artery narrowing on the coronary arteriogram is often used as a reason for doing coronary bypass surgery or balloon dilation. The argument is that the severe narrowing may cause heart attack and death, which can be prevented by balloon dilation or bypass surgery. However, long-term follow-up of patients with normal heart pumping shows no higher death rate in those with more severe narrowing than in those with mild coronary artery narrowing. (See figure 3.20.)

Survival in patients with normal pumping function and even severe disease of all three coronary arteries is comparable to that in patients with mild narrowing of the coronary arteries. For this reason, the severity of narrowing on the coronary arteriogram is not a justification for balloon dilation or bypass surgery. On the average in groups of patients, these procedures do not reduce the incidence of heart attacks or death in patients with coronary artery disease who have normal heart pumping function. The explanation for these observations is as follows: Heart attack most commonly occurs due to plaque rupture at sites of mild to moderate narrowing that are not severe enough to restrict blood flow or cause symptoms, an abnormal exercise test, or an abnormal ECG prior to the rupture. These mild lesions are rich in

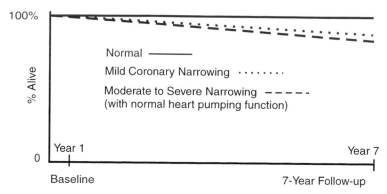

Figure 3.20. Survival Related to Severity of Coronary Artery Narrowing. Adapted from Little, Clinical Cardiology 1991; 14:868–874.

cholesterol with a thin fibrous covering that is easily ruptured, leading to thrombosis and blockage of the artery, with an associated heart attack or sudden death. More advanced, severe narrowing causes chest pain. However, in the presence of low cholesterol, severe narrowings become more stable and therefore are less likely to undergo plaque rupture or cause a heart attack.

In addition, the severe narrowings frequently stimulate the development of new vessels, or collaterals, that carry blood to the heart muscle beyond the partially blocked artery, as described in part 1 of this book. When such narrowings progress to complete blockage, heart attacks usually do not occur because the new vessels, or collaterals, carry blood to the heart muscle, preventing damage. For example, in the FATS study discussed in part 2, two-thirds of the cardiovascular events were due to plaque rupture of mild to moderate narrowings of less than 70 percent diameter narrowing. The more severe narrowings that did progress to complete blockage were usually not associated with heart attack or death due to the development of collaterals.

Most heart attacks or coronary deaths are caused by plaque rupture of mild to moderate narrowings that are loaded with cholesterol and covered by a thin, fibrous cap. Therefore, bypass surgery or balloon dilation would not be expected to prevent heart attacks or death since progressive disease with recurrent plaque rupture continues unless progression is stopped by vigorous cholesterol lowering. Hence, chest pain due to coronary heart disease that can be controlled by cardiovascular drugs and vigorous reversal treatment does not require balloon dilation or bypass surgery.

The primary approach to stable coronary heart disease, either with or without symptoms, should be reversal treatment. Bypass surgery and balloon dilation should be reserved for the uncommon patient who is refractory to reversal treatment and for the sudden unstable plaque rupture resulting in severe chest pain or impending heart attack that does not respond to medical treatment.

Costs of Reversal Treatment, Balloon Dilation, and Bypass Surgery

Today, the most common sequence of diagnostic and treatment steps for coronary heart disease is: (1) exercise treadmill testing with ECG monitoring; (2) stress imaging of blood flow in heart muscle using standard radionuclide technology; (3) coronary arteriography; and (4) balloon dilation or bypass surgery. As reviewed earlier, there are major limitations in the technology and clinical paradigm of this approach based principally on invasive procedures. (See table 3.8.)

Not only is the effectiveness of such procedures limited, but the estimated total costs (for all professional and technical components) are high:

✓ standard exercise testing, $800;
✓ stress imaging using standard radionuclide technology, $2,500;
✓ coronary arteriography, $10,000;
✓ balloon dilation, $17,000 times a 1.3 factor for 30 percent repeat procedures due to recurrence of narrowing;
✓ coronary bypass surgery, $43,000 times a 1.15 factor for 15 percent graft failures requiring repeat bypass surgery.

In contrast, the cost of PET plus reversal treatment includes:

✓ diagnostic PET, $2,500;
✓ cholesterol-lowering drugs, $1,800 per year;
✓ clinic visits, laboratory monitoring of liver function, and cholesterol levels, $2,000 per year.

The total annual costs for noninvasive reversal treatment based on PET as well as for balloon dilation and bypass surgery based on conventional testing methods are provided in table 3.9.

Table 3.8. Limitations of Current Standard Technologies in Coronary Heart Disease

Patients encountering errors in standard exercise tests	40–60%
Coronary arteriograms showing no significant narrowing	25–40%
Visual overestimates of severity on arteriograms	30–60%
Overestimates of improvement by balloon dilation	180%
Patients with recurrence of narrowing after balloon dilation	30–40%
Potential overutilization of bypass surgery, balloon dilation	30–44%
Patients with coronary heart disease not on reversal treatment	75–85%

SOURCE: Circulation 1994; 90:1,558.

Table 3.9. Annual Costs of Reversal and Standard Treatments for Coronary Heart Disease

Diagnosis and Treatment Plan	Annual Cost per Patient
PET plus reversal treatment: diet, medications, lifestyle change	$ 6,300
Standard exercise test, arteriogram, balloon dilation	35,000
Standard exercise test, arteriogram, bypass surgery	62,750

The American Heart Association has estimated the cost per year of lives saved by various treatments for coronary heart disease. The cost per year of life saved by use of cholesterol-lowering drugs is estimated at approximately $4,000. By comparison, the cost per year of life saved by bypass surgery is estimated to be approximately $9,000. Other studies have also shown cholesterol-lowering drugs to be the most cost-effective treatment for coronary heart disease.

In the 4S trial from Scandinavia, the group of patients treated with cholesterol-lowering drugs had a 32 percent decrease in the number of hospitalizations, a 34 percent decrease in the number of days spent in the hospital, and a 32 percent decrease in accumulative hospital costs per patient compared with those undergoing standard cardiovascular treatments including bypass surgery and balloon dilation.

These data indicate the diagnostic effectiveness of cardiac PET and the treatment effectiveness of reversal treatment. Cardiac PET provides noninvasively the most accurate, least expensive definitive diagnosis for coronary heart disease and is the optimal technique for determining its severity and following its progression or regression. PET combined with reversal treatment is the basis for the comprehensive management of coronary heart disease with the best outcomes and lowest cost.

Economics, Ethics, and Politics of Cardiovascular Disease

Although medical care in the United States is considered optimal for those with access to it, the cost for achieving optimal outcomes is high. Not only does this inefficiency of high cost for good outcomes involve high-cost procedures; it also is associated with excessive diagnostic tests that are not definitive, unnecessary procedures, and the practice pattern of "doing everything to all patients." Current reimbursement policies and insurance coverage provide strong economic incentives for such inefficient practice patterns. The field of health care is therefore focusing on containment of costs, effectiveness of outcomes, elimination of unnecessary tests or procedures, alternative treatment modalities that are less expensive but still effective, and alternative clinical pathways that are less costly. These issues in health care reflect a fundamental problem long familiar to industry and to business, that is, the problem of cost versus quality of product.

Most current approaches to this problem in health care have used potentially counterproductive strategies of discounted fees; restricted access; increased volume to offset lower per-procedure cost; second-opinion requirements from like-minded specialists; restrictive preapproval requirements for diagnostic testing that ignore real patient needs, preventive approaches, and new technologies, like PET, that offer better solutions; and even omission of services, particularly new services such as reversal treatment documented to be effective. These "clamp-down" approaches may ultimately hinder optimal solutions to the problem because they disallow innovation and flexibility for developing new clinical practice strategies, protocols, and technologies that would provide higher-quality care at lower cost than heavily discounted traditional practices.

It is therefore important to consider reversal treatment as an alternative to the current standard practice of balloon dilation or bypass surgery in the management of stable coronary artery disease. However, currently only 25 to 30 percent of patients who have established coronary artery disease documented by balloon dilation or coronary bypass surgery undergo intensive cholesterol lowering and risk-management programs, despite the benefits of decreased cardiac events. Analyzing why regression treatment is not more widely used requires consideration of broad practice patterns in cardiovascular medicine now being scrutinized in an environment of cost and outcome consciousness.

The best illustration of economic incentives in cardiovascular medicine is balloon dilation. This procedure has a 30 to 40 percent failure rate within six months and does not prevent heart attacks or deaths. It was not tested scientifically until the recent RITA-2 Trial, which showed more deaths and heart attacks with balloon dilation than without it. However, balloon dilation is the most widespread cardiovascular treatment procedure used for coronary heart disease because reimbursement for this procedure is high, as it is for bypass surgery. By comparison, there are twenty-six good scientific studies demonstrating the value of cholesterol lowering. Yet, only 25 to 30 percent of patients undergoing balloon dilation or bypass surgery receive cholesterol-lowering drugs. The only explanation for these practice patterns is the economic incentive for doing procedures in our health care delivery system. There is no reimbursement for intensive reversal programs that require as much or more time and skill—though of a different kind—as cardiovascular procedures do.

The time and skill required to explain reversal treatment to a patient with coronary heart disease, and to motivate the patient sufficiently to ensure success, is not reimbursed. Current standards of practice are set by professional committees of cardiovascular practitioners. While these guidelines are intended to maintain high-quality standards of cardiovascular care, they also serve to maintain the current economic incentive for invasive procedures in cardiovascular practice.

The basic economic, ethical, and political issue is the fundamental conflict of interest between the business of cardiovascular medicine based on current expensive procedures or standard practices and more effective, less costly, newer approaches using reversal treatment. Cardiologists, individually and as a professional group, generally take the position that cholesterol lowering and medical management are not effective enough as primary treatment to substitute for balloon dilation or bypass surgery. This point of view is supported by tradition, training, patient expectations, fear of coronary heart disease, a limited mechanical view of coronary artery narrowing, and a large health care industry whose bottom-line economic survival depends on these procedures.

The problem can be restated in another way. If reversal treatment were used as the primary approach to managing coronary heart disease, a large number of hospitals might be forced to close for financial reasons and a large number of cardiologists would make substantially lower incomes. The health care industry might lose jobs, and health care professionals, including physicians, might face substantial decline in incomes. Currently, in fact, a substantial consolidation of all medical care is occurring. Unfortunately, this current consolidation is not based on new innovative technologies or new treatment approaches. Current consolidation focuses principally on packaging discounted volume services using traditional approaches and procedures to coronary heart disease. This repackaging approach actually impedes the development of newer, more effective technologies and approaches that would provide more effective outcomes at lower costs.

Therefore, the economics, ethics, and politics of cardiovascular medicine raise real dilemmas and paradoxes. The most valid solutions will come from people with atherosclerosis who want optimal care at lowest cost. However, this goal requires that people with atherosclerosis (1) understand the basics about atherosclerosis and particularly coronary heart disease, (2) have the interest and self-discipline to control their own health, (3) call upon their physicians to provide interactive care, which they, the consumers, demand after gaining adequate knowledge about treatment options and how best to communicate with physicians. This book provides that information.

Managing Your Physician

Many people would like to manage their own cardiovascular problems without a physician. Others would like to rely passively and completely on their physician for solving the problem; they do not want to take any personal responsibility whatsoever. On the whole, the majority of patients prefer to control their own lives and resolve their cardiovascular problems with essential but minimum input from a physician. Doctors cause substantial disruption of their schedules and concern over procedures and expense. A number of popular self-help books attest to this point of view.

However, cardiovascular disease is a real killer. Everyone would like to prevent, stabilize, or reverse it with the greatest likelihood of preventing deaths, heart attack, disability, or the need for major procedures or surgery. Current medical knowledge provides individuals with the means to assume nearly complete control of their health management. Breaking the smoking habit, eating very low-fat food, losing excess weight, exercising on a regular basis, and managing stress are powerful therapeutic steps that everyone can undertake. (This book provides the necessary information in simple terms based on good science and good medical practice.) In addition, modern science has developed powerful, safe, lifesaving pharmacologic agents that are "natural" drugs in the sense that they augment the beneficial effects of the self-determined steps listed above.

The objective is to take advantage of new scientific discoveries about atherosclerosis, food, smoking, antioxidant vitamins, exercise, stress management, *and* appropriate cholesterol-lowering and cardiovascular drugs to maximize well-being and survival. This approach also optimizes the quality as well as quantity of life by increasing exercise tolerance, providing a sense of well-being and relief of symptoms.

You must acquire sufficient knowledge about cholesterol lowering and cardiovascular drugs to manage and effectively engage your physician. Since many doctors do not understand, use, or get reimbursed for reversal treatment, they may not be a good source of detailed knowledge or motivation for people seeking answers to their questions about medical care. (This book provides that knowledge.) Ideally, someone with coronary heart disease or high risk for it will not passively rely on a physician for treatment. Rather, he or she will employ the physician as a consultant to provide specialized assistance with appropriate cardiovascular drugs used in the context of a comprehensive self-determined reversal plan. You should not be afraid of or ignorant of these cardiovascular drugs. They should be used, in conjunction with risk-factor management under individual control, to counteract a lethal process—atherosclerosis.

The first step toward managing your physician, especially your cardiologist, is to understand generally what is on the cardiologist's mind, what are the motivations, problems, and pressures behind the white coat. Remember, physicians and cardiologists are just like everyone else. They are equipped with special training and skills to carry out the tasks outlined by their professional society as "good" medical practice. They become preoccupied with daily concerns and with schedules that may be too busy or not busy enough. The stream of consciousness in the mind of a typical cardiologist would likely include the following concerns: "I have too much to do, and not enough time, I don't understand this problem, why doesn't this patient get better, the system doesn't work, where are all the lab reports, what I was taught in medical school has little to do with practicing medicine, this patient talks forever, this paperwork drives me crazy, I better check with someone else, no matter what I do I can get sued, I'll get sued if I don't do bypass surgery and something happens to the patient, I will get sued if I do bypass surgery without trying reversal treatment first, I don't have time to spend with this patient, who won't give up smoking anyway, I'd better do whatever my colleagues are doing, in all this hassle I deserve to get paid a lot, the reimbursement system is crazy, I am reimbursed for procedures, not for spending time with patients."

Since the reimbursement system rewards procedures more than time spent with patients, the physician has the choice of doing as many procedures as possible or turning over a large volume of office or consultative visits at a maximum of ten to fifteen minutes per patient. By not choosing either of these options, the physician has to live with a lower income than his or her colleagues who play by the rules of reimbursement. In effect, every cardiologist faces a conflict of interest: on the one hand, there is a financial incentive for doing invasive procedures; on the other hand, not doing procedures in favor of reversal treatment is better for the patient but is not reimbursed.

In addition, certain patient "characteristics" complicate the physician's thinking, regardless of whether or not they are true in an individual case. Patients demand: an immediate fix to the medical problem, guaranteed outcome, no effort or disruption of lethal living habits, infinite time and patience from the physician, no waiting in the doctor's office, no side effects of treatment, easy parking, Solomon's wisdom and knowledge—all of it for free or at less cost than cigarettes or a new suit or a new car or a new dishwasher. Moreover, patients think: "The company should pay for it, the government should pay for it but without taxes, anybody but me should pay for it, while I continue to eat high-fat foods, smoke, lie around, and make no effort to improve my health." Doctors perceive that patients believe: "If something goes wrong it is somebody else's fault, I will sue if it doesn't turn out well, bad things just don't happen, and my disease is not my responsibility." These fragmented thoughts of patients reflect some of the negative but real concerns of physicians. In fact, most physicians and their patients do their best to work together within a complex social setting involving life and death, well-being, money, status, and power over lives or lifestyle. However, these attitudes are common enough to influence strongly the patterns of medical practice.

The aim of this book is to give people the knowledge to manage their own health and utilize their physician as a consultant on the addition of cardiovascular drugs to their reversal regimen. Under certain limited circumstances, it may be essential for the physician to also perform balloon dilation or coronary bypass surgery, which the person with coronary heart disease should clearly understand—the reasons for the procedure, the risks, the outcomes, and the need for reversal treatment anyway. Many people may require only this book and a prescription from a willing physician who has no more time or interest than providing cardiovascular and cholesterol-lowering drugs. Other people may want or need a greater level of direct exchange with a physician, who is particularly interested, skilled, or trained in providing reversal treatment.

A physician who falls into the latter category should do the following:

✓ Spend time with the patient at onset and follow-up.
✓ Review basic concepts in coronary heart disease.
✓ Emphasize that atherosclerosis is diffuse throughout arteries.
✓ Communicate the idea that without reversal treatment, progression will continue, with risk of heart attack and death.
✓ Review heart images and status of patient.
✓ Cover the benefits and risks of the alternatives: reversal treatment, balloon dilation, and bypass surgery.
✓ Provide a personal food plan, with each meal adapted to the individual's habits.
✓ Prescribe cholesterol-lowering drugs, perform lab tests, adjust drug dosages, and monitor side effects as necessary.
✓ Establish an exercise routine tailored to the individual.
✓ Give the patient positive reinforcement through clinic visits, phone calls, and overall accessibility.

However, the physician is not reimbursed for spending time with patients to accomplish the above list. Therefore, someone wanting this input should expect to reimburse the physician directly for such time and expertise. Doing your homework—such as reading this book and learning about heart disease, what to do about it, and what to ask your cardiologist—is an important first step. Preparation and knowledge in advance of consulting your physician will enhance the level of effective interaction and care that you will receive: you will ask better questions, get better answers, understand them better, and receive better care. It is a fundamental axiom that a physician, like anyone else, will deal more carefully with a client who is informed, asking the right questions and expecting rational answers. If the physician is unwilling or unable to engage in a rational discussion of those questions, the client-patient should find another doctor who will.

In the spirit of goodwill between cardiologist and patient-client, when should the client be tolerant and when should the client be demanding, what questions should be asked and when? The client-patient should be tolerant of issues that are not important to health. For example, do not be demanding or upset about the traffic or parking, even about waiting in the doctor's office for one to two hours sometimes because the doctor is late (it is usually not the doctor's fault—things happen on a tight schedule), about the hospital losing your record (it is not the doctor's fault), about his or her help-staff being harried (it is not their fault that the doctor is late), about needle sticks for lab work, about nickel-and-dime amounts in the bill. While the client-patient's time may be as valuable as the doctor's, it is understood that the multiplicity of a physician's duties and emergency or unexpected problems of other client-patients require certain concessions from waiting client-patients. The client-patient's impatience with these secondary issues detracts from more important issues. A client-patient who complains about such problems will turn the physician's attention toward them and away from the primary focus: keeping the client-patient alive and healthy. As a client-patient, decide what is really most important to you and focus on that in the time available with your doctor.

Do be demanding about explanations of procedures. Why are they necessary? How accurate are the tests? What are the outcomes? If balloon dilation or bypass surgery is recommended to prevent a heart attack or prevent death, ask to see the data showing that these outcomes result from the procedure proposed for you as an individual patient. Alternatively, show the cardiologist the data in this book and ask for a justification of his or her recommendations as a reasonable exception to the general conclusions reached here. If you want to take charge of your own well-being, ask to undergo reversal treatment first and sign a consent form to that effect. Also, understand that there is always a risk of some adverse event occurring, no matter what treatment is chosen.

It is important to remember that physicians are not reimbursed for expertise, for spending time with patients, for motivating them to do whatever it takes to implement successful reversal treatment. If the client-patient wants optimal objective advice or treatment, paying for that time and expertise without insurance reimbursement is the best way to get objective, valuable time, advice, and support. Questioning the cost of the physician's time may be self-defeating since it seems to encourage the doctor to stop spending time with the client-patient and do some procedure instead. On the other hand, questioning a procedure is appropriate in view of current outcome data and high costs of the procedures.

The important points to remember from this discussion are to: (1) understand the basics about atherosclerosis, (2) determine how much responsibility or control you want in managing your own health, (3) approach the physician accordingly as a consultant for integrating cardiovascular drugs into a self-management program with greater or lesser input from the physician depending on your individual needs.

PART 4

The Gould Guidelines to Prevent or Reverse Vascular and Coronary Heart Disease

✓ The Gould Guidelines—What's New and Different?

✓ Cholesterol and Coronary Heart Disease—A Review

✓ Goals of Reversal Treatment

✓ Fat-Free Foods—Pleasure and Utility

✓ Types of Food—Fat, Protein, and Carbohydrate

✓ Fats, Oils, and Cholesterol

✓ Protein

✓ Carbohydrates

✓ Overall Guidelines for a Food Plan of Less Than 10 Percent Fat

✓ Weight and Hunger

✓ Essential Fatty Acids

✓ Food Labels

✓ Food "Zigzags," Food Breaks," and "Average" Cholesterol/Fat Consumption

✓ Food "Substitutes" and Processed Foods

✓ Menus

✓ Antioxidant Vitamins and Aspirin

✓ Types of Cholesterol-lowering Drugs

✓ Special Problems and Combinations of Cholesterol-lowering Drugs

✓ Angina, or Chest Pain, of Coronary Heart Disease

✓ Estrogens and Coronary Heart Disease

✓ Daily Workout Routines

✓ Stress Management

✓ Who Needs Reversal Treatment?

✓ Common Problems and Their Solutions

✓ Limitations of Reversal Treatment

✓ Weighing the Alternatives

✓ How Dr. Gould Implements His Program for Preventing or Reversing Vascular Disease

This section describes the overall principles and the definitive program for preventing or reversing vascular and coronary heart disease. As a cardiovascular scientist and specialist, I developed these guidelines from an extensive analysis of scientific publications (listed in part in the "Sources of Information and Bibliography" section of this book) and from my own clinical observations over thirty years of medical practice. I call them the Gould Guidelines since they are quite different from the recommendations of the American Heart Association, the National Cholesterol Education Program, and programs of other physician-authors. They are more vigorous and incorporate more scientific evidence without being influenced by the economic incentives of invasive procedures. My guidelines integrate the most advanced information on food and lifestyle with lifesaving, safe medicines for cholesterol lowering proven to dramatically reduce the risk of death or heart attack, and the need for bypass surgery or balloon dilation procedures. The Gould Guidelines are practical, individualized, enjoyable, applicable in daily living, effective, scientifically based, economical, and actually fun. Moreover, they are free of the limitations that have restricted the success of other programs. Not only have I personally tested the guidelines, but I have used them with hundreds of my patient-clients. Each component of preventive-reversal treatment is developed in detail in this book, including a section (in part 3) on how to manage your physician in addition to actively managing your own cardiovascular health.

Many readers may at outset consider these guidelines "too hard, too difficult" to follow. But they will be pleased to learn about the experience of a client-patient of mine, himself a physician. After our initial review of his reversal program, he said to me, "This is impossible; Gould, you live on another planet." One year later, jubilant, pain free, active, twenty pounds lighter, reassured by seeing markedly improved blood flow flooding through his heart muscle on his follow-up PET scan, he said, "You know, once you start and get used to it, this [program] is easy. I love to live this way; I love the food. I didn't believe it was possible at first; I didn't believe I could feel so good, better than I've ever felt in my life."

Most people, but not everyone, feel that way when they achieve the goals outlined here. However, no outcome can be guaranteed for any treatment of coronary heart disease. Some people are simply unable to adhere completely to these lifestyle guidelines but can benefit from doing the best they can in addition to taking cholesterol-lowering and cardiovascular medications. This program is also designed to benefit these people as much as possible. Although markedly reduced by reversal treatment, there remains some risk of uncontrolled chest pain, heart attack, stroke, death, the need for balloon dilation or bypass surgery, just as these procedures themselves carry a definite risk of these and other adverse outcomes. Neither I nor the publisher can be responsible for a reader's personal health. By following the guidelines presented here, readers can assume control of and responsibility for their own well-being along with their physician-consultant.

The Gould Guidelines—What's New and Different?

✓ *Practical, easy, fast.* These guidelines can be followed by people in all walks of life and of all ages, regardless of their lifestyles, time schedules, and economic resources. This program can work for you if you have heart disease, a positive test of some kind, high risk factors, or simply want to adopt a healthy lifestyle.

✓ *Individualized, flexible.* These guidelines do not impose a fixed or rigid program to which all people must adhere. Rather, the reversal program adapts basic principles to each person's individual needs and lifestyle, at the office, at home, and when traveling or dining out.

✓ *Enjoyable, satisfying.* Healthy food and healthy living are fun. They do not involve deprivation, restrictions, sacrifice, or hunger. This program succeeds because it makes people feel good, puts them in control of their lives, and emphasizes living well.

✓ *Integrated into daily living.* This program integrates the principles for preventing or reversing vascular disease into everyone's daily living. It does not require prolonged retreats, retirement, or leisure time of the well-to-do. While one to three weeks at a health spa, lifestyle seminar, or beauty farm may be a healthy vacation, its benefits usually vanish on returning to the pressures of daily living.

✓ *Weight control.* These guidelines show you how to control your weight without being hungry; to eat as often and as much as you want and enjoy a wide variety of delicious food without calorie counting. The trick is choosing what to eat, not how much or how often.

✓ *The double whammy.* These guidelines integrate the most advanced information on food and lifestyle with lifesaving, safe medicines for lowering cholesterol. The elements of this reversal program have been proven to dramatically reduce the incidence of death, heart attack, bypass surgery, or balloon dilation. Encouraging basic human urges for optimal lifestyle combined with modern medicines provide maximal advantage against the relentless killing and disability of vascular disease.

✓ *Effective, immediate results.* Numerous scientific studies have demonstrated the clinical benefits of this type of treatment for the commonest cause of death and disability in the United States—vascular disease. The benefits of each component of the program have been shown to start within weeks, build steadily, and continue throughout a lifetime.

✓ *Scientifically based alternative medicine.* Successful application of this program is a valid alternative to the current, widespread techniques of coronary bypass surgery and balloon dilation. More clinical studies on the el-

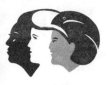

WOMEN'S
HEALTH
INITIATIVE

(716) 829-3128

Jeff — I am sending this
to you first, please pass
it along to drew and hi
I have marked a few pages
on the back cover area.

Dad

ements of this program have been carried out than all the studies of bypass surgery or balloon dilation collectively, with substantially better outcomes in terms of preventing subsequent heart attacks and death. As an established scientist and professor of medicine and cardiology, I have personally carried out many of the studies, personally analyzed extensive scientific data, personally developed these guidelines, and demonstrated their application in my daily personal life and daily clinical practice as an advanced, verified alternative to bypass surgery and balloon dilation. Nothing in these guidelines is unscientific or unorthodox. Rather, they are based on accepted scientific methods with innovative results that challenge the core of traditional but outdated practice paradigms based on invasive procedures. This challenge comes from a recognized cardiovascular scientist and clinician within the cardiology profession, not from some far-out guru or fringe element.

✓ *Economical, a "health democracy."* This program is for everyone who wants to prevent or reverse vascular disease, regardless of economic status. It does not require an expensive retreat, multiple medical consultations or procedures, specialized equipment or facilities, group interaction, or classroom formalities. It can be implemented as a take-charge-yourself program integrated with traditional medical care of commercial health insurance, the preferred provider organization, the health maintenance organization, the self-insured, the uninsured, those with and those without substantial financial resources. The cost of this program, including cholesterol-lowering drugs and their medical supervision, is substantially less than the charges for most lifestyle retreats or health spas.

The Gould Guidelines to prevent or reverse vascular disease are unique in integrating lifestyle and lifesaving medications to maximal effect. Other programs involve too much fat or too much carbohydrate in the food, too rigid a regimen, too extreme restrictions, too much time, too much cost, too much emphasis on one or another component of reversal treatment, too much compromise, too much "guruism," or too much hype without adequate scientific validation. The Gould Guidelines have a solid foundation in modern science and medicine, and are formulated as simple principles that everyone can apply to prevent or reverse vascular disease.

Cholesterol and Coronary Heart Disease—A Review

The role of cholesterol in heart disease was described in detail in part 1. However, because of its importance in understanding and applying this reversal program, cholesterol and coronary heart disease are briefly reviewed again here.

Coronary heart disease is a diffuse process of cholesterol deposition, scarring, and calcification (hardening of the arteries) throughout the major coronary arteries supplying blood flow to heart muscle. In figure 4.1, a cross-

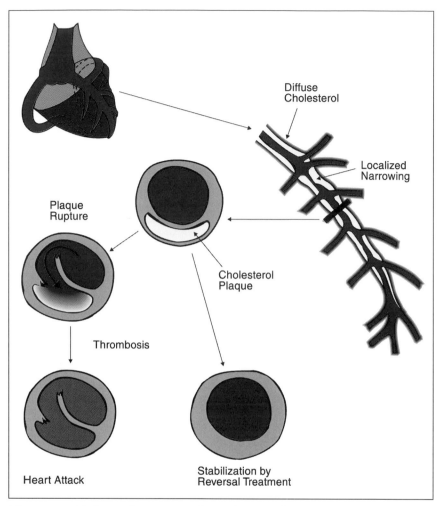

Figure 4.1. Cholesterol, Heart Attacks, and Reversal Treatment

sectional view of an affected artery shows the cholesterol deposited in the arterial wall, covered by the inner lining of the artery through which the blood flows.

The fibrous lining, or cap, over the cholesterol deposit may break at the shoulder where it attaches to the arterial wall. This tendency to break at the shoulder is due to high mechanical stress and inflammation at the edges of the cholesterol deposit. When the fibrous cap over the cholesterol deposit breaks (plaque rupture), the blood in the artery is forced by blood pressure to flow under the fibrous cap. The ruptured cap is lifted up into the artery and causes a narrowing that impedes blood flow. The blood mixes with the cholesterol deposit and immediately clots. This blood clot propagates into the narrowed artery and may completely or partially block it, thereby causing a heart attack, sudden death, or unstable, severe chest pain. Plaque rupture usually occurs at sites of cholesterol deposition that only mildly narrow the artery (by 50 percent or less). It explains why an individual may be active without any accompanying symptoms, not even during the most intense exercise, but have a heart attack several hours later caused by sudden plaque rupture.

Goals of Reversal Treatment

Although not clearly defined, there is variable susceptibility to coronary atherosclerosis for a given level of risk factors. In addition to traditional risk factors, dietary fat causes progression of atherosclerosis separate from levels of blood cholesterol measured after fasting. Some people with severe risk factors appear resistant to coronary heart disease, whereas many other people are susceptible to heart disease with only modest or no identifiable risk factors. When such susceptible people develop coronary heart disease, their condition may continue to progress even with "normal" cholesterol levels. A vigorous effort to lower cholesterol and restrict dietary fat intake is necessary to get these levels lower than conventional "normal" ranges as the most effective way to stop progression or reverse the disease.

Therefore, for persons with coronary heart disease at high risk, this program does not accept "normal" cholesterol levels as a goal. It aims to reduce total cholesterol and LDL as much as possible to well below the "normal" range and to increase HDL as much as possible. The specific cholesterol levels achieved are based on medical judgment, the response of each person, and on side effects for each individual. At target levels (presented in the accompanying box), progression of disease, heart attacks, sudden death, and the need for balloon dilation or bypass surgery are uncommon. Several special points about these goals need to be emphasized, as discussed below.

Six Steps for Preventing or Reversing Vascular or Coronary Heart Disease

1. Stop smoking.
2. Eat foods that are very low in fat (10% of calories), low in cholesterol, and low in carbohydrates in order to reach lean body weight.
3. Take cholesterol-lowering drugs: statins, gemfibrozil, niacin, or resin powder (aim for total cholesterol <140, LDL <90, HDL >45).
4. Take antioxidant vitamins.
5. Do moderate exercise daily.
6. Manage stress.

Combining Very Low-Fat, Low-Carbohydrate Foods and Cholesterol-lowering Medications

Treatment by very low-fat foods alone or by cholesterol-lowering drugs only, stops progression or causes regression in 40 to 50 percent of the treated subjects, depending upon the study. There is a comparable decrease in the cardiovascular events of death, heart attack, bypass surgery, or balloon dilation. However, low-fat foods *alone* or cholesterol-lowering drugs *alone* have a substantial remaining risk of coronary events. Treatment by a combination of very low-fat foods and cholesterol-lowering drugs is supported by scientific data. The twenty-four-hour exposure of coronary arteries to atherogenic material is minimized by two steps. The first is by eating low-fat foods, which eliminates the surge in blood lipids that occurs after a fatty meal and lasts eight hours. The second step is by taking lipid-active drugs, which minimize fasting LDL cholesterol levels and maximize HDL levels. On a combined regimen of both very low-fat foods and cholesterol-lowering drugs, or of double drug treatment, the atherosclerotic process is reversed or progression stopped in over 90 percent of people, with a corresponding decrease in cardiovascular events.

In patients with "normal" or only mildly elevated cholesterol levels, stabilization or regression also occurs with marked cholesterol lowering by eating low-fat foods and taking cholesterol-lowering drugs. The abnormal function of the endothelial lining of arteries caused by elevated cholesterol or coronary atherosclerosis starts to heal within three months. Even within days to weeks after undertaking this program, there are usually decreased symptoms, increased exercise capacity, and heightened sense of well-being. For people with chest pain due to coronary heart disease, standard cardiovascular drugs are also used with cholesterol-lowering drugs to minimize symptoms. These cardiovascular drugs include nitrates, beta blockers, calcium channel blockers, and angiotensin converting enzyme (ACE) inhibitors. Balloon dilation or bypass surgery is usually not necessary, since the response to this integrated vigorous treatment is so consistent and effective in most people.

Adverse Effects of a High-Carbohydrate Diet

In many people, particularly those with coronary heart disease, the triglycerides increase and HDL cholesterol decreases in response to low-fat, vegetarian, high-carbohydrate foods. Since low HDL, particularly with high triglycerides, incurs substantial risk of coronary events, my guidelines do not recommend a high volume of high-carbohydrate vegetarian foods. Such diets may incur excessive carbohydrates for adequate protein from beans or grain sources, with adverse effects on HDL, triglycerides in blood, and weight.

Reduction in carbohydrate and weight loss lower triglycerides in blood and raise HDL. An optimal food plan achieves lean body weight by both *carbohydrate and fat reduction*, with adequate protein from no-fat, low-carbohydrate sources, and volumes of vegetables for fiber and phyto-nutrients. These protein sources include no-fat dairy products, such as no-fat yogurt, no-fat cheese, skim milk, no-fat cottage cheese, egg whites, veggie burgers, or soy protein, supplemented on an optional basis with some breast of turkey, and chicken, fish, or buffalo/venison. The protein sources can vary according to individual taste, but daily cholesterol intake should be limited to 60 to 80 milligrams per day or below and fat to 10 percent of total daily calories.

A low-fat, high-volume carbohydrate diet may cause some weight loss because total calories are reduced by fat restriction. However, typically, weight does not continue falling to optimal lean body weight due to excessive calories from the high-volume carbohydrates required for adequate protein intake. For carbohydrate-sensitive individuals, food should consist of a limited volume of carbohydrate, adequate no-fat protein sources, and volumes of vegetables. The amount of carbohydrate eaten depends upon weight. For overweight people, carbohydrate intake should be markedly reduced. For lean people, high carbohydrate intake may be necessary to maintain adequate weight. The benefits of low-fat, low-cholesterol foods are widely recognized. However, less well recognized are the adverse effects of high-carbohydrate foods even if low in fat. These adverse effects are excess body weight and the associated effect of excess weight on increasing LDL, decreasing HDL, and increasing triglycerides. Low HDL and excessive triglycerides substantially increase cardiovascular risk. For the carbohydrate-sensitive person, excess carbohydrate intake and associated excess weight may be as potentially harmful as excess fat and cholesterol. Therefore, the Gould Guidelines utilize less than 10 percent of calories as fat, no-fat low-carbohydrate protein sources whenever possible, and low-volume carbohydrate intake sufficient to reach and maintain lean body weight.

Dietary Protein Deficiency

People on a self-imposed, low-fat, high-carbohydrate, vegetarian diet commonly do not consume enough protein, typically only 10 to 20 grams of protein per day. Inadequate dietary protein is frequently associated with profound fatigue, impaired concentration, lack of stamina, and personality change. Low protein intake also lowers HDL. Once adequate dietary protein is restored, these symptoms disappear within days. In addition, when protein is maintained as carbohydrate and weight are reduced, the high triglycerides also decrease and HDL increases while continuing the same fat restrictions to less than 10 percent of calories.

Decreased HDL on Low-Fat Foods

Some people who are lean and have normal or low triglycerides may decrease the HDL as well as LDL cholesterol on a low-fat diet. A modest fall in HDL on a low-fat diet may be normal and not associated with cardiovascular risk. However, if the HDL falls too low (below 35 mg/dl), it is appropriate in patients with known coronary heart disease to use statins, niacin, and/or gemfibrozil to increase levels of HDL, in addition to exercising regularly, maintaining lean body mass, and not smoking. Finally, weight loss in overweight people has been shown to increase HDL.

Maximizing Results through a Comprehensive, Individualized Approach

Since cardiovascular disease is a major killer and cause of disability, this reversal program uses a vigorous approach, combining all of the major therapeutic steps available, such as very low-fat foods, cholesterol-lowering drugs, smoking cessation, exercise, and stress management. The goal is to maximize regression or stop progression and minimize the risk of heart attack, death, chest pain, stroke, or the need for balloon dilation or bypass surgery. These components of the program are individually planned for each patient, depending on his or her time constraints, work demands, lifestyle, and personal preferences. This tailoring to individual needs optimizes compliance and therefore outcomes.

Each patient is encouraged to develop knowledge, motivation, and active self-maintenance of his or her reversal treatment. The physician and the physician's staff demonstrate how the principles of reversing coronary heart disease apply to the patient's particular situation and provide follow-up reinforcement, motivation, and monitoring by a variable mix of outpatient clinic visits, home lifestyle improvements, and intensive telephone or written follow-up locally or at a distance. This intensive follow-up communication includes exchange with the private physician according to individual needs.

There is no single, fixed regimen, diet, or method to which all individuals must conform. Multiple subspecialty consultations, special equipment or facilities, group interaction, classroom meetings, unnecessary clinic visits, excessive time demands, or disruption of busy schedules are avoided in this program. Alternatively, it integrates essential lifestyle changes and medical management into daily living at home and work. Other programs utilize one-to three-week stays at a health spa or beauty farm for weight loss and physical conditioning. Such programs are time consuming, expensive, and may not address the essential needs of healthy living habits throughout the year. The reversal program, by contrast, can usually provide results in a minimum amount of time with follow-up support to encourage the patient-client commitment and follow-through required for success.

Each individually designed food regimen is integrated with one or more lipid-active drugs in order to achieve a total cholesterol below 140 mg/dl, LDL below 90, HDL 45 or greater, and lean body mass. With an individualized approach, most patients can achieve these goals, enjoy a great variety of delicious food without being hungry, and profoundly reduce the risk of myocardial infarction, death, bypass surgery, or balloon angioplasty, even with severe advanced coronary heart disease.

Fat-Free Foods—Pleasure and Utility

Fat-free foods are not a restrictive diet. They are not only healthy but also a source of pleasure, social exchange, and utility. One chooses a mode of eating that is satisfying, enjoyable, and makes one feel good in preference to some other mode of eating. These choices may be healthy, life-sustaining food or may be unhealthy and self-destructive. The motivations behind food choices are complex, driven by genetics, hormones, upbringing, traditions, habits, physical activity, social pressures, food availability, emotions, stresses, and essentially all the behavior and activity of living. Food behavior is therefore a deep-seated part of our personality. It is inherent in our self-image.

Food habits in some individuals are fixed and unalterable, whether healthy or not. However, in most people, some aspects of food behavior are surprisingly flexible and adaptable. Food habits are influenced through a sense of well-being and pleasure that can be developed and refined for optimizing health. Healthy food habits interact with many other aspects of living, such as weight control, appearance, physical activity, and social exchange, all of which create a positive feedback cycle.

Some food habits are more adaptable or changeable than others. For example, typical "evening" people, who are at their best late in the day and at their worst in the morning, usually dislike breakfast. Putting food into their already-queasy morning stomach is nauseating; therefore, they usually skip breakfast. That trait is basic and not easily changed. Some people need three square meals per day. Others want only one meal per day. Still others eat five to eight times per day, an eating pattern called "grazing." Some people eat in response to success or in response to stress or depression. There are fast-food freaks, meat hounds, steak-and-potatoes people, vegetarians, carbohydrate addicts, and others with no regular food preferences, which is itself a pattern of food behavior.

Of these food habits, those involving time of day, volume of food, frequency of eating, interactions with personality, stress, physical activity, and so forth, are the most inherent in personality. These characteristics are the most difficult to change. However, perhaps because of the wide range of food types available and experience with them, the most flexible of all food habits is the sense of taste determining what one eats. Low-fat eating is most successful when it adapts to most of an individual's other inherent food habits and personality. The basic food habits relating to food volume, frequency of eating, time of day, social circumstances should be maintained or encouraged. The only change is what kind of foods are eaten—no-fat or very low-fat, moderate or low-carbohydrate. The essential idea is to adapt low-fat foods to the individual, not the individual to some rigid uniform "diet" scheme. This approach requires a basic guiding set of principles, outlined below, which can be adapted to most lifestyles. Low-fat foods may be fast-fix meals, between-meal snacks, elegant dining, or travel cuisine (where food choices are limited).

For the physician or counselor discussing food with someone, it is therefore essential to listen, to understand the individual's food habits, lifestyle, personality, and food interactions, and to suggest specific steps and foods that fit that individual's living habits. Follow-up reinforcement, discussion, refinement, and suggestions are also essential until the individual has successfully developed the practical knowledge and taste to modify the food choices toward healthier low-fat content.

The same individualized approach may be used for modifying carbohydrate consumption in order to achieve additional weight control. It is useful for developing regular exercise habits that burn calories, contribute further to weight loss, lower the LDL cholesterol, and increase the HDL cholesterol. An individualized approach is also essential to deal with specific stresses that often impact food habits.

Hunger reduces control over the selection of foods and the quantity of foods eaten. A hungry person will "eat anything in sight," overeat, and likely depart from low-fat, moderate- to low-carbohydrate intake. Therefore, a basic rule is to avoid getting hungry. Some individuals never get hungry on one meal per day. Others need to graze frequently or eat three major meals as well as snacks. However, to avoid excess fat and carbohydrate that adversely affect cholesterol levels and weight, snacks should be principally protein combined with vegetables, salads, or modest amounts of fruit. Then, weight loss without hunger often creates a mild euphoria.

Protein foods suppress appetite. Sweets or carbohydrates tend to stimulate more carbohydrate craving. Suboptimal protein in food often creates carbohydrate craving. A successful approach for avoiding hunger and associated overeating is to snack on protein food regularly one to two hours before lunch and one to two hours before the evening meal. Such snacks might include two no-fat mozzarella string cheese sticks and an apple, grapes or tomatoes, a cup of no-fat fruit yogurt, cottage cheese mixed with mustard or fruit, or a protein-powder, skim milk, or fruit drink. These protein snacks suppress appetite, which allows rational control in selecting low-fat food at the coming meal.

For many individuals, feeling full after a meal is an important element of satisfaction that improves adherence to low-fat foods. For such people, it is appropriate to eat large volumes of vegetables with appropriate daily requirements of protein from low-fat or no-fat sources. The meal should include five to six different kinds of vegetables and low-fat protein foods. A variety of no-fat seasonings is available, including butter substitutes. The meal can include vegetable purees, soups, and large portions of single or mixed nonfat protein sources.

Such protein sources might include a cup or two of cottage cheese (good mixed with mustard and certain vegetables), three to four mozzarella string cheese sticks, or a handful of grated cheese melted over vegetables, all of the no-fat variety. Augment these nonfat dairy products with fish, turkey, or low-cholesterol, low-fat meats or meat substitutes, such as veggie burgers. A small serving of some favorite carbohydrate, such as pasta, or a small serving of potatoes may be eaten as a special treat but not as a main-course volume food, for it will add calories, weight, and cholesterol. As one becomes accustomed to the taste of low-fat food with adequate protein, control of carbohydrates also becomes easier.

This approach to low-fat eating does not count calories or mete out portions of various foods. It is at once simpler yet more effective.

In addition to being connected with individual personality, food is a powerful symbol of social interchange, friendship, family ties, love, business—that is, interpersonal relations. For such occasions, the richness of the food is often symbolic of the importance or intensity of the social interchange. Therefore, social pressure to serve or consume rich food may be substantial. However, in recent years the awareness of healthy eating has become sufficiently widespread that individuals requesting low-fat foods are not only accepted but admired. The food industry, restaurants, community leaders, and families are recognizing the value of healthy, low-fat foods.

For dinner at home with family or guests, thoughtfully prepared, gourmet, low-fat meals reflect the care, esteem, and "heart" of social exchange. Guests trying to maintain their own low fat intake will be pleased when their hosts offer low-fat options; not only is this a sign of the hosts' thoughtfulness, but it also reinforces the guests' eating habits. To the old adage that "the route to a man's (or woman's) heart is through their stomachs" can be added "without killing them with too much fat."

For restaurant dining, the solution is simple: order low-fat foods, such as steamed vegetables, grilled fish or turkey, salads without dressing. Ignore the menu and tell the waiter what you want, and most restaurants will gladly oblige. Even fast-food outlets are now advertising low-fat foods. Given the wide availability and high demand for low-fat foods, there should be some acceptable dietary options at virtually all social occasions. The secret to maintaining low-fat food intake at such times is simply to stay focused on proper food choices without being distracted by social environment.

Most people are successful with a low-fat eating plan when the major dietary changes they have made lead to real immediate rewards. These rewards are substantial. They include weight loss, more energy, fewer symptoms, lower cholesterol, control of one's life and future health. Minor incremental changes in eating habits have little impact since the rewards are too small. Here, "major change" means what one eats, that is, what one tastes, not all of the other more deep-seated food habits inherent in personality. As noted earlier, these other food habits are characteristics of an individual personality and should be recognized, integrated, and reinforced to support the one key change in what one eats—no-fat, low-carbohydrate foods. The Gould Guidelines for food are as follows:

1. Eat no-fat or very low-fat foods. Eliminate margarine, oils, butter, and all identifiable fat. Any food with more than 1 to 2 grams of fat per serving should be avoided.

2. Get adequate protein from nonfat sources, particularly nonfat dairy products, but also including occasional fish, turkey, or chicken breast, yolk-free eggs, and veggie burgers.

3. Reduce or eliminate the large-volume carbohydrate sources, such as rice, bread, potatoes, pasta, pastries, sweets, fruit juice, and bananas in order to reach ideal weight, reduce triglycerides, and increase HDL. Substitute protein, vegetables, and up to three fruits per day for the fat and carbohydrate eliminated from food. After reaching lean body mass, increase these carbohydrates just enough to maintain weight.

4. Fill up on large amounts of vegetables—raw, steamed, or "stir-fried" without oil.

5. Never get too hungry. Snack often if needed. If hungry, eat large amounts but only of the right kinds of food, principally vegetables and nonfat protein with some fruit. Add rice, bread, potatoes, or pasta in modest amounts only when ideal weight is reached.

6. Appropriate shopping plays an essential role in successfully maintaining low-fat foods. People usually do not do grocery shopping when they are hungry, and can make rational food choices if they focus on low-fat items. *Shopping* for the right no-fat or low-fat meals is more important than cooking or preparation. Purchasing the right foods makes the preparation easy. Preparation is simple and quick after appropriate shopping.

7. Read labels on food products for fat content. There is an enormous range of good no-fat or low-fat food now marketed.

8. "Zigzag" once per month with a favorite food that is not part of the new low-fat eating plan: a steak, hamburger, rich sauces, whole milk, a chocolate sundae. Using the "zigzag," a person avoids the empty feeling of "giving up forever what I really liked." It also frequently leads to the discovery that the fatty, rich, dream food doesn't taste so good anymore. Low-fat food has created greater taste sensitivity and

refinement. At this point, fatty, rich food tastes "muddy," "thick," even unpleasant.

9. Think of low-fat, low-carbohydrate food as a special pleasure, a taste refinement, a "natural food." It enriches life, it creates a "lightness of being" and an "ease of living" that permeates all aspects of life.

10. Be flexible in food habits. For example, most breakfasts consist of orange juice, cereal, toast, bagels, jam, and/or a Danish—even a no-fat one. However, this breakfast is principally carbohydrate, high in calories, prevents weight loss, and commonly increases triglycerides and decreases HDL. As listed in the menu section later in part 4, a better breakfast with less carbohydrate, fewer calories, and more protein could be apples and no-fat cheese, tomatoes and no-fat cottage cheese, no-fat yogurt or cottage cheese with fruit, egg white omelet with vegetables, tomatoes, or no-fat cheese.

An inverted triangle standing on its tip symbolizes the ideal food regimen. (See figure 4.2.) At the top are vegetables, comprising the greatest volume of food eaten. Next comes protein, also an essential component of one's diet. Third is fruit, eaten with protein such as no-fat cheese or cottage cheese; an average of about three fruits per day is recommended, with more allowed for lean people. At the next-to-last level of the triangle are bulk carbohydrates such as bread, pasta, rice, potatoes, pastries, sweets; their quantities are limited to achieve lean body weight. Finally, at the tip of the triangle, fat should be the smallest component of one's food.

Types of Food—Fat, Protein, and Carbohydrate

Food has a powerful influence on health. What you eat, interacting with other risk factors, substantially determines the development of coronary heart disease. For people with coronary heart disease, following a good eating plan is a major component of reversal treatment, along with reducing other risk factors and taking cholesterol-lowering medications.

There are three principal mechanisms by which food influences coronary heart disease. The first is the effect of food on cholesterol levels measured in blood obtained after fasting for eight hours, as routinely done in clinical laboratories. The second mechanism is the surge of cholesterol components and related fats in blood that begins immediately after eating and lasts eight hours. The third is the role of food on body weight. Increased fasting blood cholesterol levels, an increased after-eating lipid surge, and increased weight are all associated with increased risk of vascular disease, its progression, and/or heart attacks. Consequently, it is important to review the various types of food and how they affect these mechanisms.

The principal components of food are fat, carbohydrate, protein, fiber,

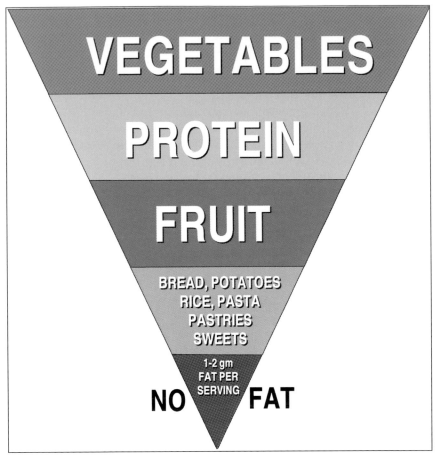

Figure 4.2. The Principles of Low-Fat, Low-Carbohydrate Foods

vitamins, and minerals. Most foods contain all or most of these components in varying proportions. However, for simplicity's sake, most foods can be viewed as consisting principally of one of these components. The simplest way of thinking about foods is to group them into a few functional categories.

These categories can serve as the basis for eating guidelines that are directly related to the labels on foods. (Such labels indicate food content as required by the Food and Drug Administration.) They may also be directly related to calorie counting for calorie-oriented readers, as will be discussed later. These simplified functional categories of food are fats, protein, carbohydrates, vegetables, snacks, and food supplements, each of which is addressed in detail below and in corresponding tables.

Fats, Oils, and Cholesterol

Fats and cholesterol are different molecules unrelated to each other chemically. Fats are long linear chains of carbon atoms connected by single (saturated) or double (unsaturated) bonds. The number of carbon atoms in the chain, the number and location of the single and double bonds determine the type and name of the fat. Cholesterol is a molecule consisting of rings of carbon atoms rather than chains.

In animals, the metabolism of fats and cholesterol is highly interrelated. In meat and animal products, fat content and cholesterol content tend to parallel each other, even though they are separate substances. The fats from animal products are principally saturated fats that are solid or semisolid at room temperature, like butter.

Plants also make fats but not cholesterol. Plant fats may be saturated or predominantly unsaturated, either polyunsaturated (multiple double bonds) or monounsaturated (a single double bond). The mono- or polyunsaturated fats of plants are liquid at room temperature and therefore called oils. Food fats are therefore generally categorized as saturated, polyunsaturated, or monounsaturated.

In mammals, most cholesterol in the body is made in the liver as opposed to externally consumed cholesterol in foods which adds to a lesser extent to cholesterol levels in the blood. The amount of cholesterol made by the liver depends principally on the amount of fat in the diet. The different kinds of fat have different effects on the various fraction of cholesterol and fats in blood. These various fats and cholesterol fractions in the blood are collectively called lipids.

The most important fractions of lipids for clinical management are the blood levels of total cholesterol, the high-density lipoprotein fraction (HDL), the low-density lipoprotein fraction (LDL), and a noncholesterol component of blood fat called triglycerides. The lipoprotein fraction refers to the chemical form in which the cholesterol circulates in blood. As reviewed earlier in this book, the LDL cholesterol is the fraction causing vascular disease, the bad cholesterol or the "low down lipid." The HDL is the fraction protecting against vascular disease, the good cholesterol or "highly defensive lipid." The HDL exerts its beneficial effect by transporting cholesterol out of the wall of arteries back to the liver, thus removing it from the circulating blood, a process called reverse transport. The triglycerides are fats associated with an intermediate risk of vascular disease that increases to very high risk when combined with low HDL.

In this program, target goals for reversing coronary heart disease or preventing it with the greatest certainty in people at high risk are a total cholesterol below 140 mg/dl, LDL cholesterol below 90 mg/dl, HDL cholesterol above 45 mg/dl, and triglycerides below 130 mg/dl.

In general, saturated fats cause an increase in LDL and HDL. In people eating an average diet with 30 to 60 percent of calories as fat, polyunsaturated fats cause a modest decrease in both LDL and HDL; monounsaturated fat is neutral or lowers LDL without lowering HDL. Oils high in monounsaturated fat are hazel nut oil (78 percent), olive oil (74 percent), almond oil (73 percent), and avocado oil (71 percent). All other oils are high in either polyunsaturated or saturated fat, most of which have undesirable effects. Accordingly, in some individuals whose HDL decreases on very low-fat food, the addition of one to two teaspoons of olive oil or hazel nut oil per day may be useful under special circumstances. However, using these oils adds approximately 4.5 grams of fat per teaspoon of oil. It is therefore important to keep other fats at a minimum. Unlike a very low-fat diet in which less than 10 percent of calories come from fat, a diet containing any of these fats in excess will increase LDL cholesterol.

Another form of fat is called a trans fatty acid. The production of margarine and vegetable shortening involves a process called partial hydrogenation of vegetable oils. It produces an adulterated type of fat that raises LDL, lowers HDL, and is therefore particularly bad in causing vascular disease.

Optimal lowering of LDL requires reducing all forms of fat in food to less than 10 percent of calories as fat. For a total of 1,800 calories consumed per day, 10 percent would be 180 calories as fat. Since 1 gram of fat is equivalent to 9 calories, 180 calories would be equivalent to 20 grams of fat. For many people, 1,800 calories per day would be too much, causing weight gain. For a weight-reducing 1,200 calories per day, 10 percent, or 120 calories as fat at 9 calories per gram of fat, would be 14 to 15 grams of fat per day. Achieving this goal requires removing most identifiable fat from one's food. How to determine the fat grams in your foods is reviewed later, in the section "Food Labels."

In addition to the goals of 15 to 20 grams of fat, the target for cholesterol intake in food each day is less than 60 to 80 milligrams for the day averaged over a week. This level of cholesterol minimizes the effect of dietary cholesterol on blood levels of cholesterol. It also allows a wide range of protein sources without the higher caloric burden that typically characterizes pure vegetarian food deriving all protein from high-carbohydrate sources such as grain food. The details of low-fat, low-cholesterol protein sources are discussed in the next section.

This program's goal of 10 percent of calories or approximately 15 to 20 grams of fat and less than 60 to 80 milligrams of cholesterol in food each day is much lower than the guidelines of the American Heart Association and National Cholesterol Education Programs, which are 20 to 30 percent of calories as fat. While the American Heart Association Guidelines may reduce the overall risk of vascular disease in the general population, as a preventive measure they do not predictably stabilize or reverse vascular disease that has already developed. In large studies of lowering cholesterol and heart disease, half of the subjects (the control groups) were treated by placebo and put on diets of 20 to 30 percent of calories as fat. Vascular disease in these control groups demonstrated progression of vascular disease and significant risk of heart attacks, strokes, and deaths. Consequently, in this prevention-reversal program, fat in food is reduced to 10 percent of calories, or approximately 15 to 20 grams per day, in order to optimize outcomes.

In some people, a very low-fat diet may not only lower LDL but also cause a normal physiologic decrease in HDL. This physiologic decrease appears to reflect a decreased need for reverse transport of LDL cholesterol, which is also low. On occasion, the HDL may fall to very low levels of less than 30 mg/dl as the LDL also decreases to low levels, below 90 mg/dl, on a very low-fat, low-cholesterol diet. The specific risks or benefits associated with both low LDL and low HDL are not known precisely. In my own clinical experience, I have seen vascular disease develop or progress with the combination of low LDL and low HDL; however, the risk appears to be substantially less than low HDL with high or even average levels of LDL. To optimize outcomes with the least risk, I aim to increase HDL as much as possible by specific HDL-raising medications, exercise, and lean body mass in addition to lowering LDL.

In people with known coronary heart disease, it is not uncommon for HDL to fall below 30 to 35 mg/dl as total cholesterol and LDL decrease due to a low-fat diet. Such people have a particularly difficult cholesterol problem: Their HDL remains normal only when their LDL cholesterol is high, thereby putting them at high risk of progressive disease, heart attacks, and death due to the high LDL cholesterol. On the other hand, when these people go on a low-fat diet, the fall in LDL cholesterol is associated with a decrease in HDL cholesterol, which in turn is associated with a high risk of progressive vascular disease and its complications. This problem is best managed by low-fat foods *in addition to* a combination of two medications: either a statin class of cholesterol-lowering drug together with regular, immediate-release niacin; or a statin together with gemfibrozil. (All of these medications are discussed in detail in the section "Cholesterol-lowering Drugs.")

Commonly, people with vascular disease have the combination of excess weight, low HDL, elevated triglycerides, and elevated LDL. These abnormalities are typically worse on a diet of high-carbohydrate foods. Such people have in a functional sense a "double defect" such that high-fat foods increase LDL and low-fat, high-carbohydrate foods increase triglycerides and lower HDL. Carbohydrate and fat restriction with weight loss lowers triglycerides, lowers LDL, and raises HDL.

In people with low HDL and elevated triglycerides, fish oil rich in omega-3 fatty acids lowers triglycerides, inconsistently increases HDL, and has differing effects on LDL depending on fat content of the diet. When substituted for carbohydrates or saturated fat of equal caloric content, fish oil lowers LDL. Moderate fish oil also reduces the after-eating lipid surge. However, a moderate to high intake of fish oil increases LDL compared with low-fat foods plus carbohydrate restriction and lean body mass. In diabetes mellitus, fish oil may increase daily insulin requirements. After weighing the net balance of these conflicting effects of fish oil, I recommend eating fish twice per week or more but do not favor taking large amounts of fish oil supplements (more than 1,000 milligrams) long term because good scientific studies have shown no sustained benefit.

However, in certain situations, higher amounts of fish oil are called for. Refractory low HDL or refractory high triglycerides respond occasionally to the combination of fish oil in doses of 4 to 8 grams per day and niacin or gemfibrozil. The potential increase in LDL due to large supplements of fish oil may then be prevented by a statin. On rare occasions, a patient is so sensitive to carbohydrate—which causes high triglycerides and low HDL, even at lean body mass—that a higher-fat diet, particularly high in fish and fish oil, is necessary to maintain weight while keeping carbohydrates low to control triglycerides. The increased LDL associated with higher fat or fish oil intake is then also reduced by a statin.

Eating fatty foods carries a significant risk of vascular disease or its progression that is completely separate from the risk associated with the levels of cholesterol measured in blood under fasting conditions. This direct effect of fatty foods is due to the surge in very low-density lipoprotein cholesterol (VLDL), triglycerides, and a poorly defined, heterogenous cholesterol fraction called chylomicron remnants. We know that this after-eating surge in blood lipids is highly atherogenic, that is, prone to cause atherosclerotic vascular disease (see the discussion in part 1). Since the surge lasts eight hours after a fatty meal, with three meals per day, the exposure of the coronary arteries to atherogenic material may be substantially more than is apparent from cholesterol levels in blood measured after fasting for eight to twelve hours, as is the custom clinically.

While the statin class of cholesterol-lowering drugs reduces blood cholesterol levels measured after fasting, these drugs used alone do not affect the after-eating lipid surge. Very low-fat foods eliminate the after-eating lipid surge and thereby reduce the exposure of the arteries to atherogenic material and the risk of vascular disease. Other than very low-fat foods, the only treatment that reduces the after-eating lipid surge is a combination of medications, specifically a statin plus niacin or statin plus gemfibrozil.

In my opinion, the benefits of eliminating the after-eating lipid surge can be observed by comparing outcomes of studies on cholesterol lowering and by clinical experience. In most cholesterol-lowering trials, a single statin class of cholesterol-lowering medication was used in addition to an American Heart Association diet of 20 to 30 percent of calories as fat. The decrease in cardiovascular events such as heart attacks, strokes, death, bypass surgery, or balloon dilation in the groups receiving statins was reduced by 30 to 60 percent compared with groups receiving a placebo and the same diet. However, in the Familial Atherosclerosis Treatment Study (FATS), double drug therapy was used, which, although not recognized at the time, reduces the after-eating lipid surge in addition to lowering LDL cholesterol. Over the twenty-four months of treatment in the FATS study, the frequency of cardiovascular events in the group receiving double drug therapy was 73 percent lower than for the placebo (control) group. Even more striking, after the first six months, cardiovascular events in the treated group were reduced by 85 percent.

In my clinical experience, I have found that using a 10 percent fat diet, combined with single, double, or triple drug therapy, leads to a profound reduction in cardiovascular risk; over 90 percent of patients are free of cardiovascular events after the first six to eight months of achieving target levels of dietary fat, blood cholesterol, and weight.

Protein

Proteins are compounds made up of amino acids that are required by the body. The recommended dietary allowance (RDA) of protein is 0.8 grams of protein per kilogram of body weight. For a person at ideal weight of 120 pounds (or 59 kilograms), the minimum recommended protein in the diet should be approximately 47 grams each day. For a person at ideal weight of 220 pounds (or 100 kilograms), the minimum RDA is 80 grams of protein. For someone in between, at ideal weight of 185 pounds (or 84 kilograms), the RDA is 67 grams.

Proteins are found in meats, fish, dairy products, eggs, beans, grains, and vegetables. Animal sources provide the most concentrated or richest sources of food protein but typically contain substantial amounts of fat and/or cholesterol. Plant sources are somewhat less concentrated sources of protein without cholesterol and little or no fat. However, plant sources of protein in sufficient amounts to meet minimum daily protein requirements typically contain large amounts of carbohydrates that add calories and weight.

Thus, prior to the widespread availability of palatable, commercially marketed, low-fat, low-cholesterol food products, people were faced with the following dilemma: how could they balance or choose between foods adequate in protein but high in fat and cholesterol, on the one hand, and foods adequate in protein and low in fat and cholesterol but high in carbohydrate, on the other? Many diet regimens have been used to resolve this dilemma at both extremes of the diet spectrum.

At one extreme is a predominantly meat diet that eliminates most carbohydrates and sugars. For an 1,800-calorie diet derived from average beef sources, the amount of beef, cholesterol, and fat consumed is substantial. Each ounce of average standard beef contains 5.6 grams of fat, 27 milligrams of cholesterol, and 82 calories. For a daily 1,800-calorie beef diet, 22 ounces of meat would be consumed with 593 milligrams of cholesterol and 124 grams of fat each day. For a daily 1,200-calorie beef diet, 15 ounces of beef would be consumed with 394 milligrams of cholesterol and 83 grams of fat each day. The benefits of these all-meat diets of relatively reduced caloric content would be weight loss and reduced insulin stimulation associated with low carbohydrate intake. The disadvantages are excessive fat and cholesterol incurring high risk of vascular disease, inadequate fiber, vitamins, minerals, other micronutrients, and essential fatty acids found only in plant foods.

At the other extreme is the strict, pure vegetarian diet including only unprocessed plant sources of protein. In order to obtain an average adequate protein intake of 60 grams each day, a person would have to eat 4.2 cups of beans with 900 to 1,000 calories from principally carbohydrate and 4.5 to 14 grams of fat depending on the type of beans. For a weight-losing diet of 1,200 calories per day, consumption of 900 to 1,000 calories with beans as the protein source would allow only 200 to 300 calories from other food; for an 1,800-calorie diet, 900 to 1000 calories from beans for adequate protein leaves 800 to 900 calories from other foods.

Such diets are highly restrictive, and many people cannot tolerate the high volume of beans required to consume adequate protein. For other sources of grain protein such as pasta or rice, the protein content is lower than the carbohydrate content. Consequently, obtaining adequate dietary protein from these sources incurs excessive calories from carbohydrate and excess weight. For example, if white rice were the only source of protein, it would be necessary to consume over 3,000 calories per day.

While some people can maintain lean body mass on such high-caloric, high-volume carbohydrate diets, others cannot; their excess weight from excessive calories puts them at increased risk for vascular disease, hypertension, diabetes, and other medical problems. If the caloric load is limited to maintain weight, the diet would be deficient in protein. Thus, the disadvantages of pure vegetarian food with only plant sources of protein are that the diet can be restrictive, can prevent certain people from losing weight or even cause them to gain weight due to excessive consumption of carbohydrate, and is often deficient in protein.

The dilemma of choosing between these dietary options is easily resolved by selecting palatable, well-labeled no-fat or low-fat foods, particularly low-fat or no-fat protein sources. These foods are widely available, comprise a range of food types, and can be adapted to suit individual tastes while still easily maintaining 10 percent of calories as fat and achieving lean body mass. This book describes the principles for adapting these low-fat and no-fat protein sources to the food habits and tastes of most people.

Table 4.1. Comparison of Nonfat, Nonmeat Sources of Protein Providing
60 Grams of Protein Each Day

Source	Amount	Cholest (mg)	Fat (gm)	Calories
Mozzarella (no fat)	6.6 oz	33	0	267
Cottage cheese (no fat)	2.3 cups	23	0	323
Yogurt (no fat)	6.6 cups	33	0	600
Skim milk	7.1 cups	29	0	614
Yolk-free eggs	2.5 cups	0	0	300
Veggie burgers	5.5 patties	0	0	382
Garbanzo beans	4.2 cups	0	14	1,056
Kidney beans	4.2 cups	0	4.5	909
Rice (white)	14.7 cups	0	6	3,234

No-Fat and Low-Fat Protein Sources

No-fat and low-fat protein sources include nonfat dairy products, yolk-free eggs or egg products, veggie burgers derived from soy protein, soy protein powder for mixing into drinks, low-fat processed meats, chicken or turkey white meat, fish, venison, buffalo, emu.

A list of nonmeat sources of protein is provided in table 4.1. More than half of these items are nonfat dairy products:

Nonfat mozzarella string cheese has 9 grams of protein and only 40 calories per ounce. It is an excellent low-cholesterol, low-calorie, high-protein source with the best protein-to-calorie ratio of any protein source. This cheese can be the main meal protein for breakfast, lunch, supper, or snacks. They are particularly good with fruit, chopped in salads, soups, and vegetables. The cholesterol per ounce is 5 milligrams, an acceptable amount. If the entire daily 60 grams of protein needed each day were obtained from six to seven ounces, the total cholesterol intake would be only 33 milligrams with 267 calories.

Skim milk has 8.4 grams of protein, 86 calories per cup (eight ounces), no fat to 0.4 grams of fat, and 4 milligrams of cholesterol. It has more calories than cheese sticks or cottage cheese due to its lactose (milk sugar) content. If the entire daily 60 grams of protein were obtained from 6.6 cups of skim milk, total cholesterol intake would be 29 milligrams each day with 614 calories. For whole milk, each cup has 8 grams of protein, 8 grams of fat, 35 milligrams of cholesterol, and 140 calories. For 1 percent milk, one cup has 8 grams of protein, 2.5 grams of fat, 10 milligrams of cholesterol, and 100 calories. Consequently, if whole milk were the sole source of daily average protein requirements of 60 grams of protein, the associated consumption of fat would be 60 grams and cholesterol 263 milligrams. Skim milk is therefore optimal, with 1 percent or 2 percent milk being acceptable as long as other fats in food are kept low enough to keep total food fat between 15 and 20 grams each day. For people who are lactose intolerant, skim milk that is 70 percent or 100 percent lactose free is a delicious alternative to regular milk. The extra calories in milk and yogurt compared with cottage cheese and no-fat cheese for comparable protein content are due to the lactose (milk sugar) in yogurt and milk.

Nonfat yogurt has high protein content of 9 to 10 grams for 90 to 100 calories per eight-ounce container (one cup), either plain or mixed with fruit. Each serving of this size has 5 milligrams of cholesterol, the same amount as no-fat mozzarella cheese.

Nonfat cottage cheese has 13 grams of protein and 70 calories for a four-ounce serving (half cup). The 5 milligrams of cholesterol per serving is acceptable. If the entire daily 60 grams of protein were obtained from 2.3 cups of cottage cheese, total cholesterol intake would be 23 milligrams with 323 calories.

Nonfat cream cheese has 4 grams of protein per one-ounce serving, with 25 calories and 5 milligrams of cholesterol. If the entire daily 60 grams of protein were obtained from 15 ounces of nonfat cream cheese, total cholesterol intake would be 75 milligrams of cholesterol with 375 calories.

Nonfat cheddar and Swiss cheeses are also available, with protein content similar to that for mozzarella cheese.

Nonfat veggie burgers, yolk-free eggs, and protein powder drinks have high protein content with no fat or cholesterol and low calories. *Veggie burgers* are made from soy protein. A typical 78-gram patty contains 11 grams of protein, 70 calories, and no cholesterol, whereas a meat hamburger of the same size has 68 milligrams of cholesterol and 16 grams of fat. If all 60 grams of protein for the day were obtained from 5.5 soy patties, total fat and cholesterol would be zero with 382 calories.

Yolk-free egg products are available in one-cup cartons containing four yolk-free eggs, each egg white providing 6 grams of protein and 30 calories, for a total of 24 grams of protein and 120 calories with no cholesterol. This egg product typically has a low sodium content, much lower than the no-fat dairy products, and is the second best protein source per calorie after no-fat mozzarella cheese with less cholesterol. These egg products can be prepared as scrambled eggs, omelets, or soufflés with added no-fat cheese, no-fat burgers, vegetables, parsley, dill, or other herbs. The soufflés are particularly good served with chopped fruit topping flavored with Grand Marnier liqueur.

Protein powder from soybeans, eggs, or from dairy products is an excellent source of relatively concentrated pure protein without cholesterol or fat. Two tablespoons of protein powder typically contain 20 to 24 grams of protein. Since the protein powder can be obtained without added carbohydrate, the

Table 4.2. Comparison of Meat, Fowl, and Fish Sources of Protein Providing 60 Grams of Protein Each Day

Source	Amount	Cholest (mg)	Fat (gm)	Calories
Beef steak	7.8 oz	210	44	639
Special lean beef	6.7 oz	175	12	357
Franks (low fat)	10.0 oz	150	11	500
Turkey (breast)	6.5 oz	143	5	291
Buffalo	6.1 oz	68	3	303
Tuna (water packed)	8.0 oz	100	4	280
Salmon	7.8 oz	78	12	374
Swordfish	8.3 oz	119	12	367
Halibut	7.9 oz	91	6.5	315

calorie content is that of protein: 4 calories per gram. Protein drinks can be made in a wide variety of ways. Two scoops of protein powder added to a glass of skim milk blended with four or five strawberries make a delicious high-protein supplement. Juices such as cranberry, apple, or orange juice or other fruit can be used. Yogurt is a good additive to thicken the protein drink. Some protein powder has carbohydrate added, which may add calories. If weight loss is important, protein powder without added carbohydrate should be used. However, it is not a good idea to have protein drinks serve as the main nutrition. They are nutritional supplements to augment low-fat, low-cholesterol foods.

It is acceptable to eat more than 60 to 80 grams of protein per day. Many people find maximal satisfaction with 100 to 150 grams of protein each day, but at this higher protein consumption, fat should be kept at 15 to 20 grams per day and cholesterol consumption at 60 to 80 milligrams or less. The higher-protein diet therefore must contain more nonmeat sources. Since protein suppresses appetite and causes satiety at lower caloric consumption than carbohydrate, it is difficult to eat excessive calories as protein.

Lowfat sources of protein from meat, fowl, and fish are listed in table 4.2. We will first consider lowfat meat sources of protein, which have less cholesterol and fat for each gram of protein than standard, untrimmed beef:

Lean beef, trimmed of all fat, has substantially less fat and cholesterol than standard, untrimmed beef. An amount of lean trimmed beef providing the daily protein requirement of 60 grams has 12 grams of fat, 357 calories, and 175 milligrams of cholesterol, too much to be the main or sole source of protein.

Low-fat franks are usually made with beef, turkey, or pork. Each 1.6-ounce frank typically has 50 calories, 6 grams of protein, 1 gram of fat, and 15 milligrams of cholesterol. An amount meeting the daily protein requirement of 60 grams has 11 grams of fat and 150 milligrams of cholesterol, too much to be the major source of dietary protein. However, low-fat franks can be eaten several times per week, with other protein coming from lower-cholesterol sources.

Turkey breast, skinned, grilled, or baked, in an amount providing daily protein requirements of 60 grams has 4 grams of fat and 143 milligrams of cholesterol. *Chicken breast*, skinned, grilled, or baked, has fat and cholesterol content comparable to that for turkey. If turkey or chicken breast were the sole source of dietary protein, cholesterol intake would be too high. However, these foods can be eaten several times per week, with other protein coming from lower-cholesterol sources.

Buffalo, or bison, has the highest protein, lowest cholesterol, and lowest fat content of the common meats. An amount meeting daily protein requirements of 60 grams has 3 grams of fat and 68 milligrams of cholesterol. Commercially marketed buffalo meat as a burger or patty is commonly prepared by adding oil to reduce its dryness. Consequently, the fat content is high. It is important to check the label on the package, order buffalo without added oil, or obtain meat cuts, not preground buffalo meat. *Venison* and *emu* are similar to buffalo in protein, fat, and cholesterol content.

Fish, particularly deep-sea fish such as salmon, tuna, haddock, sole, swordfish, are good sources of protein. The protein, fat, and cholesterol content of fish is comparable to buffalo. Some fish, particularly salmon, have a higher fat content than buffalo or no-fat dairy products. Even if salmon (or one of the other fattier fish) were the sole source of the daily 60 grams of protein, it would add only 12 grams of fat per day. In addition, the fat added is an omega-3 fish oil, which does not have the same adverse effects as animal fats. The fattier fish have substantially less cholesterol than the leanest beef. Therefore, fish can also be eaten several times per week, with other protein coming from lower-cholesterol sources.

Meats, fowl, or fish should be grilled, baked, or sautéed, not fried. Serving size should be four to eight ounces, and frequency during the week will vary depending on what other protein sources are eaten. Food plans with the lowest fat, lowest cholesterol, and lowest carbohydrates would exclude meats, fish, or poultry and derive their protein from no-fat dairy products, veggie burgers, yolk-free egg products, and protein powders. A more flexible regimen would add fish, fowl, buffalo, or equivalent two to four times per week as alternative protein sources providing part of the daily protein requirements but remaining within the average daily limits of 15 to 20 grams of fat and less than 60 to 80 milligrams of cholesterol. A still more meat-oriented diet would use only fish, fowl, buffalo, or equivalent for all of the daily protein needs. In this instance, for approximately 60 grams of protein consumed each day from fish, fowl, or buffalo, the fat content remains within the 15-to-20-gram limit per day, but the daily cholesterol intake ranges from just over the 60-to-80-milligram goal to about 150 milligrams of cholesterol, which is still much less than the average 300 milligrams or more of the typical unrestricted diet.

Therefore, the ideal balance with greatest flexibility and range of protein sources is fish, fowl, buffalo, or equivalent two to four times per week, with the balance of protein coming from the other nonfat, nonmeat sources. However, this approach to food planning is flexible and easy enough to accommodate those who want to exclude all meat, fowl, or fish and those who want to eat only these items as sources of protein.

Ideally, the daily protein requirement should be eaten relatively evenly throughout the daily meals with other food. For people who need three meals per day, approximately 20 grams of protein per meal are ideal. The reason is that protein tends to satisfy hunger, suppress appetite, and reduce the amount of carbohydrate with each meal. Carbohydrates tend to increase insulin levels and stimulate appetite several hours after eating, with a tendency to crave more carbohydrate and calories. For people who eat only two meals per day, protein should be divided relatively equally between these two meals. Eating one large late meal is not ideal since people become very hungry before the one meal and end up losing control and overeating at mealtime, consuming excess carbohydrates in particular.

Tables 4.1 and 4.2 compare various protein sources, showing the amount of protein, total calories, fat, and cholesterol that will provide 60 grams of protein per day. For greater or lesser protein requirements each day, the protein amounts and the corresponding calories, fat, and cholesterol and calories are proportionately larger or smaller.

Carbohydrates

The intake of bulk carbohydrates and starches such as bread, potatoes, rice, pasta, cereals, sugar, alcohol, and fruit should depend on weight. If a person is overweight, most starches except beans should be eliminated, with the aim of weight loss at one to two pounds per week until lean body mass is achieved. Excess calories, even as fat-free starches, may increase or maintain excess weight and higher than desirable cholesterol levels. If you are already lean, carbohydrate may be necessary to maintain weight as fat is removed from the diet.

The elimination of excess carbohydrate to achieve lean body mass in my guidelines is a major departure from most other diets. However, reduction in the volume of carbohydrates is important since people with low HDL and high triglycerides may demonstrate marked increased in triglycerides and fall in HDL on a low-fat, high-volume carbohydrate vegetarian diet. If grains and vegetables are the only source of adequate protein, carbohydrate intake and calories may be high enough to prevent some people from reaching lean body mass and optimal cholesterol lowering, with adverse effects on HDL and triglyceride. My modified semivegetarian diet with alternative good protein sources described here usually achieves desired weight and keeps HDL high and triglycerides low.

Unlike fat grams and protein grams, the number of grams of carbohydrate is not a useful way of determining the amount of carbohydrate to consume each day. Each gram of carbohydrate is equivalent to 4 calories, just as one gram of protein is equivalent to 4 calories; by comparison, 9 calories are in each gram of fat. The proportion of each food contributing to total calories can be easily determined.

For an 1,800-calorie diet, an average daily requirement of 60 grams of protein would include 240 calories as protein ($60 \times 4 = 240$), which is 13 percent (240/1,800) of the total calories. On this diet, 20 grams of fat would contribute 180 calories ($20 \times 9 = 180$), which is 10 percent of total calories. Starting with total calories (100 percent) and subtracting 13 percent of calories as protein and then subtracting 10 percent of calories as fat leaves 77 percent of calories as carbohydrate. The grams of carbohydrate would be calculated as follows: total calories of 1,800 minus 180 calories as fat minus 240 calories as protein equals 1,380 calories from carbohydrates, which at 4 calories per gram is 1,380/4, or 345 grams of carbohydrate. Thus, in low-fat foods, the proportion of carbohydrate is high, and the calorie content is determined principally by the grams, or volume, of carbohydrate.

How many grams of carbohydrate should be eaten is highly variable depending on individual sensitivity to weight gain or loss. Some people need high calories such as 2,500 to 3,000 calories or 600 to 800 grams of carbohydrate just to maintain lean body mass. Heavily trained athletes may have to double these amounts and proportionate amounts of protein and fat in order to maintain the balance of protein, carbohydrate, and fat. However, many, if not most, adults gain weight on 1,800 calories. To lose weight, most people need to reduce caloric intake to between 1,200 to 1,000 calories, corresponding to 200 to 300 grams of carbohydrate.

Because of this great individual variability in the amount of carbohydrate needed to achieve and maintain lean body build, a target number of grams of carbohydrate is not useful. When one is eating principally low-fat food, the best guide to volume of carbohydrate is the individual's weight. For overweight people, the first step is to eliminate entirely the large bulk sources of carbohydrate until reaching desired weight reflecting lean body mass. These large bulk sources of carbohydrate include rice, bread, potatoes, pasta, cereal, candy, pastries, alcohol, fruit juices, and bananas. While vegetables, dairy products, and other low-fat foods may contain some carbohydrates, the amount is low enough that weight will fall if the large bulk sources are eliminated. The optimal rate of weight loss is an average of one to two pounds per week.

Once target weight is reached, nonfat carbohydrate should be reintroduced in the diet, but only in amounts that will hold weight constant at the target level. Excess carbohydrates cause weight to increase, which is an indication that carbohydrates in food should be readjusted downward. If weight falls below target, more nonfat carbohydrates should be added to the food. Depending on weight loss needed and/or rate of weight loss achieved, this elimination of bulk sources of carbohydrates may be moderate. For example, one small to moderate-sized serving of rice, bread, pasta, potatoes, cereal, alcohol, juices, or bananas each day as a special treat, while otherwise adhering to the regimen, is reasonable. However, the cumulative calories of fruit juice, bananas, cereal, bread, pasta, and wine, for example, are simply too much for most people and cause weight gain.

Fruit is a source of the simple carbohydrate sugar. In excess, fruit adds too many calories and causes weight gain. On the other hand, up to three fruits per day as snacks or main meal food is very refreshing, easy to eat, and does not add excessive calories. Note that fruit should always be eaten with nonfat cheese or some protein in order to suppress appetite later. Fruit is better than fruit juices because, like vegetables, it contains the fiber and bulk to fill up the stomach. If fruit is a mainstay of one's diet, weight is the best guide to the amount. For people who don't like fruit, eating equivalent amounts of some other carbohydrate is reasonable but always with protein and within weight guidelines.

Overall Guidelines for a Food Plan of Less Than 10 Percent Fat

The accompanying box summarizes this food regimen in simple terms. Here is an eating plan that involves no counting of calories, and which can be boiled down to six easy steps:

1. Reduce or eliminate obvious fats.
2. Eat 60 to 80 grams of protein each day from low-fat or nonfat sources.
3. Eliminate bulk carbohydrates until reaching lean body mass and then add back enough to maintain body weight.
4. Eat vegetables as the physical bulk of food in addition to protein.
5. Read labels for food content discussed in detail in a later section.
6. Snack when hungry.

In this food program, no one should get too hungry since hunger causes people to lose control over what they eat. Whenever hunger strikes, a snack of protein in some form, protein with fruit, or protein with vegetables should be eaten. The protein food suppresses appetite and produces satiety at a lower caloric consumption than bulk carbohydrates. For most people, it is

---

Examples of No-Fat, High-Protein, Low-Carbohydrate Breakfasts

✓ Yolk-free scrambled eggs or omelet, plain or with cheese, veggie burgers

✓ No-fat mozzarella cheese with tomatoes, apples, grapes, pears, or no-fat pretzels

✓ No-fat cottage cheese with chopped fruit or green, yellow, or red peppers, mustard, tomatoes, vegetables, herbs

✓ No-fat yogurt with mustard or with fruit, or mixed with no-fat bran cereal

✓ Protein powder milk shake or fruit juice shake blended with fruit

✓ Vegetables—carrots, cauliflower, broccoli, celery, zucchini, raw or steamed, topped with no-fat cheese, grilled chicken, or fish

✓ Avoid bread, cereal, bagels, pastries, muffins, sausage, bacon

---

easy to overeat and consume excessive bulk carbohydrates. However, it is harder, and therefore less likely, for most people to overeat protein because it produces a greater sense of fullness and satiety. (In the accompanying boxes, examples of low-fat menus are provided for breakfast, lunch, supper, snacks, travel food, warm and hot meals.)

Examples of Lunch and Supper Salads or Cold Plates

✓ Vegetable salad with chopped no-fat cheese

✓ Mixed vegetable-fruit salad with no-fat cheese

✓ Apple, grape, fruit salad with chopped grilled chicken, turkey, tuna, or salmon

✓ Vegetable-pasta salad with no-fat cheese or chopped chicken, turkey, fish, or no-fat frankfurters

✓ Salad with tabouleh, tomatoes, turkey, and parsley

✓ Fruit salad with no-fat yogurt or no-fat cottage cheese

✓ Bean salad with parsley, chopped vegetables, turkey

✓ Tomatoes with no-fat mozzarella

✓ Tomatoes with no-fat cottage cheese with mustard

✓ Spinach or field lettuce with no-fat cheese or chicken

✓ Couscous with raisins, apple, orange, celery, turkey

✓ Red beets and carrot salad

✓ Fine chopped carrots, corn, pea salad

✓ Dilled green beans, corn, carrots, and tuna

✓ Fava beans with red, green, and yellow peppers

✓ Grilled salmon, broccoli, asparagus, peas

✓ Jicama-carrot salad with raisins

Examples of Quick Meals, Snacks, and Travel Foods

✓ Mozzarella cheese sticks with apples, grapes, or tomatoes

✓ Cottage cheese with tomatoes or fruit

✓ Egg whites or yolk-free egg substitutes as omelet or scrambled with no-fat cheese, veggie burgers

✓ No-fat yogurt flavored with fruit

✓ Mixed fruit-vegetable salad with no-fat cheese, cottage cheese, yogurt, chopped grilled chicken or fish

✓ Vegetables and mixed greens, salads with chopped cheese, chicken, or fish

✓ No-fat bran mixed in yogurt, skim milk

✓ Protein powder shake made with fruit juice or skim milk

✓ Decaf coffee dissolved directly in hot skim milk without water

Weight and Hunger

Excess weight may have a marked effect on cholesterol levels. On average there is a significant fall in cholesterol on achieving lean body weight. In people with coronary heart disease, achieving a lean body weight allows lower doses of cholesterol-lowering drugs to achieve the low cholesterol levels necessary for predictable reversal or stabilization of coronary heart disease.

Achieving lean body weight typically produces a sense of well-being with increased energy and a sense of accomplishment. The optimal rate of weight loss for women and men on a low-fat, low-carbohydrate eating plan is

Guidelines for Food with Adequate Protein, Less Than 10 Percent of Calories as Fat, and Weight Control

No fat	Avoid oils, whole milk products, eggs (except egg whites), most red meat, fatty salad dressings, fast food, fatty cereals, sauces, fried food
Protein	Choose from the following sources of no- or low-fat protein: yogurt, cottage cheese, mozzarella string cheese, other cheese, skim milk, fish, beans, nonfat processed meats, buffalo, turkey or chicken breast, yolk-free eggs, veggie burgers
Carbohydrate	Reduce consumption of rice, bread, pasta, potatoes, cereal, alcohol, fruit juice, bananas, pastry, candy
Vegetables	Eat a variety of fresh vegetables as the bulk of one's food
Snacks	Snack regularly but include protein sources with every meal and snack
Labels	Read labels for no-fat products, particularly cheese, salad dressing, milk products, protein sources, cereals

Examples of Lunch and Supper Hot Meals

Vegetables:

✓ Broccoli, cauliflower, brussels sprouts, zucchini, tomatoes, green beans, carrots, cabbage, turnips, squash, red beets, celery, peas, garbanzo, black, red and white beans, corn, spinach, kale, greens

✓ Steamed, microwaved, grilled, stir-fried, baked, pureed

✓ Three to five types with each meal

Served with

✓ No-fat shredded or melted cheese, no-fat cottage cheese, or no-fat yogurt mixed with mustard or herbs, tomato sauce, no-fat grated parmesan, no-fat sour cream sauce with herbs

✓ Turkey or chicken breast, buffalo, venison—grilled, broiled, baked, steamed, or sautéed in wine or lemon juice

✓ Salmon, tuna, swordfish, haddock, sole, snapper—grilled, broiled, baked, steamed, or sautéed in wine or lemon juice

✓ Veggie burgers, no-fat weiners, no-fat bologna

✓ Small amount of pasta, potatoes, bread, or rice

Examples of Salad or Vegetable Dressing

✓ No-fat ready made

✓ Balsamic vinegar

✓ Honey mustard and lemon juice

✓ No-fat yogurt, no-fat sour cream with herbs

---

typically four to six pounds in the first two weeks, then one to two pounds per week thereafter. The decrease in weight may be steady or may occur in steps with plateaus of stable weight for several days or weeks between the downward steps.

Weight loss at greater than two pounds per week may be associated with fatigue or weakness, particularly if food is deficient in protein. Being hungry during weight loss or eating foods deficient in protein or deficient in essential fatty acids may also cause headaches, light-headedness, "fuzzy" feelings in the head, a lack of mental sharpness, drowsiness or fatigue, as discussed earlier. In addition, hunger causes loss of control over food choices, with a high likelihood of eating any food available that may have a high-fat, high-sugar, or high-carbohydrate content, typical of readily available snack foods. Therefore, it is essential to eat enough protein to avoid getting hungry and to avoid these symptoms. Enough protein in food is specifically 50 to 80 grams per day for lighter (120 pounds) or heavier (200 pounds) people, eaten as main course meals or frequent snacks of principally protein food with some fruit or vegetables.

Weight loss without hunger and with adequate protein often produces euphoria and unusual sharpness of thinking. On the other hand, too much hunger can cause lack of concentration and a "fuzziness" in mental function or fatigue. Therefore, an essential principle to successful weight loss is avoidance of hunger by eating large enough meals or between-meal snacks whenever one starts to get hungry. The secret is what one eats, not how much or how often. Protein tends to suppress appetite and carbohydrate craving. Sugar and carbohydrate tend to stimulate appetite several hours after being eaten, leading to more sugar and carbohydrate consumption. This hunger cycle then makes weight control difficult. Choosing or planning regular snacks of protein, vegetables, and some fruits that minimize fat and excess carbohydrate allows weight control without hunger. A snack containing substantial protein, eaten one to two hours before a regular meal, dulls the appetite so that control of food during the meal is much easier. Therefore, eating protein snacks between meals is a good idea.

Essential Fatty Acids

Some people reduce the percentage of calories as fat in their diet to below 10 percent. At a level of 5 percent of calories as fat or less than 10 to 15 grams of fat each day, a deficiency may occur in certain fats called essential fatty acids, which cannot be made by the body but must be obtained in food. Two essential fatty acids, linoleic and alpha-linolenic acid, are required for synthesis of a wide variety of compounds essential for normal body function, called arachinoids, eicosanoids, prostaglandins, thromboxanes, and leukotrienes. These two essential fatty acids are found principally in plants, particularly soybeans and specific nuts or seeds.

The recommended dietary allowances (RDA) published by the National Research Council do not make recommendations on minimum daily requirements of essential fatty acids. The reason is a lack of data and the difficulty of identifying essential fatty acid deficiency in a population other than that of patients with malabsorption syndromes or total intravenous feedings (parenteral alimentation). The United Kingdom Reference Nutrient Intakes suggest minimum consumption of 1 percent of calories from linoleic acid and 0.2 percent from alpha-linolenic acid. For a 1,500-calorie diet commonly needed to achieve lean body mass, approximately 1.67 grams of linoleic and 0.33 grams of alpha-linolenic acid would be minimum requirements based on these criteria. For an 1,800-calorie diet, 2 grams of linoleic and 0.4 grams of alpha-linolenic would be the minimal requirements by these criteria.

Soybean oil, walnut oil, corn oil, grapeseed, sunflower, and cottonseed oil contain over 50 percent linoleic acid. Soybean oil, walnut oil, canola, and rapeseed oil contain 7 to 11 percent and linseed oil contains 53 percent alpha-linoleic acid. Only soybean and walnut oils have significant balanced amounts of both linoleic and alpha-linolenic acid in proportion to their essential requirements by the body. Alternatively, two body compounds synthesized from one of the essential fatty acids (alpha-linolenic acid), called docosahexaenoic (DHA) and eicosapentaenoic (EPA), can be acquired from seafood, specifically omega-3 fish oil. In view of the ubiquity of the two essential fatty acids in Western diets, essential fatty acid deficiency is considered rare in adults; if it occurs at all, it is seen only, and uncommonly, in those with severe malnutrition, untreated abnormalities of fat absorption in the gut, or prolonged incomplete fat-free intravenous feeding.

However, I have seen sixteen lean patients on self-imposed, well-documented diets of less than 5 percent of calories as fat (less than my guidelines of 10 percent of calories as fat) for one to three years who had clinical symptoms consistent with essential fatty acid deficiency. These symptoms included mild but definite temporary recent memory loss, difficulty concentrating, episodic somnolence during the day, light-headedness on standing up, low blood pressure, visual scotoma, decreased visual acuity, and/or sexual dysfunction. One, several, or all of these symptoms first appeared while the patients were on very low-fat diets and disappeared on increasing sources rich in essential fatty acids.

In addition to these symptoms, four of these sixteen patients had their first episode of irregular abnormal heart rhythm without alcohol exposure or identifiable cause and without recurrence after increasing their essential fatty acid intake. Nine of these patients had their first episode of overt passing out (called vasovagal syncope), preceded by symptoms of similar but less intense near fainting reactions, all of which disappeared on increasing sources of essential fatty acids without other identifiable changes in food, weight, or medications. Two people developed flaking soft nails that became normal after they increased their intake of essential fatty acid sources. None had the typical fatigue, elevated triglycerides, and low HDL commonly due to excess carbohydrate and inadequate protein.

Therefore, in my opinion, clinically relevant essential fatty acid deficiency may occur in otherwise well-nourished, active, well individuals on very low-fat diets of less than 5 percent of calories as fat. Any treatment powerful enough to heal is also powerful enough to harm if it is misused or its side effects are not understood. Hence, a very low-fat food plan must be implemented properly, with no less than 10 percent of calories as fat and a source of essential fatty acids.

For people on very low-fat foods, I recommend specific sources of essential fatty acids. Soybean oil contains 51 percent linoleic and 6.8 percent alpha-linolenic acid. One teaspoon of soybean oil containing approximately 4.7 grams of oil provides 2.4 grams of linoleic acid and 0.38 grams of alpha-linolenic acid, the minimum requirements to prevent clinical essential fatty acid deficiency based on the criteria of the United Kingdom Reference Nutrient Intakes and consistent with discussion of the recommended dietary allowances of the National Research Council. One form of soybean oil is soya lecithin containing 1.2 grams of oil per capsule, so that four capsules each day would provide this minimum requirement.

One teaspoon of walnut oil provides 2.4 grams of linoleic acid and 0.25 grams of alpha-linolenic acid. One to two teaspoons of walnut oil ingested per day provide the minimal requirements for essential fatty acids. It is the only oil besides soybean oil with balanced equivalent amounts of both linoleic and alpha-linolenic acids in approximate proportion to their essential requirements. Walnut oil tastes delicious and is available in most grocery stores. Walnut kernels contain 28 grams of linoleic acid per 100 grams of kernels, so that the minimum requirements of 2 grams of linoleic acid would be provided from 7 grams of walnut kernels or one to two tablespoons of walnut kernels.

One teaspoon of corn oil, grapeseed, sunflower, or cottonseed oil provides the same amount or more of linoleic acid since all contain over 50 percent linoleic acid. However, these oils lack the alpha-linolenic acid. Alpha-linolenic acid can be obtained from a teaspoon of linseed oil, grapeseed oil, or canola oil containing approximately 2.4 grams, 0.5 grams, and 0.5 grams of alpha-linolenic acid respectively. Alternatively, fish or fish oil could be used as sources of EPA and DHA instead of oils containing alpha-linolenic acid, from which the body synthesizes these compounds.

One fish meal per week is reportedly associated with a 50 percent decrease in risk of primary cardiac arrest in patients without known heart disease after adjustment for confounding other risk factors. This level of fish intake is the equivalent of only 0.2 grams of fish oil per day. Although the study reports these observations have limitations, it suggests that very small amounts of fatty acids may be beneficial. At the other extreme, a high consumption of the essential fat linoleic acid (greater than 12 percent of calories) leads to a decrease in HDL cholesterol associated with higher risk of atherosclerosis.

Therefore, for people *consuming less than 10 percent of calories as fat*, I recommend that the small amount of fat consumed contain a daily source of essential fatty acids by one of several alternative regimens as follows:

- ✓ One teaspoon (4.7 grams fat) of soybean oil or four soya lecithin capsules each containing 1.2 grams of oil, either of which provides 2.4 grams of linoleic and 0.38 grams of alpha-linolenic acid, the minimum essential fatty acids requirements.
- ✓ One teaspoon (4.7 grams fat) of walnut oil providing 2.4 grams of linoleic and 0.25 grams of alpha-linolenic acid in addition to a fish meal once per week or a fish oil capsule once per day or an extra teaspoon of walnut oil to increase the alpha-linolenic acid intake.

✓ One teaspoon (4.7 grams fat) of canola oil containing 1.22 grams of linoleic acid and 0.47 grams of alpha-linolenic acid in addition to the small amounts of linoleic acid in vegetables since vegetable oils are rich in linoleic acid, or two teaspoons of canola oil.

Food Labels

There are many no-fat, no-cholesterol foods currently on the market. It is simple to read the labels on food products for fat and cholesterol content since the Food and Drug Administration (FDA) rules require accurate labeling. There are no-fat, no cholesterol salad dressings, butter substitutes, mayonnaise, cheese, and other protein sources, as discussed above. Some food products have 1 to 2 grams of fat per serving, which is acceptable as long as the total fat consumed is less than 15 to 20 grams per day.

Food labels list the content of protein, fat, cholesterol, carbohydrate, sodium potassium, vitamin A, calcium, and calories. The protein tables (tables 4.1 and 4.2) can be used to estimate proteins, fat, cholesterol, and caloric content of common fresh food products that are not labeled. Using food labels together with these protein tables provides a simple, accurate way of quickly analyzing the contents of each meal and the total amount of protein, fat, and cholesterol consumed each day without counting calories or carbohydrate grams. Examples of food labels follow, as well as how to use them.

Example 1. Creamed Spinach (Frozen)

Nutrition Facts
Serving Size 1/2 Cup (125 g)

Amount per Serving
Calories 156, Calories from Fat 108

	% Daily Value
Total Fat 12 g	17%
Saturated Fat 4 g	20%
Cholesterol 15 mg	5%
Sodium 380 mg	15%
Total Carbohydrate 8 g	3%
Dietary Fiber 2 g	6%
Sugars 2 g	
Protein 4 g	

Vitamin A 50%	Vitamin C 8%
Calcium 10%	Iron 4%

In addition to this label of contents, there is a table on every food label giving the Percent Daily Values of each food based on a daily consumption of 2,000 or 2,500 calories:

Percent Daily Values are based on a 2,000-calorie diet. Your daily values may be higher or lower depending on your calorie needs:

	2,000	2,500
Calories	2,000	2,500
Total Fat	less than 65 g	80 g
Sat Fat	less than 20 mg	25 g
Cholesterol	less than 300 mg	300 mg
Sodium	less than 2,400 mg	2,400 mg
Total Carbohydrate	300 g	375 g
Dietary Fiber	25 g	30 g

Calories per gram:
Fat 9, Carbohydrate 4, Protein 4

Spinach is a vegetable with no cholesterol and negligible fat content. However, in this commercial frozen food preparation, 12 grams of fat for each half-cup serving size has been added as "seasoning" to make creamed spinach. A half cup of fresh spinach solids contains only 48 calories derived from 4 grams of protein (16 calories) and 8 grams of carbohydrate (32 calories). Twelve grams of fat with 15 grams of cholesterol contain calories ($12 \times 9 = 108$) that have been added to each half cup of spinach; total calories per serving is 156 ($48 + 108 = 156$). A half-cup serving is not very large for most adults; they would commonly eat a full cup of creamed spinach at one meal, thereby consuming 24 grams of fat, 30 milligrams of cholesterol, and 312 calories. This load of fat, cholesterol, and calories would come from only one vegetable, creamed spinach, at one meal. With other foods comparably fixed and three meals per day, the fat, cholesterol, and calorie load becomes enormous, causing excess weight, high cholesterol levels, and high risk of heart disease.

In this program, any food with more than 2 grams of fat per serving, or a cumulative fat load of more than 15 to 20 grams of fat each day, and more than 60 milligrams of cholesterol each day should be avoided as a regular daily food item. As an alternative to this creamed spinach, eat fresh spinach as a salad or lightly steamed. For those who must have creamed spinach, fix it with no-fat yogurt, no-fat cream cheese, no-fat whipped cream, no-fat condensed milk, and/or no-fat soups.

In my opinion, the table of daily requirements listed in food labels gives daily requirements of calories, fat, cholesterol, and carbohydrate that are much too high for most people. For most people, but particularly middle-aged adults, eating these amounts of calories, fat, cholesterol, and carbohydrate will cause weight gain, cholesterol levels that are too high, and increased risk of vascular disease.

My belief that these recommended daily amounts of fat, cholesterol, and calories are excessive is based on the fact that in large scientific studies, coronary heart disease progresses, with continuing heart attacks and excessive death, in control groups of people eating according to the American Heart Association Guidelines, which call for even less fat and less cholesterol than the recommended amounts on the food labels.

Many people eat more than the recommended amounts on food labels, perhaps explaining the widespread, massive problems of obesity and related diseases in this country. Excessive, high consumption of food, like other habits such as smoking, is driven by advertising, social custom, stress, and multiple other facets of living. Aside from individual rights to live as desired, consume freely, and have any personal appearance without restriction, excess weight is a health problem associated with increased death rates, particularly from vascular diseases and some cancers. Reading food labels helps one choose healthy foods that taste good, and consume a reasonable volume to ward off hunger and to maintain lean body mass.

Example 2. Chicken BBQ

Nutrition Facts
Serving Size / Meal

Amount per Serving
Calories 314, Calories from Fat 18
Total Fat 2 g
   Saturated Fat 0.5 g
   Polyunsaturated Fat 0 g
   Monounsaturated Fat 1.5 g
Cholesterol 35 mg
Sodium 290 mg
Total Carbohydrate 55 g
   Dietary Fiber 6 g
   Sugars 38 g
Protein 19 g

This food label indicates an acceptable amount of protein, fat, cholesterol, and calories for one meal. If the entire daily average protein allotment of 60 grams were obtained by eating three of those frozen dinners, the cholesterol consumption would be 105 milligrams ($3 \times 35 = 105$). This amount of cholesterol is just one-third of the 300 milligrams recommended on the food label. However, as indicated earlier, these recommended daily amounts are excessive. For this program for reversing vascular disease, the 105 milligrams of cholesterol is more than the 60 milligrams each day which I recommend. Consequently, some other low-fat, low-cholesterol source of protein should be eaten at two other meals, while this frozen dinner is satisfactory for one meal of the day. In the food label, sugars are counted under total carbohydrates.

Example 3. Soy Protein Burger

Nutrition Facts
Serving Size 1 patty (78 g)

Amount per Serving
Calories 70
Total Fat 0 g
  Saturated Fat 0 g
Cholesterol 0 g
Sodium 360 mg
Potassium 390 mg
Total Carbohydrate 6 g
  Dietary Fiber 3 g
  Sugars 0
Protein 11 g

The soy protein burger has high protein, no fat, no cholesterol, low carbohydrate, and low calorie content for the amount of protein provided. Therefore, it is an ideal protein source. Moreover, it is easy to fix and tastes good. It can be served as is with vegetables, spiced with mustard, ketchup, chutney, chopped up in chili, soups, or scrambled yolk-free eggs or omelets.

Example 4. Whipped Butter

Nutrition Facts
Serving Size/tablespoon (9 g)

Calories per Serving 63
  Fat Calories 63
Total Fat 7 g
  Saturated Fat 5 g
Cholesterol 20 mg

Sodium 0
Total Carbohydrate 0
Protein 0

Butter is meant to be excluded from this food program because it is so high in fat and cholesterol. However, some people crave the taste of butter. The label of whipped butter suggests a compromise. Regular butter has 11 grams of fat and 30 milligrams of cholesterol in each tablespoon. One tablespoon of whipped butter contains 7 grams of fat and 20 milligrams of cholesterol. It is easier to spread thin than regular butter. If thinly spread on bread or crackers, enough to give a good taste, one tablespoon of whipped butter will last about seven days; each thin spread of whipped butter contains about 1 gram of fat, 2 to 3 milligrams of cholesterol, and 9 calories. These amounts are acceptable from a health standpoint. However, multiple thick slabs of regular butter on dry food is unhealthy. For vegetable seasoning, sprinkle on no-fat butter substitutes, which taste the same as butter without the fat and cholesterol.

People with heart failure or high blood pressure need to limit their salt intake, commonly to 2,000 milligrams or less. While nonmeat, nonfat protein sources may contain modest amounts of sodium, the amount of sodium associated with average daily protein requirements of 60 milligrams from these sources is usually less than 1,200 milligrams. As long as other sources of salt are limited, this amount of sodium is acceptable.

The most important way to use the food label is to check out protein, fat, and cholesterol contents. Add up total protein, fat, and cholesterol from food labels and from tables 4.1. and 4.2 and then compare these totals with the goals of at least 60 to 80 grams of protein, 15 to 20 grams of fat, and less than 60 to 80 milligrams of cholesterol. Weight is a guide to what's left, specifically the volume of carbohydrate.

To quickly and easily assess each day's food consumption, you can start with the rule of nines for protein. Each glass of milk, each low-fat mozzarella cheese stick, each cup or carton of yogurt, each soy burger patty, each half cup of no-fat cottage cheese, each half-cup carton of yolk-free egg product, each quarter chicken or turkey breast, fish or buffalo, approximately 2 ounces (a small half-palm-sized piece), has approximately 9 to 12 grams of protein. Having decided on adequate protein sources, you then add up the amount of protein, which should be at least 60 to 80 grams. Then add up the amount of cholesterol to be sure it is less than 60 to 80 milligrams each day. The remaining foods for the day are mostly vegetables or two to three fruits with no-fat cheese. For people trying to lose weight, the bulk carbohydrates should be eliminated or eaten in minimal amounts. For people needing to maintain weight, more carbohydrates and no-fat protein need to be added to food.

Food "Zigzags," "Food Breaks," and "Average" Cholesterol/Fat Consumption

Human nature is such that many people do not like the idea of "giving up forever" some rich, fatty, favorite food. Consequently, I advise that if you so desire, you eat once a month whatever rich, fatty, favorite food you have eliminated from your regular daily meals. At that one meal you may consume three to four times the optimal daily amounts of calories, fat, and cholesterol. However, on other days of the month, stay with the proper foods, holding down fat, cholesterol, and also calories if needed for weight loss. The one zigzag or food break is not particularly harmful if, during the rest of the month, you stick with healthier foods. Allowing one "food break" per month commonly improves adherence during the rest of the month. People also realize that having adapted and refined their taste capacity for lower-fat foods, the rich, fatty, formerly favorite food now tastes heavy, thick, or "muddy" and doesn't taste so good anymore.

Food "Substitutes" and Processed Foods

There are a number of food substitutes, particularly "artificial sweeteners," fat or butter substitutes, egg "substitutes," and lactose-free milk. In this same general category are no-fat foods (processed to remove fat), decaffeinated coffee, vitamin- or calcium-fortified milk, veggie burgers, low-fat packaged meats. Virtually every food that is commercially packaged is processed to some extent, some more than others.

Many people consider these types of foods, food additives, or food substitutes to be "unnatural" and somehow bad for the body because they are foreign, are not found or grown "naturally," and may even contain toxins or drugs that harm us. In this context, the concept of nature or natural implies minimal "interference," processing, or alteration by humans or human-generated processes of "better," "safer," "healthier," "natural" foods, or "country foods."

While concern over "food pollution," like air and water pollution, is a healthy attitude, it is important to remember that nature's ways are not always benign. Nature's ways are heavily influenced by genetic predisposition, as is the risk of vascular disease. Once vascular disease strikes, the natural course of events for many people is pain, disability, and premature death. In the absence of a well-structured human society, nature's course of events is usually a short, hard life with a violent, painful end from trauma, infectious disease, natural disasters, bad weather, or starvation. With the advantages of structured human society, enough food has evolved to too much food, excessive eating, lack of physical exertion, addiction to tobacco, hypertension, and a variety of other risk factors different from those of less structured, less complex, more "natural" societies. Now, the natural course of life is commonly too much food, too much fat, excessive weight, lack of exercise, vascular disease, disability, and death.

If people simply ate less, did regular hard physical exercise, did not smoke, did not like or buy rich fatty food, then there might be no need for specialized, processed low-fat, low-calorie foods. However, the "natural course" of human societies is greater consumption, excess food, high-risk living habits. For example, before approximately 1900, there was little widespread heavy consumption of beef. With improved cattle management, greater customer demand, more efficient production and shipping, beef consumption has dramatically increased. So has the consumption of tobacco, which, with other risk factors, causes vascular disease.

Now, large segments of society are discovering the downside of eating large amounts—excessive amounts—of the wide variety of affordable foods that are available, along with other consumption-related risk factors. The downside is vascular disease, obesity, hypertension, and chronic disability for many years of life.

Although the average life span has increased to over eighty years, for many people with a genetic predisposition, combined with these risk factors, disability or premature death from vascular disease is common. For other people with vascular disease, the possibility of an unexpected, seemingly random death due to this condition is frightening; it may become the major subliminal fear of many people as other health concerns come under their control.

However, vascular and coronary heart disease is not random. It is predictable, fairly well understood, and a disease of choice, of lifestyle habits interacting with genetic predisposition. By making different lifestyle choices, an individual can largely overcome this familial predisposition; moreover, by taking cholesterol-lowering medications, where appropriate, a person can more predictably prevent or reverse vascular disease.

In the context of this evolution of societal food and living habits, low-fat, low-cholesterol, or processed foods become the next refinement in control of the factors that disable and kill us. The demands of time, competition, social custom, psychological stress and reward, concentrated, prolonged sedentary work for most people—all require different kinds of foods and different kinds of disciplines than were required in the early part of the century, in order to optimize health and longevity. Low-fat, low-cholesterol, and/or processed foods should be viewed as a rational improvement, a beneficial evolution, a refinement of our lifestyle, an adaptation to the current social environment that makes us healthier.

From this viewpoint, such foods are a "natural" development; they are far more "natural" than the artificially fat-loaded, lethal, excessive eating-living habits of a former generation that has largely died in an epidemic of vascular disease. Unfortunately, many people still have not learned the downside of excessive consumption and high-risk living habits as evidenced by widespread obesity and continuing vascular disease as the greatest cause of disability and death in developed countries.

Practically speaking, the low-fat, low-cholesterol foods have no significant recognized harmful effects. Similarly, for the sugar and fat substitutes. The taste of low-fat foods or food substitutes is variable, some people liking one but not others. Some foods once thought to be "healthy" are no longer considered so. For example, at one time margarine was thought to be less harmful than butter. However, the trans fatty acid content of partially hydrogenated vegetable oils in margarine is now recognized as contributing to vascular disease. Tofu is commonly considered healthy since it is a plant protein source. However, tofu may contain substantial amounts of fat which in excess contribute to vascular disease. An even more widespread misconception is that if fat is reduced, unlimited carbohydrates can be eaten. This myth is the basis of several low-fat, pure vegetarian diets that fail to limit carbohydrate intake. In a large number of people, such diets increase obesity, increase triglycerides, increase insulin levels, worsen diabetes, lower HDL, and contribute to vascular disease, as reviewed earlier.

The misunderstanding about low-fat foods or food substitutes may be even more inappropriate. Yolk-free eggs are real eggs, not egg substitutes, but the yolks have been removed. Lactose-free milk is real milk, but the lactose, or milk sugar, has been cleaved to a simple sugar by an enzyme similar to that which the body produces normally to break down the lactose. Lactose-free milk tastes sweeter than "regular" milk because the lactose has already been broken down to the more easily absorbed simpler sugar.

In general, regulation of food products and their labels is reasonably strict in this country, more so than elsewhere. Consequently, labels on processed foods are a useful guide, and the low-fat, low-cholesterol foods are healthy valuable additions to our cuisine. Their benefits in preventing or reversing vascular disease far outweigh any recognizable potential adverse effects.

Menus

The following menus help illustrate the application of these food principles in daily living. Menus for a full week are provided, which should be sufficient for any individual to get off to a good start on the eating plan.

Day 1

Breakfast. Scrambled eggs, yolk free, from one carton equivalent to four eggs, with salt and pepper and chopped veggie burger mixed in, heavily topped with a layer of grated, no-fat cheddar cheese. One glass of skim milk fortified with extra calcium. A multivitamin, vitamin E (400 units), vitamin C (500 milligrams).

Lunch. Two apples with three sticks of low-fat mozzarella string cheese and a cup of no-fat fruit yogurt, a glass of skim milk.

Afternoon snack. A large, skim milk, decaffeinated latte made by adding one tablespoon of decaffeinated instant coffee directly to a large mug of hot skim milk.

Supper. A large serving of broccoli and cauliflower steamed in fat-free chicken bouillon broth, topped with no-fat Parmesan cheese. Two soy veggie burgers with mustard. A large spinach salad with mushrooms, sliced tomatoes, and a dressing made from white or red balsamic vinegar mixed with one teaspoon of walnut oil and one teaspoon of crumbled feta cheese with peppercorn. For dessert, a half cup of no-fat frozen yogurt. A multivitamin, vitamin E (400 units), vitamin C (500 milligrams).

Day 2

Breakfast. One cup of no-fat cottage cheese with grapes, chopped peaches, chopped pears, or chopped strawberries. One glass of calcium-fortified skim milk. Vitamins as above.

Lunch. A large bowl of no-fat vegetable soup into which has been added three cut-up cheese sticks, chopped soy veggie burgers, or chopped low-fat wieners. A green salad with the vinegar dressing above, or a creamy dressing made with no-fat yogurt, no-fat sour cream, mustard or curry, chopped parsley, and herbs.

Afternoon snack. A protein drink made from skim milk, two tablespoons of protein powder, strawberries, and a half cup of fruit yogurt mixed in a blender.

Supper. Grilled turkey or chicken breast with asparagus, carrots, and zucchini. A small green salad with honey, mustard, and lemon juice dressing. For dessert, chopped fruit with Grand Marnier. Vitamins as above.

Day 3

Breakfast. An entire grapefruit, peeled and in sections, in a half cup of cottage cheese, and an orange with two cheese sticks, a large skim milk decaffeinated latte. Vitamins as above.

Lunch. A bowl of no-fat chili beans with chopped soy veggie burgers. A large mixed-greens and vegetable salad with vinegar dressing.

Afternoon snack. One cup of no-fat fruit yogurt, perhaps two cups if hungry.

Supper. A large plate of four steamed vegetables (select from red, yellow, green peppers, broccoli, cauliflower, squash or zucchini, celery) covered with a thick layer of no-fat cottage cheese (one cup), a generous amount of hot, fat-free tomato sauce (one-half to one cup), and finally a thick layer of fat-free Parmesan cheese. A small fruit salad of grapefruit and orange sections. For dessert, two no-fat cookies and a chocolate coffee latte made by adding one tablespoon of instant decaffeinated coffee and one tablespoon of no-fat powdered chocolate to a large mug of hot skim milk. Vitamins as above.

Day 4

Breakfast. One cup of no-fat fruit yogurt, mixed with a half cup of no-fat or low-fat grain cereal with added fruit, grapes, chopped peaches, strawberries, or blueberries. A glass of calcium-fortified skim milk. Vitamins as above.

Lunch. Grilled swordfish without oil on a bed of steamed vegetables asparagus and carrots. A small green salad with vinegar dressing.

Afternoon snack. One apple with two low-fat mozzarella string cheese sticks.

Supper. A large mixed-vegetable, bean salad (select from canned or dilled garbanzo beans, red beans, white beans, celery, corn, red, green, or yellow peppers) with vinegar dressing, and a side dish of one cup of cottage cheese mixed with one tablespoon of mustard, peppered with chopped chives and parsley. For dessert, a blueberry fruit tart made with low-fat crust. Vitamins as above.

Day 5

Breakfast. An omelet made as follows: In a bowl, mix and whip with a fork one carton of yolk-free eggs and one half cup of skim milk. Pour the mixture into a hot Teflon skillet coated with a small amount of Pam. Add salt and pepper to taste, chopped parsley, bits of no-fat cheese or chopped low-fat wieners. Fold over when done and serve. One glass skim milk. Vitamins as above.

Lunch. A large protein milk shake made with one and a half to two glasses of skim milk blended with two scoops of protein powder, a cup of fruit yogurt, and four to five strawberries or other fruit. A green salad with vinegar dressing.

Afternoon snack. Ten to fifteen small cherry tomatoes and two low-fat mozzarella cheese sticks.

Supper. A large plate of vegetables (green beans, peppers, peas, cauliflower, asparagus) steamed in no-fat chicken bouillon broth, covered with sauce made of pureed broccoli and herbs or no-fat yogurt, no-fat sour cream, and herbs with a touch of mustard. One-half cup to one cup of cottage cheese on the side with salt, pepper, mustard mixed with sliced tomatoes. For dessert, no-fat frozen yogurt. Vitamins as above.

Day 6

Breakfast. A large bowl of cherry red tomatoes or sliced tomatoes with three low-fat mozzarella string cheese sticks or one cup of cottage cheese with salt, pepper, and a touch of mustard mixed in. One glass of skim milk. Vitamins as above.

Lunch. A large fruit salad made of chopped apples, peaches, celery, raisins, grapes with chopped grilled turkey, chicken breast, or water-packed tuna mixed with a dressing of no-fat yogurt, no-fat sour cream, no-fat mayonnaise, honey, mustard, and lemon juice.

Afternoon snack. Two low-fat mozzarella string cheese sticks with two large fat-free pretzels.

Supper. Omelet soufflé or "oven puff" made as follows: In a bowl, blend three cartons of yolk-free eggs (for two people) with three-fourths cup milk, three-fourths cup flour, salt to taste; pour into a Teflon oven pan (two to three inches deep). Preheat oven to 450°F and bake for fifteen minutes until puffed up and brown on top. Cut into thirds and serve topped with a bowl of chopped fruit, strawberries, blueberries, peaches, kiwis, soaked in Grand Marnier. Finish meal with a chocolate-decaffeinated latte as above. Save the remaining third for breakfast. Vitamins as above.

Day 7

Breakfast. Leftovers from the previous supper: warm the one-third omelet soufflé in the microwave for one and a half minutes on high; top it with a large serving of the fruit soaked in Grand Marnier. A cup of decaffeinated skim latte. Vitamins as above.

Lunch. Grilled salmon without added oil on a bed of steamed vegetables with a green salad and vinegar dressing.

Afternoon snack. A protein drink from one glass of cranberry juice, one to two scoops of protein powder, one-half cup fruit yogurt, and several strawberries or other fruit blended in.

Supper. Couscous cooked with raisins, walnuts, apples, celery, with low-fat wieners or chopped veggie burgers, orange slices, and mustard added. For desert, fruit and low-fat Gouda cheese from Holland. Vitamins as above.

For people with little time or interest in "variety," eating the same favorite lunch each day avoids having to choose where to go or what to eat. Similarly, a favorite breakfast that is fast, simple, and the same every day may be preferable to the different breakfasts and lunches suggested above.

Antioxidant Vitamins and Aspirin

In the development of atherosclerosis, the LDL, or "bad" cholesterol, is altered to an oxidized form. This oxidized form of LDL stimulates inflammation and development of atherosclerosis in the arterial wall, as discussed in part 1. Antioxidant vitamins retard the oxidative breakdown of LDL cholesterol to this undesirable form. Vitamin E is an antioxidant vitamin associated with reduced progression of coronary artery narrowing. A dose of 800 units of vitamin E per day has been shown to significantly retard the oxida-

Table 4.3. Daily Doses of Antioxidant Vitamins

Vitamin	Dose	Frequency
Vitamin E	400 units	Twice daily
Vitamin C	500 mg	Twice daily
Multivitamin		1 or 2 capsules daily

tion of LDL cholesterol more effectively than a dose of 400 units. A typical multivitamin contains 60 milligrams of vitamin C and 30 units of vitamin E, which are the minimum daily requirements. However, these amounts are not large enough to achieve the antioxidant effects of pharmacologic doses. Vitamin C is also an antioxidant associated with decreased heart attacks and death. Accordingly, this program utilizes vitamin E (400 units) and vitamin C (500 milligrams), each taken twice daily. (See table 4.3.) The purpose of these antioxidant vitamins is to minimize oxidative alteration of LDL cholesterol and retard progression of coronary atherosclerosis. Taking more than 500 milligrams of vitamin C at one time results in excess vitamin C being passed unused through the urine.

Recently, low levels of folic acid have been associated with elevated levels of a substance in blood called homocysteine. There is a modest association between levels of this compound in the blood and vascular disease in the arteries to the brain, legs, and, to a lesser extent, the heart. The association is not strong enough to predict coronary artery disease, and measuring levels of this substance in the blood is of limited use clinically for evaluating atherosclerosis. Whether taking folic acid supplements alters these associations between homocysteine and vascular disease is not known. However, standard multivitamins meet the daily requirements of folic acid as well as vitamin B_6 and B_{12}, all of which maintain low levels of homocysteine.

Aspirin improves the function of the lining of arteries. It retards the stickiness of blood elements called platelets that cause clotting and thrombosis (see discussion in part 1). It also decreases the activity of cells causing inflammation, erosion, and rupture of atherosclerotic plaques that lead to thrombosis. Taking aspirin reduces the risk of heart attacks, strokes, and cardiovascular deaths. For individuals with coronary heart disease or with high risk factors who *do not have adverse reactions to aspirin*, this program recommends taking one regular or coated aspirin or one baby aspirin each day. The main adverse reactions to aspirin are gastrointestinal problems, including upset stomach (gastritis), ulcers, or bleeding from the gastrointestinal tract. Taking buffered or enteric-coated aspirin may reduce these potential adverse side effects but not consistently. Some people cannot take regular aspirin in any form due to the gastrointestinal side effects.

Types of Cholesterol-lowering Drugs

In general, cholesterol-lowering drugs are used for people with coronary heart disease, those with markedly elevated cholesterol at high risk for coronary heart disease, or for other specific circumstances. Going on a low-fat food plan and breaking the smoking habit without taking cholesterol-lowering drugs is preferable for persons without known coronary heart disease, those at lower risk, or those who have only modest cholesterol abnormalities. Cholesterol-lowering drugs should never be used as a substitute for low-fat food in an attempt to modify cholesterol levels while continuing a high-fat, high-calorie intake. This approach won't be successful because cholesterol-lowering drugs cannot alter the surge in the triglycerides and low-density cholesterol fraction in the blood after a fatty meal. For optimal benefit in stopping the progression of or reversing vascular disease, it is necessary to reduce fat in food and control weight as well as take cholesterol-lowering drugs.

For people with diagnosed coronary heart disease, the optimal regimen consists of very low-fat foods combined with cholesterol-lowering drugs in order to reduce total cholesterol levels to 140 mg/dl or below, or LDL to 90 mg/dl or below, and increase HDL to 45 mg/dl or higher. The aim is to partially reverse or stop progression of disease with a 90 percent probability or greater. Taking two or three cholesterol-altering medications may be necessary to augment the effects of low-fat food in people with severe cholesterol abnormalities and coronary heart disease. These cholesterol-lowering drugs require a physician's prescription and follow-up laboratory and physician evaluation on a regular basis, typically once per month for three months after a dose change and every five to six months thereafter.

The following discussion covers four classes of commonly used cholesterol-lowering drugs: statins, cholestyramine, niacin, and gemfibrozil. (For recommended daily doses, see table 4.4.) The effectiveness of these drugs has been proven in the large studies reviewed in part 2.

Statins

The drugs in this class are used to reduce synthesis of cholesterol in the liver. After a person starts on any of the statins or changes the dosage, the physician needs to check liver enzymes and the cholesterol profile each month for three months; then, if necessary, the dosage is adjusted at one- to two-month intervals. The final dose is highly variable. It will be whatever dose is necessary to achieve total cholesterol of less than 140 mg/dl or LDL below 90 mg/dl; it also takes into account any side effects, which, if significant, may be grounds for reducing dosage of the drug or even changing it. The final dose is typically not related to weight or gender. The statins include:

✓ *Atorvastatin (Lipitor)*. This drug is typically started at a daily dose of

Table 4.4. Daily Doses of Cholesterol-lowering Medications

Drug[a]	Daily Dose
Atorvastatin	10–80 mg
Simvastatin	10–40 mg
Pravastatin	20–40 mg
Cholestyramine	8–24 mg
Lovastatin	20–80 mg
Fluvastatin	20–40 mg
Colestid	5–30 g
Niacin	250–1,000 mg three times each day with meals
Gemfibrozil	600 mg twice daily before meals

[a]The first seven drugs principally lower LDL but increase HDL somewhat. The last two (niacin and gemfibrozil) principally increase HDL and lower triglycerides.

10 milligrams and increased up to 80 milligrams as need to control cholesterol levels. It should be taken at supper to minimize stomach irritation, an occasional side effect, or at bedtime.

✓ *Simvastatin (Zocor)*. Start with 10 to 20 milligrams every evening, increasing up to 80 milligrams or possibly 160 milligrams as needed to control cholesterol levels. Simvastatin may be taken with the evening meal to minimize gastrointestinal side effects or at bedtime.

✓ *Lovastatin (Mevacor)*. The starting dose is usually 20 milligrams taken every evening with food and increased up to 80 milligrams to control cholesterol levels. For optimal effects, it is essential to take lovastatin with the evening meal, not on an empty stomach.

✓ *Pravastatin (Pravachol)*. The daily dosage is 20 to 80 milligrams. For optimal effects, pravastatin should be taken on an empty stomach at bedtime.

✓ *Fluvastatin (Lescol)*. Take 20 to 80 milligrams per day. Fluvastatin can be taken with or after the evening meal.

Potential side effects of the statin class of cholesterol-lowering drugs include transient elevation of liver enzymes without permanent damage to the liver if the dose is reduced or drug is stopped or changed. Accordingly, after starting a statin or increasing the dose, liver-function tests and cholesterol levels should be checked monthly for three months and every four to six months thereafter. If liver enzymes increase to 2.5 times normal baseline levels, the drug should be stopped for two weeks and be started at a lower dose. Lesser increases in liver enzyme tests do not require stopping the drug. The statins may also occasionally cause inflamed, aching muscles, called myositis, which may require discontinuation of the drug, reduction in dose, or change to another statin. Very rarely, a severe form of muscle inflammation called rhabdomyolysis may occur, with marked muscle weakness, dark urine, and a modest risk of kidney damage. This condition is reversible if the drug is discontinued.

A reaction to one of the statins does not necessarily indicate that the same reaction will occur with another statin. Commonly, the body also adapts, so that mild muscle aching disappears with continuation of the drug. Alternatively, it may be stopped for two weeks and restarted in the same dose, commonly without recurrence of muscle aching.

Cholestyramine (Questran or Colestid)

This drug binds bile acids in cholesterol synthesis. In the bowel, the cholestyramine–bile acid complex is not absorbed into the blood but passes through the bowel and out of the body with the feces. Cholestyramine is available as a powder or as a tablet. The dose is one to four scoops, packages, or tablets of powder taken three times per day with each meal. It may be mixed with juices or protein shakes as a convenient vehicle for intake. Potential side effects are gastrointestinal symptoms of bloating, gassiness, or constipation. It is important to emphasize that cholestyramine binds other drugs that are taken at the same time. Therefore, cholestyramine and other drugs have to be taken at different times during the day, at least three hours apart. For this reason, it may be necessary to take cholestyramine only twice per day, with other drugs taken at another time.

Niacin

Niacin is one of the oldest, most established lipid-altering drugs. In the regular, immediate release form, its principal effect is to increase HDL and lower triglycerides, with modest effect on LDL and total cholesterol. It must be started in low doses of 100 to 250 milligrams to avoid the side effects of flushing and itching. These side effects are reduced by taking niacin with food, eaten both before and after taking the niacin. An aspirin each day also helps reduce side effects. The dose is increased in 100- to 250-milligram steps at weekly intervals, up to one gram taken three times per day with meals. This slowly increasing dose enables the body to adapt, so that therapeutic doses can be taken without the itching and flushing. Other potential side effects include increased liver enzymes, which require reduction in the dose. Immediate-release niacin tends to cause more flushing and itching than the slow, sustained-release preparation.

Niacin is a powerful drug, and patient reactions to it are highly variable. With attention to potential adverse effects, it may be very useful. Slow-release niacin and regular immediate-release niacin are functionally different drugs. Although both preparations reduce triglycerides to the same extent for comparable doses, they produce substantially different effects on HDL and LDL. In most patients, slow-release niacin principally lowers LDL with little effect on HDL. In a minority of patients, it may increase HDL substantially or may decrease HDL substantially by its effects on blocking cholesterol metabolism. Regular immediate-release niacin tends to increase HDL more than slow-release niacin, even at lower doses. However, as noted, it causes more flushing and itching, but has fewer side effects on the liver. Side effects of both of these preparations, but particularly slow-release niacin, include elevated liver enzymes, worsening diabetes, gout, a skin condition called acanthosis nigrans, gastrointestinal symptoms, significant fatigue, and a poorly defined but definite malaise that in some few people consistently parallels taking or not taking the drug.

Since the beneficial and adverse effects of niacin are highly variable, it requires a therapeutic trial for a given individual with appropriate explanations and physician supervision. Some people respond to small doses of only 100 milligrams two to three times daily, and some people require 3 grams per day. The commonest dose to achieve target effect is approximately 500 milligrams three times daily with food.

Gemfibrozil (Lopid)

The recommended dose of this drug is 600 milligrams twice per day. Its principal effect is to lower triglycerides and to some extent increase HDL. It may not be as effective as niacin in some people but is easier to take, and does not cause flushing and itching. Potential side effects include inflamed or aching muscles, called myositis. A rare side effect, particularly when combined with statins, is a condition called rhabdomyolysis, which is a particularly severe form of muscle inflammation with elevated muscle enzymes, and dark urine. This side effect is generally reversible after the drug is discontinued.

The physician should normally be checking liver enzymes and cholesterol levels every month for the first two to three months on a drug and every four to six months thereafter. With a viral infection, such as the flu that persists with weakness and nausea, the liver enzymes should be checked again to identify an uncommon syndrome called the "cholesterol flu." On rare occasion, the virus causing the flu may further transiently inhibit cholesterol synthesis in the liver. The consequence is a profound fall in total cholesterol to 50 to 60 mg/dl and an increase in liver enzymes. In these circumstances, the cholesterol-lowering drugs should be stopped for two weeks. They may then be started again at the same previous dose level and liver enzymes rechecked. The one exception is niacin, which has to be restarted at a lower dose and increased in gradual steps as when first started. The reason is that the body loses its tolerance for niacin after two weeks, so that sensitivity to flushing or itching may recur. After the viral infection is cleared, liver enzymes typically remain normal when the original full dose of cholesterol-lowering drugs is resumed.

Many people with vascular disease or high risk for developing it prefer to avoid cholesterol-lowering drugs as "unnatural" or potential toxins that hurt the body. But without the correct intervention, vascular disease is a progressive lethal process. Low-fat foods *alone* or a statin-class cholesterol-lowering drug *alone* will reduce by approximately 30 to 60 percent the risk of heart attacks, strokes, death, or the need for bypass surgery or balloon dilation. However, with either treatment alone, there remains a 40 to 70 percent risk of having one of these adverse cardiovascular events.

In order to maximize the benefit or minimize the risk of such events, this reversal treatment utilizes the combination of both cholesterol-lowering drugs *and* very low-fat foods. Based on my thirty years' clinical experience and my interpretation of scientific reports, I am convinced that the effects of cholesterol-lowering drugs and very low-fat foods are additive and together substantially increase the probability of optimal outcome more than either low-fat food or cholesterol-lowering drugs above. Once the goals of this comprehensive reversal program are achieved for six to twelve months, the reduction in risk is over 90 percent. However, no outcome is guaranteed for any treatment. Some risk of heart attack or death remains, as with bypass surgery, balloon dilation, or any other treatment known.

This reversal program and particularly the cholesterol-lowering drugs and low-fat foods are compatible with other cardiovascular drugs typically used in patients with coronary heart disease. These drugs include beta blockers, nitrates, calcium channel blockers, diuretics, digoxin, potassium supplements, and blood pressure medications.

Special Problems and Combinations of Cholesterol-lowering Drugs

For patients with vascular disease, excess weight, elevated triglycerides, elevated LDL, and either normal or low HDL, the essential treatment steps are low-fat, low-carbohydrate foods, lean body mass, and a statin drug in doses to reach target cholesterols of 140 mg/dl or below, LDL 90 mg/dl or below, HDL 45 mg/dl or above, and triglycerides of 100 mg/dl or below. If, at an LDL level of 90 or below, the triglycerides remain too high (over 150 mg/dl) and HDL normal or low (below 40 mg/dl), the combination of a statin and niacin or a statin and gemfibrozil are useful as determined and supervised by the physician. Such people may achieve a low LDL, low total cholesterol, and low triglycerides on low-fat food and a statin drug but with persisting low HDL.

Essential steps for increasing HDL include smoking cessation, lean body mass, low carbohydrate content of food to maintain body weight, regular exercise, adequate dietary protein, and a second or third medication. In such patients, the addition of regular-release niacin may increase HDL but not predictably. Sustained-release niacin commonly does not increase HDL but usually decreases LDL further. Although considered to be primarily a triglyceride-lowering agent, gemfibrozil may in some patients increase HDL substantially, particularly when combined with niacin, even if triglycerides are not elevated.

On occasion, refractory low HDL or refractory severe elevation of triglycerides responds to two medications (niacin and gemfibrozil together) or three medications (a statin, niacin, and gemfibrozil in combination). These regimens require close management by the physician and a warning about muscle inflammation (myositis) and rhabdomyolysis. However, these complications are rare. There is a far lower risk of side effects with combinations of drugs than the risk of cardiovascular events with uncontrolled cholesterol levels. Finally, the refractory low HDL or refractory high triglycerides respond occasionally to the combination of fish oil—in dose(s) of 4 to 8 grams per day—and niacin or gemfibrozil. The potential increase in LDL due to fish oil may be prevented by a statin.

The occasional patient is so sensitive to carbohydrate that it causes high triglycerides and/or low HDL, even at lean body mass, that is resistant to medications; in such cases, a higher-fat diet may be necessary to allow reduction in carbohydrate. The increased LDL that may be associated with higher fat intake is then reduced by a statin.

The combinations of medications (a statin plus niacin or a statin plus gemfibrozil) markedly reduce the after-eating surge in lipid fractions that contributes to vascular disease. Although the *Physicians Desk Reference* (*PDR*) warns against combining statins with niacin or with gemfibrozil, clinical experience and several reviews indicate benefits and safety of double or triple drug therapy. For patients with coronary artery disease with sufficient lipid abnormalities to require two or three of these drugs, the risk of cardiovascular events with uncontrolled lipids is far greater than the relatively uncommon risks of serious side effects from combined drugs. However, whenever using combination therapy, physicians should explain the risks and benefits to their patients and maintain good communication with them, making arrangements for patients to call the medical staff at any time to ask questions or to report adverse effects or untoward symptoms.

As the benefit of progressive cholesterol lowering has been documented, several scientific studies and clinical practice have demonstrated the benefit of higher doses of the statins. Consequently, acceptable doses of these medications have progressively increased. Commonly, adverse reactions to one of the statins are not seen with other statins and are not necessarily related to relative cholesterol-lowering effects. Each of the statins—atorvastatin, simvastatin, lovastatin, pravastatin, and fluvastatin—has an important role depending on adverse reactions and extent of cholesterol lowering needed. Transient muscle pain is not uncommon, but it disappears when the drug is discontinued for several days and commonly does not recur upon restarting or changing the medication.

I cannot emphasize strongly enough that for optimal outcome, weight and food control are essential for managing coronary heart disease even with the use of lipid-active drugs. Low-fat foods are critical for reducing the postprandial lipid surge, which is not affected by any of the statins used alone. People with lean body mass, achieved by low-fat, low-carbohydrate foods, have improved survival, lower cholesterol, a lower after-eating surge in atherogenic lipids, less angina, greater exercise capacity, lower blood pressure, lower levels of stress hormones, and greater energy levels compared with people who carry excess weight.

Angina, or Chest Pain, Due to Coronary Heart Disease

The marked decrease in cardiovascular events associated with cholesterol lowering and low-fat foods is well established. It is important to emphasize that vigorous cholesterol lowering causes an equally profound decrease in angina, or chest pain, due to coronary artery disease. In scientific studies, there is an inverse relation between LDL lowering and abnormalities on the electrocardiogram during exercise stress. Approximately 65 percent of abnormal changes on the exercise electrocardiogram completely resolve after four to six months of treatment with a statin.

Exercise-induced angina may be worse after a high-carbohydrate meal or high-fat meal due to decreased coronary flow blood flow capacity caused by elevated blood sugar and elevated triglycerides after a meal. Even a single high-fat meal has significant adverse effects on function of the endothelial lining of arteries that lasts four to eight hours after the meal. This endothelial function of arteries improves within days to months after starting low-fat foods or statins. The reduction in angina associated with low-fat, low-carbohydrate foods, weight loss, and correction of lipids is due to many factors. These factors include improved endothelial function and vasodilatory capacity due to lower cholesterol and lower triglycerides, lower blood sugar, lower tendency for blood clotting, and lower weight which reduces cardiac workload. When appropriate antianginal drugs are also included, most angina can be controlled medically and managed long term without balloon dilation or bypass surgery. However, sometimes even these measures do not work, and such procedures are necessary.

The most important fact to remember about angina is that it does not always require an invasive procedure to prevent myocardial infarction or death. In the general population of patients with established coronary artery disease, exertional angina or abnormal ischemic changes by ECG recorded during daily activities, or even marked changes on the exercise ECG, do not predict cardiovascular events (see discussion in part 3). Angina is also highly variable, even occurring at rest but then improving spontaneously or with more vigorous medical treatment, again without associated cardiovascular events. Furthermore, as extensively reviewed in part 3, invasive revascularization procedures have not been documented to prolong survival or prevent myocardial infarction; groups undergoing these procedures do no better than control groups treated by other means. The following observations may help physicians and patients in managing angina and reserving revascularization for truly refractory chest pain that is unresponsive to optimal medical management.

Not uncommonly, in hypertensive patients, chest pain, or angina, at rest or during exercise is caused by unrecognized blood pressure spikes. While physicians commonly consider the blood pressure spikes as caused by the angina, in my experience it is the other way around: the blood pressure spikes more commonly cause the angina, particularly at rest, at night, in the early morning, or with exercise. This kind of resting and exertional angina is commonly misinterpreted as unstable angina and leads to balloon dilation or bypass surgery.

Usually, such angina associated with blood pressure spikes is not optimally controlled by nitroglycerin or its long-acting versions, which are large artery dilators not generally recommended for controlling blood pressure. In my experience, beta blockers alone or in combination with nitroglycerin preparations may eliminate the exertional component of angina but not the resting episodes associated with blood pressure spikes. However, good blood pressure control with ACE inhibitors usually reduces the blood pressure smoothly and eliminates the resting angina also.

There are several different mechanisms for angina. Exertional angina is due to flow-limiting stenoses of the large coronary arteries. Some angina may be due to spasm of the coronary arteries with vasoconstriction that narrows the artery transiently. The form of transient rest angina associated with blood pressure spikes is more likely due to increased workload on the heart, inadequate blood flow to the thick heart muscle seen with high blood pressure and due to microvascular disease causing arteriolar vasoconstriction like that leading to hypertension. Different drugs are required for each of these probable mechanisms.

Although usually effective for relieving angina, vasodilators of any kind clearly cause angina or worsening angina both at rest and with exercise in some patients. Either one or all vasodilators may have this effect—nitrates, calcium channel blockers, niacin, oral dipyridamole—just as intravenous dipyridamole may increase angina. Such patients usually have extensive collaterals, either large arteriographically visible collaterals or fine angiographically invisible collaterals known to be present because of normal regional ventricular function in areas of totally occluded arteries. Vasodilators, particularly calcium channel blockers, commonly cause a phenomenon called myocardial steal in such patients. In myocardial steal, blood flow from an open artery through newly grown collateral vessels to the blocked artery (see part 1 on collaterals) decreases since the open supply artery cannot provide enough blood flow for both arteries after the vasodilator.

In these instances, angina usually responds to beta blockers alone and particularly to vigorous cholesterol lowering. The resulting improvement in endothelial microvascular function can increase blood flow through collaterals by 50 percent or more. Progressive angina with increasing doses of these vasodilators may be an indication for stopping them in order to determine if angina improves as a result of eliminating myocardial steal. Unnecessary revascularization procedures may then be avoided.

Some patients prefer a balloon dilation or bypass surgery based essentially on a strong emotional response to "fix" the narrowed artery. This wish should be respected. However, such patients should also undertake a vigorous reversal regimen to prevent progression of disease and heart attack. In managing patients with coronary artery disease, I carefully review the benefits and risks of medical versus surgical treatment, emphasizing that no outcome can be guaranteed by either choice. A formal consent form defining these benefits and risks for both options is signed. However, if limiting angina progresses suddenly or continues to worsen after two to three months of optimal, vigorous medical management, balloon dilation or bypass surgery may be necessary, as occurs in a small minority of patients.

On occasion, milder stenoses unequivocally progress relatively rapidly as determined by PET imaging, coronary arteriography, or by progressive symptoms in patients who cannot control lipids or other risk factors due to adverse effects of drugs or inadequate self-discipline. Progression in severity of coronary artery narrowing is a predictor of cardiovascular events. In such circumstances with demonstrated failure of controlling lipids and risk factors for whatever reason, progression of a proximal stenosis of a large artery supplying a large amount of myocardium may be grounds for carrying out a balloon dilation procedure or bypass surgery even without angina or with worsening angina. Although there are no data on outcomes in such patients, the risk of coronary events with active progression of milder stenosis due to documented uncontrollable risk factors is high enough to consider balloon dilation or bypass surgery. However, such instances are uncommon exceptions owing to the consistent effectiveness of a focused, comprehensive, noninvasive program for stabilizing or reversing coronary atherosclerosis.

Estrogens and Coronary Artery Disease

Premenopausal women have substantially less risk from atherosclerosis than men. This difference between men and women and risk of atherosclerosis persists until the seventh decade of life. In the seventh to eighth decades, the risk of atherosclerosis and particularly coronary heart disease in women equals that of men. Although other, less well-defined factors are involved, these differences are thought to be largely due to the higher estrogen levels in women.

Estrogen administration in women after menopause has important benefits, particularly for preventing coronary heart disease and osteoporosis. Estrogen treatment increases the good HDL cholesterol and decreases the bad LDL cholesterol. It decreases a substance in blood involved with blood clotting called fibrinogen, thereby reducing the risk of thrombosis. Estrogen also improves the function of the endothelial lining of arteries, making them vasodilate better than when estrogen is low. Women who take estrogen have a 50 percent reduction in coronary heart disease and other forms of atherosclerosis compared with those who do not. This benefit is seen in older women into the eighth decade of life, as well as younger postmenopausal women.

There are some side effects associated with taking estrogens. Breast swelling and tenderness may occur. Intermittent menstruation or vaginal bleeding may return. Both of these side effects are somewhat dose-related and are usually managed by reducing the dose. Estrogen treatment alone without progesterone in women who have not undergone a hysterectomy may increase the risk of adenomatous or atypical hyperplasia (a potentially precancerous overgrowth) of the lining of the uterus. There is also an increased risk of endometrial cancer. The risk of these more serious side effects is eliminated by the concomitant use of progesterone, either daily or on a monthly cycle.

Therefore, for women who have not undergone hysterectomy, estrogen treatment should always be accompanied by progesterone as well. Combined estrogen plus progesterone treatment of postmenopausal women has favorable effects on HDL, LDL, fibrinogen, endothelial function, and reduces the risks of developing coronary heart disease or other manifestations of atherosclerosis. Women who have had a hysterectomy can take estrogens alone without risk of endometrial cancer. There is no measurable increase of breast cancer with estrogens alone or with estrogens-progesterone combined.

The usual daily dose of conjugated estrogen, which is the therapeutic form, is 0.625 milligrams alone or, combined with medroxyprogesterone, 2.5 milligrams. For women who develop ankle swelling or breast tenderness, this dose may be cut in half. For cyclic use of progesterone, the dose is 10 milligrams per day for twelve days per month and no progesterone for the remainder of the month, while taking estrogen throughout the month. If side effects develop on these doses, they should be reduced.

Daily Workout Routines

Physical activity develops or maintains cardiovascular fitness. People are highly variable in what physical activity they like or are willing to do, as well as the duration and the circumstances. Some individuals need the support of a personal trainer, a workout class, or a schedule in a gym. Others prefer to work out alone at home, where they are not distracted by other people and do not have to spend time traveling to a facility. Any activity is useful, such as walking, jogging, bicycling, rowing, repetitive light weights, sports, swimming, calisthenics, yoga that involves tensing muscles, or physical labor including vigorous housework, gardening, construction, virtually anything involving physical activity.

The three essential criteria for a successful program of physical activity are to (1) determine individual preferences for the type and time of activity, (2) aim to do that activity for at least thirty to sixty minutes per day for five to six days per week, (3) do something every day, even if the complete workout routine cannot be completed. When only ten minutes are available on some days, you should do an activity for those ten minutes. Do whatever you can, even if briefly, because regularity establishes the habit.

The time of day for a physical workout should be when you are most awake and strongest. It should be in the a.m. for "morning people." Waiting until one is too tired from the day's work commonly results in skipping the workout. A workout in the afternoon or evening is ideal for "evening people." However, late-afternoon hunger or an early evening meal may curtail a late-day workout. For such people, avoiding hunger by having a mid-afternoon protein snack is particularly important, improving adherence to a workout routine in the late afternoon.

Repetitive light weight lifting provides an excellent workout with minimum joint injury, produces significant benefits for increasing the good HDL cholesterol, and can easily be done at home without going to a special facility. In some form, light weight lifting can be done by most people, even the very elderly. Weight machines and rowing machines are sophisticated forms of repetitive light weight lifting that provide controlled workout conditions of great flexibility, variety, and interest. With hard or exhaustive weight conditioning, a day of alternative aerobic activity or a day of rest between the harder weight workouts prevents excessive fatigue in people prone to this limitation.

Individual dumbbells or wrist and ankle weights are the most easily managed. They should be three to twenty-five pounds in weight each, depending on one's age, ability, prior conditioning, gender, and strength. Start with lighter weights and do thirty to forty repetitions of each of the routines for the major muscle groups. For lighter women or the elderly, a good starting weight for each dumbbell is three to eight pounds. For stronger women and men, ten to twenty pounds for each free dumbbell are best. Choose an initial weight with which it is a real effort to do twenty to thirty repetitions. Then build up repetitions over two to four months to fifty to seventy times for each muscle group before graduating to the next higher weight. The ultimate goal for each of the larger muscle groups of the legs is 100 or more repetitions. Note that only an experienced weight-conditioned athlete should use a dumbbell of twenty-five pounds or over. Even for such athletes, increasing the number of repetitions up to fifty or seventy with the twenty-five-pound hand weights is better than increasing the weights with only fifteen to twenty repetitions.

The routine for each major muscle group should include arm curls, overhead lifts, toe lifts, half knee bends, push-ups, leg kicks, and sit-ups. (See figures 4.3 and 4.4.) Half knee bends avoid knee trauma that may occur with deep knee bends. Mixed routines are particularly useful in providing the

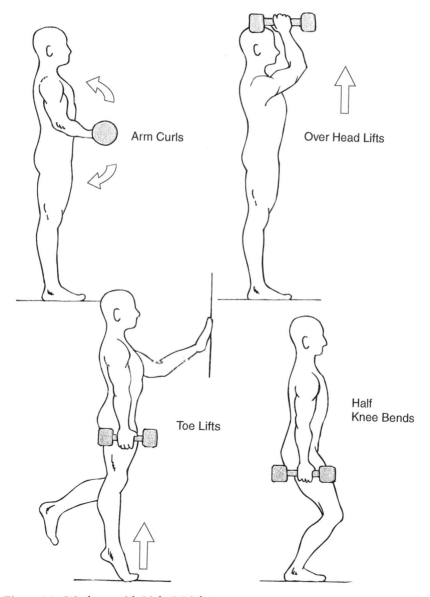

Figure 4.3. Workout with Light Weights

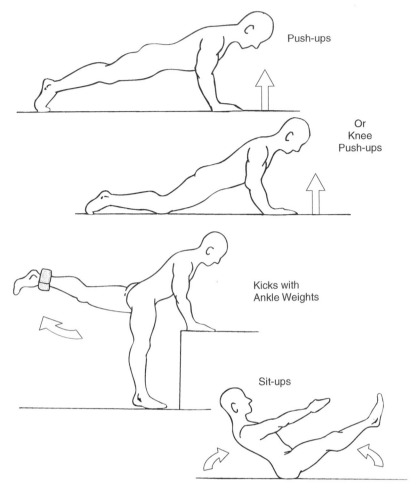

Push-ups

Or
Knee
Push-ups

Kicks with
Ankle Weights

Sit-ups

Figure 4.4. Workout with Light Weights, Continued

variety that some people need. A fifteen- to twenty-minute round of weight repetitions, a fifteen- to twenty-minute brisk walk, followed by another round of weights provides a good workout. Alternatively, you might do a longer weight routine with more repetitions, taking twenty to twenty-five minutes to go through a complete set for each muscle group, rest briefly, and then repeat the entire set.

I developed a particularly efficient exercise (as part of a complete routine) for both arms and legs using dumbbells. Depending on the individual, it can be an easy or reasonably intense workout. For lack of a better descriptive term, I call it the Gould maneuver. It seemed outlandish and made me laugh when I first tried it, but I have been so pleased with the results that I am including it here. You begin the maneuver by doing repetitive half knee bends with two dumbbells at your side as in figure 4.5. When well warmed up or

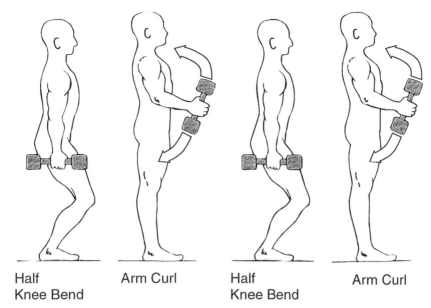

Half   Arm Curl   Half   Arm Curl
Knee Bend   Knee Bend

Figure 4.5. Workout with Light Weights—The Gould Maneuver

even a little fatigued in the legs after 100 to 200 half knee bends, you add an arm curl as you straighten your legs after each half knee bend. For this arm curl, hold the dumbbells with your palms parallel to your side rather than palms up like most arm curls. In this position, you avoid hitting your legs with the dumbbells. Doing half knee bends and arm curls is like rowing in a vertical position but requires greater effort with the major muscle groups. For an easy workout, use light weights and twenty to thirty repetitions. For an exhaustive workout, use twenty-five-pound weights and 200 repetitions, integrated into other exercises.

Travel often interrupts workout routines. However, most hotels have a workout room or are situated where a brisk walk is possible. Virtually all hotel rooms have a chair or table that can serve for repetitive weight lifting routines. Therefore, it should be possible to maintain the exercise habit and one's muscle tone even during extended travel.

The essential point is to do some focused physical activity daily. It must be integrated into essential living habits—of eating, sleeping, dressing, working, and playing. For individuals with coronary heart disease or at high risk for it, the living habits relating to food and physical activity are basic conditions for feeling well and for reversing or preventing the progression of coronary atherosclerosis. They are essential for survival itself and optimal quality of life.

While many people like to focus on calories burned, heart rate, speed, duration, or other measures of exercise intensity, these variables depend completely on individual capacity, which is determined by age, gender, prior training, interest, weight, disability, medications, and many other factors. Consequently, there is no one standard that applies to everyone. The only major requirement is to do some physical exertion on a regular basis, preferably at least four to five times per week.

People with medical limitations, particularly coronary heart disease, are often uncertain about how much exercise to do, particularly after a heart attack. If you have this problem, consider enrolling in a monitored physical rehabilitation program prescribed by your physician. A treadmill exercise stress test will probably be done to assess your capacity or potential adverse effects of exercise. An exercise program will then be designed based on your capacity at this initial assessment. Not only does a rehabilitation program optimize safe physical conditioning after a heart attack, but, even more important, it helps you overcome your fear of exercise after a heart attack. This fear is really not necessary since the body does better with exercise than without and will give signs of its distress when exercise is excessive, prompting you to slow you down.

At some point people with coronary heart disease need to undertake exercise routines on their own without fear. They need to learn the signs of their body that indicate a problem with or during exercise. These signs include: chest pain, light-headedness, excessive difficulty in breathing, heart irregularity, or profound fatigue. Exercise should be done at some level of intensity just short of these distress signals. Repetitive training at this level usually leads to progressive improvement in exercise capacity. For people with severely scarred or damaged hearts and heart failure, exercise routines must be integrated with cardiovascular medications prescribed by a physician.

Stress Management

The relation between stress and coronary heart disease is important but unclear. Part of the problem is how stress is defined and how it is measured since it is highly subjective. What is stressful for one person is not stressful for another.

Some observations favor a causal relation between certain types of stress and atherosclerosis. Clearly, in some people with coronary heart disease, emotional stress causes or exacerbates chest pain. Stress also implies conditions that disfavor good risk-factor management. When under stress, people are more likely to smoke, eat unhealthy food, skip their exercise, and have their blood pressure go up. All of these changes exacerbate coronary heart disease.

Some types of stress also trigger hormonal and metabolic changes in the body. These metabolic and hormonal changes may increase cholesterol levels, blood pressure, the intensity of inflammation in the cholesterol plaque, and the tendency for arteries to spasm and form blood clots. All of these adverse responses make atherosclerosis worse and increase the risk of heart attacks. Primates on a high-fat diet that are exposed to the stress of fear have more severe atherosclerosis than comparable control animals on the same high-fat diet without this stress. These observations and studies in humans suggest that stress involving fear, anger, and lack of control of environmental circumstances contributes to atherosclerosis.

However, the effects of stress appear to be mediated principally through other recognized risk factors. The Type A personality is associated with decreased levels of the good protective HDL cholesterol and higher risk of coronary heart disease. When HDL levels are accounted for, the Type A personality per se is no longer associated with coronary heart disease. Thus, there is no strong scientific evidence that stress itself, independent of other risk factors, causes or accelerates atherosclerosis in most people. Rather, stress causes abnormalities in known risk factors for heart disease. In medical studies, cholesterol lowering through diet and medications decreases the frequency of death and heart attacks without stress management. On the other hand, stress management may contribute significantly to controlling other risk factors.

The stress of working hard or being busy does not increase the risk of atherosclerosis as long as other risk factors are controlled. If the stress of being busy results in smoking, eating high-fat food, and inactivity, the risk of atherosclerosis will be increased because of these other risk factors. Since stress is often associated with poor control of these recognized risk factors, stress management is an important part of this comprehensive reversal program.

An essential element of successful stress management is its integration into daily living. As with low-fat food and regular exercise, stress management needs to fit within the daily activities of working, eating, sleeping, social exchange, and so forth. A two-week retreat may relieve the stresses of daily living; however, it may not help for the rest of the year. You may not have the time or financial resources for a two-week retreat. You may not even have the time for an hour of meditation and an hour workout. Therefore, the approach to stress management outlined here focuses on simple daily practices that take little time. Follow the six simple steps for stress management presented in the accompanying box, and integrate them with the workout routines described earlier. These steps recognize and take advantage of basic physiologic body reactions or reflexes that have been scientifically demonstrated. They are suitable for people on a very busy schedule as well as those who operate at a more leisurely pace.

The focus of this stress management is to optimize adherence to a program that minimizes the known risk factors for atherosclerosis. Therefore, stress management strongly interacts with low-fat food, regular exercise, no smoking, blood pressure control, and cholesterol-lowering drugs.

Stress Management on a Tight Schedule

Step 1. Work out, then relax and remember

✓ Work out for 30 to 60 minutes each day.

✓ Lie on floor, totally relax after workout.

✓ Focus on breathing (regular, slow).

✓ Concentrate on breathing, relaxing for 5 minutes.

✓ Remember this feeling of total relaxation.

Step 2. Make time for relaxation

✓ Hold calls, appointments three times per day.

✓ Put feet up, get comfortable, close eyes.

✓ Recall total relaxation after workout, focus on it.

✓ Concentrate on breathing, relaxing for 5 minutes.

Step 3. Walk your way to relaxation

✓ Concentrate on a relaxed loose gait.

✓ Swing arms freely, keeping hands, shoulders loose.

✓ Focus on walking and on a relaxed body.

✓ Walk this way for a few minutes every hour.

Step 4. De-stress your body whenever you're tense

✓ Make your muscles relax, go loose.

✓ Relax clenched fists, shoulders, jaws.

✓ Breathe regularly, slowly.

✓ Repeat for 5 minutes several times per day.

Step 5. Deal with stress and fatigue to ward off food cravings and overeating

✓ Recognize stress, fatigue, hunger separately.

✓ Ask yourself, Am I stressed, fatigued, or hungry?

✓ For stress, focus on relaxing, breathing.

✓ For fatigue, rest, nap, or sleep more.

✓ For hunger, eat protein-fruit-vegetables, eat slowly, concentrate on tasting food.

Step 6. Remember

✓ Your life is the first priority; take care of it.

✓ Working incurs stress; work but de-stress.

✓ De-stress every day, not just on vacation.

✓ Stress and fatigue cause food cravings; de-stress, sleep, and don't overeat.

Who Needs Reversal Treatment?

Everyone with coronary heart disease can profit from reversal treatment. A definitive diagnosis of coronary heart disease should be the basis for lifelong use of cholesterol-lowering drugs and very low-fat foods. The following criteria are suitable for a definitive diagnosis of coronary heart disease:

- ✓ heart attack or stroke
- ✓ coronary atherosclerosis by arteriogram, intracoronary ultrasound, or PET imaging
- ✓ balloon dilation or bypass surgery
- ✓ family history of premature coronary artery disease associated with elevated cholesterol
- ✓ positive PET scan showing mild or severe abnormality of blood flow to heart muscle
- ✓ risk factors for atherosclerosis, such as elevated cholesterol, low HDL, elevated triglycerides, smoking habit, family history of atherosclerosis, high blood pressure, diabetes
- ✓ cerebrovascular or peripheral vascular disease by Doppler-ECHO tests.

Diabetics with coronary heart disease have a very high risk of coronary events. However, they may respond particularly well to reversal treatment. In the 4S study discussed in part 2, major coronary events occurred in 48 percent of diabetic patients treated with standard management. In the diabetic patients treated with the cholesterol-lowering drug simvastatin, major coronary events were reduced to 25 percent. This improvement was greater than in nondiabetics.

With reduced carbohydrate intake and weight loss, adult-type diabetes as well as vascular disease becomes less severe. Reductions in carbohydrate consumption and weight often allow reduction in the dose or elimination of diabetic medications or insulin. This improved metabolic status of diabetics on reversal treatment markedly improves their survival and reduces atherosclerotic complications. Therefore, diabetics with coronary heart disease are particularly good candidates for reversal treatment.

Mild coronary artery narrowing on the coronary arteriogram is not a reason for excluding patients from the reversal program. Plaque rupture and coronary thrombosis arise from mild, early, cholesterol-rich plaques that cause little narrowing. Coronary atherosclerosis may be documented by mild narrowing or only irregularities in the wall of the artery on an arteriogram or by mild abnormalities on a dipyridamole PET scan. Such patients should be treated vigorously. If chest pain due to coronary heart disease is controlled medically, even severe coronary artery narrowing may be managed primarily by vigorous reversal treatment, since there is lower risk of coronary events from stable severe lesions than unstable mild ones. If chest pain cannot be controlled by intense medical management and reversal treatment, balloon dilation or bypass surgery is indicated. Standard stress testing cannot be relied on alone for definitive diagnosis of coronary heart disease because of the poor diagnostic accuracy of the two most common tests: standard ECG stress testing and standard imaging of blood flow in heart muscle. Hence standard stress testing cannot be the *sole* basis for *lifelong* reversal treatment with cholesterol-lowering drugs.

There are some cardiac conditions (listed below) where cholesterol lowering as part of reversal treatment has not been specifically studied. However, for these conditions the available data suggest that bypass surgery or balloon dilation as the initial primary treatment has limited benefit, no benefit, or potentially adverse effects. For stable angina, in independent, randomized, separate, large scientific trials, vigorous cholesterol lowering decreases the frequency of deaths and coronary events more than bypass surgery or balloon dilation does. It is therefore reasonable to consider vigorous cholesterol lowering as primary initial therapy without balloon dilation or bypass surgery in the following circumstances:

✓ Severe three-vessel coronary artery disease and normal ventricular function with chest pain controlled by medical treatment.
✓ Unstable or progressive chest pain due to coronary heart disease that stabilizes with medical treatment.
✓ Clinically stable patient who has just suffered a heart attack.

In the Veterans Administration study of male patients with severe, unstable coronary heart disease, emergency bypass surgery caused more deaths than traditional antianginal medical treatment in patients with normal heart pumping function. Since neither bypass surgery nor balloon dilation decreases the number of deaths any more than medical treatment does, in my practice I treat most patients with the above conditions with a vigorous reversal program. Treatment includes immediate cholesterol lowering by low-fat foods and cholesterol-lowering drugs in addition to nitrate vasodilators, beta blockers, antiplatelet drugs, heparin, antioxidant vitamins, and whatever else is indicated clinically. Under some of these circumstances, exercise training should be temporarily curtailed.

Most such patients in these "unstable" categories stabilize, become pain free, improve exercise tolerance under supervised exercise conditions, and do well without further coronary events. Some of the more severe narrowing of the coronary arteries may, in subsequent months, block completely without causing a heart attack due to development of collaterals (see discussion in part 1). This complete blockage may be without symptoms or with some mild worsening of chest pain for several days or weeks after several months without angina. Where increased chest pain follows a period of improvement, it may be necessary to increase the dosage of antianginal drugs such as beta blockers and nitrates until collaterals fully open or develop more completely over the next several weeks, after which symptoms again resolve.

Such instances of slow blockage of severe narrowing occurring with very low cholesterol levels do not usually cause a heart attack. The FATS trial reviewed in part 2 provides strong support of this point of view. However, progressive worsening or severe recurrent angina despite intense reversal treatment and cardiovascular medications may indicate that a balloon dilation or bypass surgery should be done.

In people with well-developed collaterals, angina may increase transiently after eating foods that raise triglycerides, even transiently. In some people, one high-carbohydrate or fatty meal that causes a triglyceride surge will cause angina within several hours after the meal. Since the severity of coronary narrowing has not changed when I have done coronary arteriography in such circumstances, the mechanism is transient impairment of endothelial function and fall in collateral flow specifically related to elevated triglycerides. Foods rich in protein do no have the same effect.

For people at these more advanced stages of coronary heart disease, reversal treatment as the primary initial approach requires medical judgment modified by individual physician and patient preferences. Excellent, open communications between physician and patient with fully informed consent are essential no matter what treatment approach is taken.

Legally, any treatment approach can be challenged, including adverse outcomes of bypass surgery or balloon dilation done without a trial of reversal treatment in patients with normal pumping function of the heart. The best way for physicians to provide optimal medical care at lowest legal risk is with careful explanation, signed informed consent, flexibility, and a willingness to try alternative treatment if a given approach does not work. Patient-clients and physicians need to understand the alternatives, the advantages and risks, and participate mutually in the decision making. Adverse outcomes may occur with any treatment alternative and usually do not indicate legal-medical fault but rather the natural course of coronary heart disease.

The exclusions or contraindications to using cholesterol-lowering drugs are best judged by the physician on a case-by-case basis. People with active liver disease, cancer, some gastrointestinal disorders, prior reaction to the drugs, or known recurrent adverse side effects should not take those of the cholesterol-lowering drugs having these effects. Other liver and gastrointestinal conditions, such as inflammatory bowel disease or diarrheal disorders with certain types of liver disease, may markedly improve with cholestyramine and/or a statin.

Based on the medical literature, cholesterol lowering is associated with

---

Seven Benefits of Reversal Treatment for Coronary Heart Disease

1. Reverses or stops progression of disease in over 90% of people
2. Decreases incidence of heart attacks, balloon dilation, bypass surgery by 90%
3. Improves coronary blood flow by PET
4. Relieves angina, increases activity level, energy, sense of well-being
5. Treats diffuse disease, throughout length of arteries
6. Heals endothelial lining of arteries
7. Serves as valid alternative or supplement to balloon dilation, bypass surgery

---

partial regression or no progression of coronary atherosclerosis in 40 to 85 percent or more of patients, depending upon the study reported. There is also a comparable decrease in future clinical events of heart attack, sudden cardiac death, balloon dilation, and/or bypass surgery. The goals of this reversal program are lean body mass and total cholesterol below 140 mg/dl, LDL below 90 mg/dl, HDL over 45 mg/dl, and elimination of other risk factors such as smoking, hypertension, and inactivity. In my experience, 90 percent of patients who achieve these goals by a combination of very low-fat foods and cholesterol-lowering drugs will experience a stabilization or regression of their coronary atherosclerosis, with a corresponding reduction of symptoms and cardiovascular events. However, as noted earlier, no treatment has a guaranteed outcome; a small risk of clinical events may remain with reversal treatment just as with any other treatment, including bypass surgery or balloon dilation.

Common Problems and Their Solutions

In my experience of implementing this program with many individuals, the following complaints and questions commonly arise. My suggested solutions or responses should help readers achieve better success with the program.

"The Food Is Boring"

Some people require a variety of food to be satisfied. There are several low-fat cookbooks on the market that provide a wide range of recipes. However, using one's own creativity in meal planning and preparation is the best option. Currently, grocery stores carry a wide range of no-fat to low-fat food products, including dressings, spices, herbs, sauces, mustard, ketchup, picante sauce, chutney, vegetables, and/or protein sources with the same range of possibilities for preparation as high-carbohydrate foods and meats offer.

To satisfy the need for a varied cuisine, it is important to draw on this wide range of possibilities and to develop one's imagination. Involvement of spouse or partner, family or friends in planning food alternatives can help broaden the possibilities even further.

"I Am Always Hungry"

Hunger causes loss of control over food, leading to overeating whatever is available, particularly carbohydrates or fatty fast-food snacks. Therefore, it is important to attack hunger by eating whenever you first feel hungry—but choose the right foods to eat.

No-fat protein snacks satisfy or suppress appetite and provide better control of food choices at the next meal. For those of you who get hungry between meals or are very hungry by the next meal, eating a regular mid- to late-morning and mid- to late-afternoon protein snack will help you stay on track with this eating plan. Protein snacks may include two no-fat cheese sticks with an apple, no-fat yogurt, no-fat cottage cheese salad, a protein-fruit shake, or raw vegetables, such as carrots, cauliflower, tomatoes (particularly the small, red, cherry tomatoes which are quick and easy to eat), all with no-fat cheese or some protein supplement.

"Do I Eat This Way Forever?"

Yes, the low-fat food habit with weight control by substituting vegetables for carbohydrates should become a lifelong habit. This is because the risk of coronary atherosclerosis returns when healthy food habits are given up. On the other hand, some zigzag in the diet is appropriate, with occasional variations to include food that is not compatible with a healthy food style. For example, a steak or chocolate mousse once per month may increase adherence to the eating plan at all other times. Those of you who need a wide variety of foods will especially appreciate these occasional breaks. However, people often find that rich foods do not taste good after they have become accustomed to a low-fat diet; now they enjoy and actually prefer low-fat foods.

"I Miss the Rich, Fatty Taste of Certain Foods"

For two to three weeks, you may temporarily miss this rich fattiness or sugary-ness in food. However, as noted above, fatty foods eaten after a period of low-fat intake no longer taste good; they are too thick or "muddy" and not particularly pleasant. At that point, the taste buds have adapted to low-fat food. The once-per-month zigzag also helps eliminate the sense of loss of the old tastes.

"I'm Having Trouble Reaching My Target Weight"

With low-fat food and substitution of vegetables for carbohydrate, weight is usually lost rapidly. Typically, in the first two weeks, four to six pounds are lost. Weight loss thereafter continues at approximately one and a half pounds per week until the target weight is achieved. However, sometimes weight will plateau for one to four weeks and then drop over a period of days or may fluctuate up and down by three to four pounds each day around an average weight loss. These fluctuations are commonly due in part to variable salt and fluid retention, as well as variable caloric intake. However, the initial body reaction to a change in diet is to preserve weight, to prevent a weight change despite the change in calories. Over one to four weeks, this initial reaction abates, and weight readjusts to the altered calories.

A long-lasting weight plateau without further weight decline while adhering to a strict low-fat food plan is usually due to the consumption of excess carbohydrates. The obvious solution is to exclude such carbohydrates as cereals, pasta, rice, potatoes, bread, bananas, sweets, and particularly alcohol, which has high caloric content. When target weight is reached, nonfat carbohydrates and/or protein should be increased just enough to maintain ideal weight.

"How Much Carbohydrate Should I Eat?"

Carbohydrates essentially provide calories that maintain weight. Excess weight prevents optimal fall in cholesterol levels, worsens tendencies toward diabetes, and is associated with cardiovascular risk. Commonly, carbohydrates in food and excess weight cause a rise in triglycerides with a fall in HDL. The amount of carbohydrate required to maintain or lose weight is highly variable with each individual. Some people require large amounts of carbohydrate with 2,000 to 3,000 calories per day simply to maintain lean body mass. Other individuals may gain weight consuming 1,200 calories consisting of only 206 grams of carbohydrate (824 calories), 60 grams of protein (240 calories), and 15 grams of fat (135 calories). Such individuals need to reduce carbohydrate to substantially lower levels by substituting vegetables for the carbohydrate. They need to reduce total caloric intake to 1,000 calories or less while at the same time eating sufficient volumes of vegetables and protein to avoid being hungry.

Therefore, the gauge for the amount of carbohydrates consumed should be body weight. When body weight is in excess of the lean body target, carbohydrates should be markedly curtailed by substituting vegetables while maintaining adequate protein until the target weight is achieved. After adequate weight reduction, just enough fat-free carbohydrates should be added in order to maintain target weight without further weight loss or weight gain. It is essential to consume 60 to 80 grams of protein to avoid fatigue and to maintain stamina.

"How Do You Relate Calories to Grams of Protein, Fat, or Carbohydrate?"

One gram of carbohydrate or 1 gram of protein equals 4 calories. One gram of fat equals 9 calories. While counting calories is beneficial to some people, the majority find it easier and more effective to make clear-cut changes, such as eliminating all identifiable fat, getting enough protein (60 to 80 grams per day), and controlling carbohydrates on the basis of weight.

"I Dislike or Can't Digest Dairy Products"

Some people feel bloated and gassy or get diarrhea from milk due to intolerance of the milk sugar lactose. The best solution is lactose-free milk, which is real milk with lactose enzyme added that has cleaved the milk sugar to a simple form that is more easily digested. This milk tastes sweeter than regular milk, is healthy and safe.

Sources of protein that can be substituted for milk products include turkey or chicken breasts, deep-sea fish, such as tuna, swordfish, haddock, sole, salmon, venison, buffalo meat, or equivalent. These meats should be grilled or sautéed in wine or juice but never fried, and without oil added. Other nondairy sources of protein include powdered protein from vegetable, egg, or no-fat milk sources that can be purchased from any health food store. The protein powder can be mixed with fruit juice and/or fruits to make a high-protein fruit shake or with skim milk to make a high-protein milk shake. These protein drinks have only moderate caloric intake, no fat or cholesterol, and, obviously, a high protein content. Egg whites or egg white cartons available in grocery stores are other excellent sources of protein, as are veggie burgers made from soy protein. Beans, pasta, or rice have a relatively low protein content, so that fairly large volumes of these foods must be consumed in order to obtain adequate protein. They therefore also incur a high carbohydrate and calorie load, which keeps weight, cholesterol, and particularly triglycerides high.

"I'm Experiencing Increased Fatigue, Decreased Stamina, and Personality Changes"

Some people eating low-fat foods experience a group of disturbing symptoms: increased fatigue, particularly in the afternoon; decreased stamina; difficulty concentrating; personality changes, especially the increased tendency to get angry or impatient. This symptom complex is typical of suboptimal protein consumption by people on very low-fat diets who eat principally vegetables or carbohydrates. It is quite common and may be debilitating. Men, especially big men whose protein needs may be 80 to 100 grams per day, are most likely to have this problem. It is corrected by increasing protein intake to at least 60 to 100 grams per day, depending on body size or weight.

Less commonly, the problem may be due to low blood sugar without the warning signal of hunger but in association with excessively rapid weight loss of more than two pounds per week. The solution is to eat more, and more often, particularly protein foods. If the problem still doesn't resolve itself, the physician needs to consider other causes, such as side effects of medications.

"My Progress Is Too Slow"

Some people readily adapt to the reversal regimen, very low-fat foods, and the cholesterol-lowering medications. Within weeks to months, they achieve the goals for cholesterol and weight. Other individuals require prolonged effort and support of physician and/or family/friends over one to two years in order to reach these goals. For excessively overweight people who need to lose 80 to 100 pounds, one to two years may be necessary at a pound-and-a-half weight loss per week. Whatever your circumstances, you should never give up. Permanent changes can be made in eating and living habits even if it does take one or more years to accomplish this task. Set specific, realistic goals on a realistic time frame.

"Does Partial Success Help Me?"

Many people are successful at lowering cholesterol and weight to some degree, but they fail to achieve the goals necessary for optimal protection against coronary events. It is essential for you and your physician to continue with all aspects of this program until target weight and cholesterol levels have been achieved. Partial success means only partial protection against cardiovascular events. Bear in mind that the process of vascular disease is relentless and predictable. Once the goals of this program are reached and maintained, the disease stabilizes and partially reverses, with a 90 percent reduction in risk of coronary events. Partial success is associated with partial benefit but remaining risk.

"Does It Matter Which Protein Powder I Use?"

Not all protein powders have the same ingredients. Many of them contain monosodium glutamate (MSG). People with a sensitivity to MSG or salt should carefully review the label on any protein powder before purchasing it. Many protein powder mixes also contain carbohydrate, which is usually not desirable since it maintains excess weight. So be sure to select a protein powder that is principally protein without carbohydrate. You will find protein powders in health food stores, although the specific types that are available will vary somewhat from one region to another. The label shows the complete contents of each can of protein powder.

"Should I Be Concerned about the Salt Content of Foods on This Eating Plan?"

Some protein powders have a high salt, or sodium, content, while others have virtually no salt. For people who are extremely salt-sensitive, egg protein can be obtained with very little sodium. For other nonfat protein foods, the cumulative sodium dose that is acceptable ranges from 800 milligrams (for the daily 60 milligrams of protein from yogurt) to 2,000 milligrams (for 60 milligrams of protein from soy burgers). Look at the labels to determine salt content.

For people who have high blood pressure, salt intake should be kept to a minimum. The same holds true for people with damaged or poorly functioning hearts; they may retain salt and fluid excessively, which causes swelling of the legs, more short-windedness, or increased symptoms of heart failure. For such susceptible individuals, nonfat protein sources with less sodium (e.g., 100 to 250 milligrams per serving, providing 8 to 10 grams of protein) are acceptable. Medications to control blood pressure and/or heart failure have to be continued under a physician's supervision.

On the other hand, many people need substantial amounts of sodium in order to maintain adequate blood pressure, particularly if they lose salt and fluids through sweating. For such people, the higher salt content of soy protein is desirable.

"Is Alcohol Allowed on This Program?"

While alcohol has been touted as protective against cardiovascular disease in the lay press, its medical use should be limited for several reasons. Alcohol is a carbohydrate high in calories that may maintain elevated triglycerides and excess weight. It is also metabolized in the liver. When taken in excess, alcohol may harm the liver. The liver is then more susceptible to the effects of cholesterol-lowering drugs, which cannot be used if the liver is severely damaged by alcohol. The cholesterol-lowering drugs are more effective in protecting against cardiovascular events than is alcohol. Therefore, alcohol intake should be limited in order to allow optimal cholesterol lowering by drugs in addition to low-fat foods. While all forms of alcohol (whiskey, beer, and wine) have a tendency to increase HDL, other methods of increasing HDL are more effective without the risks to the liver seen with high alcoholic intake.

Accordingly, for patients who do not normally drink alcohol, this program does not encourage its use. For individuals who regularly consume alcohol, one glass of wine per day should be the maximum, since the side effects of greater intake far outweigh the potential benefits. There is little hard scientific data indicating that red wine is better than other forms of alcohol. Whether red wine has additional antioxidants of medical importance has not been proven, whereas all forms of alcohol may have some effect on increasing HDL.

"What about Coffee?"

Coffee and caffeinated drinks have not been shown to increase the risk of cardiovascular disease. However, they tend to produce a "coffee high" followed by the fatigue of a coffee-deprived "low." These energy "highs and lows" may be associated with a variety of food cravings. Late-afternoon fatigue is often interpreted as a food craving, which makes adherence to the program more difficult. Hence heavy caffeine use should be curtailed. Many people miss caffeine for several weeks after its discontinuation. However, after overcoming caffeine withdrawal, they adapt and feel better, with a more uniform energy level throughout the day. Decaffeinated beverages are preferable for the social or habitual "coffee breaks" during the day. A particularly good café latte can be made by heating a cup of skim milk in a microwave oven without boiling the milk, and then adding one tablespoon of decaffeinated coffee powder. The result is a rich-tasting café latte undiluted by water that also provides substantial protein from the skim milk. Decaffeinated coffee and tea are jokingly named "why bother" drinks. I always counter that these are PWP drinks (pleasure without pain).

"What If My Liver Enzymes Are Increased by the Cholesterol-lowering Medications?"

The increase in liver enzymes should be at least two and a half to three times the normal upper limits before it is necessary to stop the cholesterol-lowering drug. The drug can then be restarted at a lower dose. Increased liver enzymes usually call for a dose adjustment or a change in drugs as determined by the physician.

The combination of a statin with slow-release niacin is more likely to increase liver enzymes than the statin alone. Under these circumstances, the dose of statin may often be continued with the dose of niacin somewhat reduced. The liver enzymes then return to normal. The benefit of this combination of drugs, particularly for elevated cholesterol and low HDL, is sufficiently great to outweigh the minor risk of side effects, which can be monitored and managed by dose reduction if they occur.

"What Is the 'Cholesterol Flu'?"

With a viral infection, such as the "flu," some people on a statin plus niacin may show a particularly sharp drop in their cholesterol levels with a rise in liver enzymes This side effect is called the "cholesterol flu." Under these circumstances, both the statin and niacin should be discontinued for approximately one to two weeks until the flu has resolved. The cholesterol-lowering drugs can then be restarted at the previous dose. The niacin dose has to be slowly built up again to avoid the side effect of flushing or itching, since niacin sensitivity returns during the one to two weeks off the drug while recovering from the virus infection.

"My Cholesterol Levels Are Increasing Even Though I'm on a Statin"

In some instances, after an initial fall in cholesterol after starting a statin drug, the cholesterol slowly increases, sometimes back to baseline levels. This slow increase of the cholesterol level is called statin escape and usually indicates that the dose of statin is inadequate. It should therefore be increased until target cholesterol levels are reached. The body sometimes adapts to initial low doses of a statin, so that it is less effective. Several increases in dose up to the maximum may be necessary; for example, atorvastatin 20 to 80 milligrams, Zocor 40 to 80 milligrams, lovastatin 80 to 120 milligrams, pravastatin 40 to 80 milligrams, Lescol 40 to 80 milligrams. Alternatively, the dose may be increased more moderately with another drug added, such as niacin or cholestyramine. Combinations of drugs are particularly effective.

If you have the problem of rising cholesterol after an initial fall while taking a statin, your physician needs to make the decisions about the dose or combinations of your medications. The initial increased doses do not indicate that you will forever need to increase dosage. The correct dosage for you needs to be determined over several months up to a year by careful trial.

"Why Are My Muscles Sore and Achy?"

On occasion, muscles may become sore and tender throughout the body or only in specific locations, such as the legs or arms or back. This may be the side effect of any cholesterol medication. It is particularly associated with the combination of a statin and gemfibrozil or a statin and niacin. In an unusual, more severe form, muscle weakness may also be present with increased muscle enzymes in blood. More commonly, a person complains of a particular set of sore muscles without rise of muscle enzymes in the blood. The specific muscles getting sore are often used in some specific activity. Runners may complain of sore thigh muscles, architects or carpenters may complain of sore hand muscles, weight lifters and swimmers may complain of sore shoulder or upper arm muscles.

In many instances, this soreness disappears while continuing the same dose as the body adapts to the drugs. Alternatively, the dose may be decreased temporarily or the drug stopped for a week and then restarted without return of symptoms. If the muscle soreness persists and is a limitation on activity, switching to an alternative statin is frequently successful in lowering cholesterol without this side effect.

Combinations of statins with gemfibrozil, or niacin with gemfibrozil, may be very effective in lowering cholesterol and increasing HDL. These combinations should be considered in patients with high triglycerides and low HDL. While the risk of muscle soreness or inflammation is somewhat increased by these combinations, these side effects are not common, are reversible, and are easily recognized. Therefore, these combinations of cholesterol-lowering drugs should be used to optimize lipid profile, since low-HDL syndromes are associated with a high risk of heart attacks, which outweighs the lesser risk of side effects of these combinations of drugs. It is important to rely on one's physician to help with these side effects and combinations of medications that may be necessary to manage the LDL, HDL, and triglyceride balance.

"Why Does My HDL Stay Low?"

Low HDL is associated with smoking, lack of physical activity, elevated triglycerides, excess weight, excess carbohydrate, inadequate protein, very low-fat diets, and with a primary genetic abnormality in metabolizing cholesterol. Treatment should eliminate all of the above by achieving lean body mass, restricting carbohydrates, increasing physical activity, and breaking the smoking habit. In addition, niacin is the most potent HDL-raising drug available. Gemfibrozil is an alternative.

Many people with elevated cholesterol and triglycerides will have normal HDL initially. However, the HDL falls as total cholesterol is reduced by either a low-fat diet or cholesterol-lowering drugs. This response to low-fat foods reveals an underlying lipid disorder.

Frequently, the HDL-raising effect of a statin may suffice to lower the total cholesterol and maintain normal HDL. However, in many people a second or third drug, such as niacin or gemfibrozil, must be added to keep the HDL as high as possible. It should be augmented by adequate exercise and correction of triglycerides by low-carbohydrate food and weight loss. In some normal people without coronary heart disease, a very low-fat diet may cause a small decrease in the HDL "naturally" or physiologically because of very low cholesterol levels (but HDL should not fall to lower than 40). It should not cause concern. The fundamental approach to this problem is to lower the total cholesterol, LDL, and triglycerides as much as possible and raise the HDL as much as possible within the limits of tolerable low-fat foods, weight, and cholesterol-altering drugs. All of these steps are necessary to raise HDL.

For some people, HDL remains low despite all efforts. In such instances, lower LDL as much as possible and accept the HDL level. The benefits of low LDL despite a low HDL are still substantial as shown by the 4S trial discussed in part 2. This point of view is based on the principle of optimizing reversal treatment in order to minimize cardiovascular risk or the need for bypass surgery or balloon dilation.

Limitations of Reversal Treatment

Potential limitations to reversal treatment for coronary atherosclerosis include inadequate modification of risk factors over the long term, the risk of interim coronary events, the side effects and expense of cholesterol-lowering drugs, and failure of patient or physician to recognize the benefits of reversal treatment.

Fear can be especially acute for some people and will impair sound judgment. Fear of dying, fear of heart attack, fear of being disabled, fear of pain, fear of the unknown, fear of losing independence, fear of being unable to support oneself and family are powerful inducements for an immediate surgical "fix" by balloon dilation or bypass surgery. This fear may lead to excessive procedures and associated costs and risks. The documented limitations of balloon dilation and bypass surgery, including their inability to prevent the progression of atherosclerosis, are greater than the limitations and risks of reversal treatment. Fear, along with anxiety and lack of knowledge, may result in a failure to do anything or to recognize the benefits of reversal treatment; their perception is that it takes too long or isn't enough. Yet reversal treatment is effective and readily managed in daily living with better survival and lower risk of heart attack than with any other treatment including balloon dilation or bypass surgery.

In my many years as a physician, I have encountered a large number of people with coronary heart disease who are good candidates for and want to undergo reversal treatment, including lifestyle changes and cholesterol-lowering drugs. However, frequently they are unable to obtain appropriate guidance and medical management from the cardiology profession, which is oriented toward invasive alternatives. If you are considering reversal treatment, ask your physician to try this approach first, reserving invasive procedures only as a last resort if the reversal treatment doesn't work.

Reduction of dietary fat to 10 percent or less of calories is one of the goals of this program. Although many people think this goal is unrealistic, in my reversal clinic, it is routinely achieved. The large number of no-fat food products now commercially available, especially the nonfat protein sources, make it easy for people to adhere to a low-fat food plan, provided their motivation is sufficiently high.

Motivation can be generated by having people review their own PET scan and gain the knowledge that low-fat food combined with lipid-lowering drugs typically relieves angina, partially reverses or stops progression of narrowing, and substantially prevents death, heart attacks, and the need for bypass surgery or balloon dilation. Family support may be an important influence as well. (By the way, children of parents with heart disease need to learn early about prevention since they are also at future risk.) In blunt terms, the basic choice is between living properly and taking cholesterol-lowering drugs, on the one hand, or being cut open, disabled, or dying an early death, on the other. When a reversal program is presented appropriately and adapted to individual needs, most people are able to stay on it indefinitely.

The risk of coronary events is always a concern while reversal treatment is under way. However, studies have shown that cholesterol lowering leads to a remarkable decrease in the incidence of heart attacks and death, and a reduced need for coronary bypass surgery or balloon dilation (see discussion in part 2). Chest pain, ECG abnormalities, or ischemia do not necessarily indicate a high risk of future coronary events either in people without prior symptoms or with only mild symptoms, in people with new-onset chest pain due to coronary heart disease, or in people with ischemic episodes during daily life, with exercise, or even with severe exercise-induced ischemia.

Therefore, these abnormal events are not a reason or justification for carrying out balloon dilation or bypass surgery for purposes of preventing heart attack and death. Neither balloon dilation nor bypass surgery has been shown to prevent heart attacks or death as much as reversal treatment, except in patients with impaired pumping function of the heart. Hence, for most patients with coronary heart disease, it is appropriate and safe to pursue a medical regimen and reversal treatment involving low-fat foods, cholesterol-lowering drugs, antioxidants, and other standard cardiovascular drugs with deferral of balloon dilation or bypass surgery. Bypass surgery and balloon dilation are an option in a minority of cases where reversal treatment is not successful or where limiting chest pain progresses despite optimal medical treatment.

The use of cholesterol-lowering drugs requires that liver function be checked by blood tests every month for three months after starting or changing the dose of a cholesterol-lowering drug. Every four to six months thereafter, blood should be checked in order to ensure continuing safety. It is occasionally necessary to discontinue these drugs because of side effects; however, such instances are relatively uncommon and substantially less than the 40 percent failure rate documented after balloon dilation and 15 to 20 percent closures of bypass grafts.

The expense of cholesterol-lowering drugs is a valid limitation. However, this cost is substantially less than the cost of balloon dilation or bypass surgery. Most commercial medical insurance plans cover costs of medications with a modest copayment fee.

As discussed in part 2, twenty-five major studies since 1990 consistently show the clinical benefits of vigorous cholesterol lowering. In comparison, despite the current widespread use of balloon dilation, there are no well-designed scientific studies in stable coronary heart disease showing decreased risk of heart attacks or death. Similarly, in long-term follow-up, coronary artery bypass surgery has not been demonstrated to reduce the risk of death or heart attacks. There are more studies showing decreased incidence of heart attacks and death by reversal treatment than by bypass surgery or balloon dilation.

Therefore, the argument that there is inadequate evidence to justify using reversal treatment as the primary step in the management of coronary heart disease is unfounded. There is substantially less scientific justification for balloon dilation or bypass surgery.

However, no outcome can be guaranteed for any treatment of coronary heart disease. Although the threat is reduced, there remains some risk of heart attack, death, stroke, balloon dilation, or bypass surgery; furthermore, these surgical procedures carry their own definite risk of heart attack, death, stroke, and other adverse outcomes.

Whether marked cholesterol lowering causes increased deaths due to suicide or trauma has been a concern in scientific studies prior to 1990. In large population studies, there may be an association between low cholesterol and accidental death, suicide, or cancer. This association can be explained by the existence of preexisting conditions which cause death as well as lower cholesterol. For example, psychiatrically depressed people are prone to accidental or suicidal deaths, as well as being anorexic with consequent low cholesterol levels. Individuals with undiagnosed cancer may have low cholesterol; after the cancer diagnosis is established, the association with cholesterol level is made. When these preexisting medical conditions are identified and removed from the analysis, lower cholesterol levels are associated with longevity without any relation to trauma, suicide, or cancer.

Furthermore, trials of low-fat or low-calorie diets do not show an increased risk of accidental death, suicide, or cancer. In the Multiple Risk-Factor Intervention Trial (MRFIT), no excessive traumatic or suicidal deaths were observed. In the Family Heart Study, the group of people on a low-fat diet showed a reduction in depression and aggressive hostility, paralleling lowered cholesterol, as compared with more depression and hostility in the control group on a standard, high-fat diet. Even very low-calorie diets in addition to low-fat diets are not associated with adverse violent deaths. In the 4S trial from Scandinavia, the group taking a cholesterol-lowering drug had no higher rates of cancer, suicide, trauma, depression, or other medical problems than the group not on the drug. Therefore, in clinical trials, there is no identifiable risk of significant adverse effects from vigorous cholesterol lowering or cholesterol-lowering drugs.

Weighing the Alternatives

People with coronary heart disease should be fully informed and give their consent to a given treatment plan. This consent should follow a discussion of traditional alternatives using balloon dilation and bypass surgery, as well as newer reversal treatment. Coronary arteriography and balloon dilation of a localized narrowing in the coronary arteries may be an alternative treatment preferred by most cardiologists. For acute, unstable coronary syndromes, such as increasing severe chest pain or evolving heart attack that is not controlled by reversal treatment, balloon dilation may be necessary. However, there is a 40 percent recurrence of coronary artery narrowing within six months after initial success with the balloon dilation. Bypass surgery may also be a viable alternative, particularly for patients with poorly contracting heart muscle that is damaged but salvageable if blood flow is restored by bypass grafts. However, bypass surgery is associated with some risk of death, heart attack, or stroke and does not retard the progression of coronary atherosclerosis.

As noted earlier, no treatment has a guaranteed outcome, and some risk of clinical coronary events remains during reversal treatment, as with bypass surgery and balloon dilation. Reversal treatment may require major changes in lifestyle in addition to the expense, inconvenience, and modest risk of taking cholesterol-lowering drugs. However, the risk of taking these drugs is lower than the risk of bypass surgery or balloon dilation. The aims of low-fat foods and cholesterol-lowering drugs are to partially reverse or stop the progression of coronary heart disease with as great a certainty as possible and to decrease the risk of death, heart attack, chest pain, bypass surgery, or balloon dilation.

Another alternative approach to treating coronary heart disease is balloon dilation or bypass surgery in addition to or followed by reversal treatment. However, reversal treatment does not prevent the recurrence of internal scarring that causes recurrence of narrowing after balloon dilation. The reason is that this recurrence of narrowing is not influenced by cholesterol lowering.

How Dr. Gould Implements His Program for Preventing or Reversing Vascular Disease

The principles for preventing or reversing vascular disease described in this book may be applied in many different ways. Optimal results combine a "do it yourself" intensity in controlling one's own risk factors with a supportive, knowledgeable physician who supervises medications and gives advice on risk factor management as necessary. In clinical practice, I implement these principles in an integrated five-step reversal program outlined below.

1. Initial Medical Evaluation

✓ History and physical examination.
✓ Review of all current medical data, including prior exercise tests, coronary arteriography, and laboratory work if available.
✓ Assessment of lifestyle, risk factors, lipid profile, diet, activity level, smoking risk, stress, hypertension, family history of coronary heart disease, and diabetes if present.

✓ Evaluation of past and current treatment, including cardiovascular medications, prior balloon dilation, bypass surgery, or recommendations for these procedures for patients needing a second or alternative medical opinion.

2. Positron Emission Tomography (PET)

Noninvasive PET is done as an outpatient service in order to rule out or identify coronary heart disease, its severity, extent of heart damage and/or salvageable heart muscle, the suitability for the reversal program, and/or the potential need for balloon dilation or bypass surgery. PET also provides baseline data for determining whether progression or regression is occurring at a later time following a period of reversal treatment.

For those without access to PET, high risk factors must be present or a definitive diagnosis of vascular or coronary heart disease must be made in order to undertake a lifelong regimen of reversal treatment. The indications for reversal treatment include previous heart attack, stroke, positive coronary arteriogram or PET scan, balloon dilation, bypass surgery, high or multiple risk factors for vascular disease or cerebrovascular (brain artery) disease as determined by exam or by Doppler-ultrasound tests.

3. Evaluation of Individual Treatment Needed

✓ Review of PET images and results with each individual.
✓ Determination of appropriate treatment including cardiovascular and cholesterol-lowering drugs, evaluation of the best psychological motivation and plan for lifestyle change, very low-fat food, exercise, smoking cessation, and stress management. For each individual, a plan is drawn up, taking into account preferences and personality. It includes food to be eaten at each meal, medications, doses and side effects, exercise routines, a motivational plan for breaking the smoking habit if necessary (nicotine patches or medications are sometimes required), and simple stress-modification routines.

4. Lifestyle Rehabilitation Reinforcement and Follow-up

Emphasis is placed on specific components of the reversal program, including self-maintenance of lifestyle change, low-fat food, exercise, smoking cessation, effectiveness and/or side effects of cardiovascular/cholesterol-lowering medications, evaluation of laboratory studies, particularly liver-function tests and lipid profile at each of the following time intervals:

✓ Extended follow-up by clinic visit, telephone, FAX, or letter every month initially for three months and then every three to four months thereafter, with analysis and adjustment of the reversal program individualized for each person with regard to food, medications, exercise, symptoms, and medical management, with personalized reinforcement sessions to optimize adherence to the program.

✓ Additional weekly or monthly clinic visits, telephone, FAX, or written follow-up as needed.

✓ Clinic visits, telephone, FAX, or written consultation for patient questions or unexpected problems as needed with easily available access to medical staff.

✓ Follow-up assessment or detailed diary by the patient or recorded by the medical staff (whichever works) of diet, exercise, risk factors, cardiovascular and cholesterol-lowering drugs, symptoms, side effects, and modifications needed in the program. Any modifications are tailored to each individual, and overall progress is monitored by cardiac staff.

5. Repeat PET Scan at One- to Two-Year Follow-up

These PET scans evaluate the patient's progress and can identify the need for an adjustment in the lifestyle rehabilitation regimen, changes in medications, or for balloon angioplasty or bypass surgery due to progression of disease. There is rarely a need for such surgical procedures, however, for progression usually occurs only in people who fail to adhere closely to the program.

Glossary

Angina. Angina pectoris, or chest pain, due to inadequate blood flow to heart muscle; caused by cholesterol buildup that narrows or blocks the artery.

Angiogram. An X-ray picture of an artery. Same as an arteriogram. *See also* coronary arteriogram.

Aorta. The largest artery in the body carrying blood flow from the heart to all other arteries of the body.

Aortic valve. The valve at the outlet of the heart that allows blood to be pumped into the aorta. It prevents blood from flowing backward into the left ventricle during the pause between heartbeats, called diastole.

Arterial spasm. The process of vasoconstriction of the artery whereby it becomes smaller with reduced blood flow.

Arteries. Blood vessels carrying oxygenated blood to the body from the heart. *See also* coronary arteries.

Atherogenic. Causing atherosclerosis.

Atherosclerosis. The process of cholesterol deposition and buildup in the wall of an artery associated with inflammation, scarring of the arterial wall, calcium deposition, and narrowing of the artery. The process causing coronary heart disease.

Atrium. *See* left atrium, right atrium.

Cholesterol. An essential component of normal body biochemistry involving lipids; excessive levels in blood cause deposition in artery walls. *See also* atherosclerosis, lipids, HDL, LDL.

Collaterals. New blood vessels growing around a partial or complete blockage of an artery. Collaterals carry blood flow to the heart muscle beyond the blocked artery, forming a natural bypass.

Contraction phase. The contraction or squeezing of heart muscle with each heartbeat, a process that pumps blood to the body.

Coronary arteries. The arteries on the surface of the heart carrying oxygenated blood to heart muscle.

Coronary arteriogram. Same as coronary angiogram; an X-ray movie that provides a view of the coronary artery. It is created by inserting a small tube or catheter into the artery for injection of an X-ray dye called contrast media that outlines the inside of the artery.

Coronary artery disease. Also called coronary atherosclerosis and coronary heart disease; it results from cholesterol buildup in the wall of the coronary arteries that may partially or completely block the artery, causing chest pain or a heart attack.

Coronary flow reserve. The capacity to increase blood flow to heart muscle during stress; normally, coronary artery flow can increase to three or four times the blood flow levels at resting baseline conditions. This capacity to increase flow is reduced by coronary artery stenosis, or narrowing, that impedes the increase in flow.

Diagnostic sensitivity. The percentage or number of people with a positive stress test out of 100 patients having proven coronary heart disease by coronary arteriography.

Diagnostic specificity. The percentage or number of people with a normal stress test out of 100 normal people who do not have significant coronary heart disease by coronary arteriography.

Diastole. The period of heart relaxation between heartbeats while the pumping chambers are filling with blood in preparation for the next heartbeat.

Diffuse atherosclerosis. Also called diffuse narrowing or diffuse coronary artery disease; it refers to cholesterol buildup along the entire length of an artery with narrowing along its whole length rather than at a localized segment only.

Dipyridamole. A pharmacologic drug given intravenously that normally causes a three- to fourfold increase in coronary blood flow, much more than is possible by exercise, thereby allowing identification of coronary artery disease earlier and with greater accuracy.

ECG. The electrocardiogram is the recording of electrical activity of the heart, showing the heart rhythm and other information about the heart such as a heart attack.

Ejection fraction. The fraction of blood in the pumping chambers that is ejected with each heartbeat, normally 50 percent or greater.

Endothelium. The thin layer of cells lining the inside of an artery.

Fasting cholesterol. Levels of blood cholesterol measured after fasting for twelve hours, the most accurate way to determine these values.

HDL. High-density lipoprotein fraction of cholesterol that reduces the risk of coronary heart disease; the good cholesterol or "highly defensive lipid."

Heart attack. Myocardial infarction, the event associated with complete blockage of a coronary artery and cessation of coronary blood flow to a segment of heart muscle, which necroses (dies) and becomes a scar.

Heart failure. A condition in which a damaged heart fails to contract adequately or pump enough blood to the body. The consequence is fatigue, short-windedness, fluid retention, and ankle swelling.

Ischemia. The effect of transient inadequate blood flow to heart muscle caused by partial narrowing or partial blockage of a coronary artery. It may be associated with chest pain or may not cause symptoms; it can cause ECG abnormalities, impaired heart contraction, and an abnormal picture of blood flow in the heart muscle. It is not a heart attack, which indicates permanent damage.

LDL. Low-density lipoprotein fraction of cholesterol that increases the risk of coronary heart disease; the bad cholesterol or "low down lipid."

Left anterior descending. The largest coronary artery coursing down the front of the heart; also called the "widow maker artery." *See also* left circumflex coronary artery, right coronary artery.

Left atrium. The smaller antechamber on the left side of the heart that receives oxygenated blood from the lungs and pumps blood into the left ventricle, helping to fill it completely before the ventricle contracts to eject blood out through the aorta to the body.

Left circumflex coronary artery. The coronary artery coursing around the left side of the heart supplying the left side and sometimes the bottom of the heart muscle with blood.

Left ventricle. The largest main pumping chamber on the left side of the heart that pumps blood out through the aorta to the body.

Lipids. Collectively, the triglycerides, the total cholesterol, and the different types of cholesterol, lipoproteins, HDL, LDL, VLDL, in blood.

Lipoprotein. A protein lipid complex in blood of several types containing cholesterol in different amounts and forms.

Pacemaker. The microscopic site in the right atrium that generates the primary electrical impulse that paces the rest of the heart and determines heart rate.

Perfusion. Blood flow in the heart muscle as opposed to blood flow in the coronary arteries coursing over the surface of the heart

Perfusion defect. An abnormal area of deficient blood flow on a picture of blood flow in heart muscle.

PET. Positron emission tomography, a technology for obtaining accurate, quantitative, three-dimensional pictures of blood flow in heart muscle or of heart muscle metabolism.

Pharmacologic stress. A substitute for exercise stress using pharmacologic drugs that are more effective for stimulating increased coronary artery flow than exercise, thereby achieving greater diagnostic accuracy.

Plaque. A localized segment of artery with cholesterol buildup in the wall covered by the lining of the artery.

Plaque rupture. The process in which the lining of the artery covering the cholesterol in the wall cracks loose and exposes the underlying cholesterol to blood in the artery, which then forms a clot or thrombosis at the site of rupture.

Platelets. Small cell-like particles in blood that instigate a blood clot in the artery when activated.

Positron radiotracer. A small amount of radioactive tracer that is taken up in heart muscle in proportion to blood flow or metabolism, thereby allowing accurate three-dimensional pictures to be obtained by a scanner sensitive to the radiotracer. In clinical PET, radiation exposure is not harmful to the body because it is very low, lower than any cardiac radionuclide study done routinely in medicine.

Progression. Increased narrowing of a coronary artery due to progressive cholesterol buildup in the wall of the artery or partial blockage by plaque rupture.

Regression. Decreased narrowing of a coronary artery with resorption or removal of cholesterol from the wall of the artery.

Relaxation phase. The period between heartbeats when the pumping chambers, or ventricles, of the heart are filling with blood in preparation for the next heartbeat.

Right atrium. The smaller antechamber on the right side of the heart that receives blood back from the body where the oxygen was used up; it pumps blood into the right ventricle,which then pumps the blood through the lungs for replenishing the oxygen removed by the body.

Right coronary artery. The coronary artery coursing around the right side of the heart to the inferior or bottom of the heart.

Right ventricle. The smaller, thin-walled pumping chamber on the right side of the heart that pumps blood through the lungs, where the blood is oxygenated.

Risk factors. Those factors that increase the risk of or cause vascular disease: smoking, family history of vascular disease, high blood pressure, high cholesterol, diabetes, excess weight, a diet of rich fatty foods, inactivity, elevated blood homocysteine.

Segmental narrowing. A localized cholesterol buildup that narrows a segment of an artery, thereby impeding blood flow capacity through the artery.

Stenosis. A localized narrowing of an artery due to cholesterol buildup or partial plaque rupture.

Sudden death. The process of dying due to sudden unexpected cessation of normal, rhythmic, coordinated heart contraction; chaotic electrical activity called ventricular fibrillation is responsible for the stopping of the heartbeat.

Systole. A heart contraction or time period of heart contraction.

Thrombosis. A clot in an artery.

Triglycerides. A fat in the blood separate from cholesterol. High triglycerides in association with low HDL cause increased risk of coronary heart disease.

Vasoconstriction. Constriction or narrowing of an artery that makes it smaller and diminishes blood flow.

Vasodilation. Dilation or enlargement of an artery that increases blood flow.

Ventricle. *See* left ventricle, right ventricle.

VLDL. Very low-density lipoprotein that increases the risk of coronary heart disease. Another bad cholesterol or "very low down lipid."

Clinical PET Facilities

The following PET Centers are specialized for heart imaging, with specific clinical software providing three-dimensional analysis of heart pictures. The first center listed utilizes PET imaging of the heart and reversal treatment for the primarily noninvasive management of coronary heart disease. Coronary arteriography, balloon dilation, and bypass surgery are used as secondary interventions under exceptional circumstances. (This program is the one that I developed, and is discussed in detail in part 4.) This center also does general PET imaging for brain and cancer problems.

In the next two PET Centers listed, my reversal program is used, and coronary arteriography, balloon dilation, or bypass surgery is commonly utilized more frequently than in my own program. The remaining PET Centers, specialized for heart studies, utilize PET as an optimal guide to these procedures with less emphasis on reversal treatment in the primary management of coronary heart disease. However, these other PET Centers are still evolving and would provide PET assessment and guidance on reversal treatment if specifically requested by client-patients. One of the centers listed offers reversal treatment but not PET imaging. The final category of PET centers are those doing general applications of PET imaging for cancer and brain in addition to the heart. These listings of PET facilities are not intended to be all inclusive but are those familiar to me.

PET Imaging with Reversal Treatment for Primarily Noninvasive Management of Heart Disease

> PET Imaging Center
> University of Texas Medical School
> and Hermann Hospital
> Houston, Texas
> K. Lance Gould, M.D.
> 713-500-6611

PET Imaging with Reversal Treatment but More Emphasis on Invasive Procedures

> Baptist Hospital
> Nashville, Tennessee
> Robert A. Hardin, M.D., 615-329-5911
> Andrew Carlsen, M.D., 615-329-0203

Buffalo Cardiology & Pulmonary Associates
Williamsville, New York
Michael Merhige, M.D.
716-634-5100

PET Imaging with More Emphasis on Invasive Procedures But Reversal Treatment Available

Bergan Mercy Medical Center
Omaha, Nebraska
Sam Mehr, M.D.
402-398-6948

Beth Israel Medical Center
New York, New York
Steve Horowitz, M.D.
212-420-4560

The Cleveland Clinic
Cleveland, Ohio
Richard C. Brunken, M.D., 216-444-2051
Dennis Sprecher, M.D., 216-444-9353
Caldwell Esselstyn, M.D., 216-444-6664
Richard S. Lang, M.D., M.P.H., 216-444-5707

Crawford Long Hospital
Atlanta, Georgia
Randolph Patterson, M.D.
Larry Sperling, M.D.
404-686-8203

Humana Hospital Medical City
Dallas, Texas
Roy Aldridge, R.T.
214-788-6649

Kennestone PET Cardiac Center
Marietta, Georgia
Claudia Ceminsky, R.N.
404-793-5803

Memorial Medical Center
Jacksonville, Florida
Rudy Geer, M.D., or
Mitch Lyle, R.T., 904-391-1547
Michael Koren, M.D., 904-730-0101

Yale/VA Hospital
West Haven, Connecticut
Robert Soufer, M.D., or
James A. Arrighi, M.D.
203-937-3427

Heart Disease Reversal Program without PET Imaging

St. Peter's Medical Center
New Brunswick, New Jersey
Dr. Narayanan Natarajan, M.D.
908-828-8017

PET Imaging with General Applications for Cancer, Brain, and Heart

Department of Medical Pharmacology
University of California at Los Angeles (UCLA)
    School of Medicine
10833 LeConte Avenue
Room 23-148 CHS
Los Angeles, CA 90095-1735
Heinrich Schelbert, M.D., Ph.D. or
Jamshid Maddahi, M.D.
310-825-3076 or
310-206-9896

University of California at San Francisco
505 Parnassus
Box 0252
San Francisco, CA 94143
Randall Hawkins, M.D., Ph.D. or
Eli Botvinick, M.D.
415-476-1521

Children's Hospital of Michigan
3901 Beaubien Boulevard
Detroit, MI 48201-2196
Harry T. Chugani, M.D.
313-993-2867

Department of Radiology
Duke University Medical Center
Box 3949
Durham, NC 27710
R. Edward Coleman, M.D.
919-684-7244

Indiana University PET Facility
Radiology/Nuclear Medicine
550 North University Boulevard
Indianapolis, IN 46202
Gary Hutchins, Ph.D.
317-274-1797

Department of Radiology
University of Iowa
200 Hawkins Drive
Iowa City, IA 52242
Peter Kirchner, M.D.
319-356-4302

Division of Nuclear Medicine
University of Michigan Medical Center
1500 East Medical Center Drive
Ann Arbor, MI 48109-0028
Richard L. Wahl, M.D.
313-936-5384
PET Facility

University of Pittsburgh Medical School
200 Lothrop Street
Pittsburgh, PA 15213
David Townsend, Ph.D.
412-647-0736

Department of Radiology
University of Southern California
1510 San Pablo #350
Los Angeles, CA 90033
Peter Conti, Ph.D.
213-342-5940

Positron Diagnostic Center
Department of Nuclear Medicine
William Beaumont Hospital
3601 West 13 Mile Road
Royal Oak, MI 48073
Jack Juni, M.D.
248-551-4132

University of Wisconsin Medical School
H6/317 Clinical Science Center
600 Highland Avenue
Madison, WI 53792
Charles Stone, M.D.
608-263-4856

Sources of Information and Bibliography

For more detailed information, readers are referred to the following bibliography categorized by topic. My textbook, *Coronary Artery Stenosis and Reversing Heart Disease*, second edition, published by Lippincott Raven, provides an extensive, technical analysis of these topics; its subject matter has been simplified here for general readers. Additional general information can be obtained through the PET Center Web site (http://pet.med.uth.tmc.edu) or by contacting me or my staff at the following:

K. Lance Gould, M.D.
PET Imaging Center, Room 4.256 MSB
University of Texas Medical School
6431 Fannin Street
Houston, Texas 77030
Telephone: 713–500-6611
FAX: 713–500-6615
E-Mail: gould@heart.med.uth.tmc.edu

References in the bibliography are provided to document newer, innovative, or essential concepts. References are not intended to be exhaustive but rather to be comprehensive, emphasizing selected critical points not generally recognized. For efficiency, references for several related subjects in the text may be listed together here under a single heading. Some subjects in the text do not have accompanying references since they provide generally accepted background information, such as how the heart works. Subjects in the text for which references are listed below specifically provide the information that is the basis for this comprehensive approach to preventing or reversing coronary heart disease. A few additional references are included in tables in the text.

Contents of Bibliography by Topic

Cholesterol and Coronary Heart Disease
Dysfunctional Coronary Arteries—A Time Bomb
Narrowed Arteries and Swirling Flow
How Prevalent Is Coronary Atherosclerosis?
Risk Factors and Coronary Artery Disease
Women and Heart Disease
Cholesterol Lowering—Does It Work?

Can Cholesterol Levels Be Too Low?
Smoking and Death
Excess Body Weight and Survival
Physical Fitness and Survival
Standard Exercise Stress Tests—True or False Answers?
How Accurate Is the Coronary Arteriogram?
High Tech for the Heart—Positron Emission Tomography (PET)
Other Tests—What Do They Show?
Does Coronary Bypass Surgery Prolong Your Life?
Balloon Dilation of Narrowed Coronary Arteries
Chest Pain: Reversal? Balloon? Bypass?
Costs of Reversal Treatment, Balloon Dilation, and Bypass Surgery
Types of Food—Fat, Protein, and Carbohydrate
Antioxidant Vitamins and Aspirin
Estrogens and Coronary Heart Disease
Stress Management

List of Journal Abbreviations

ACC Current J Review	American College of Cardiology Current Journal Review
Acta Med Scand	Acta Medica Scandinavia
Am Heart J	American Heart Journal
Am J Card Imag	American Journal of Cardiac Imaging
Am J Cardiol	American Journal of Cardiology
Am J Physiol	American Journal of Physiology
Ann Int Med	Annals of Internal Medicine
Arch Int Med	Archives of Internal Medicine
Arch Path lab Med	Archives of Pathology and Laboratory Medicine
Br Med J	British Medical Journal
Cath Cardiovasc Diagn	Catheterization and Cardiovascular Diagnosis
Circ Res	Circulation Research
Clin Cardiol	Clinical Cardiology
Coronary Art Dis	Coronary Artery Disease
Eur Heart J	European Heart Journal
J Am Coll Cardiol	Journal of the American College of Cardiology
J Clin Invest	Journal of Clinical Investigation
J Intervent Cardiol	Journal of Interventional Cardiology
J Nuc Med	Journal of Nuclear Medicine
JAMA	Journal of the American Medical Association
Magn Reson Med	Magnetic Resonance Medicine
New Engl J Med	New England Journal of Medicine
Prog Cardiovasc Dis	Progress in Cardiovascular Disease

Bibliography by Topic

Cholesterol and Coronary Heart Disease

Berliner JA, Navab M, Fogelman AM, Frank JS, Demer LL, Edwards PA, Watson AD, Lusis AJ. Atherosclerosis: basis mechanisms. Oxidation, inflammation, and genetics. Circulation 1995; 91:2,488–2,496.

Brown BG, Zhao XQ, Sacco DE, Albers JJ. Lipid lowering and plaque regression. New insights into prevention of plaque disruption and clinical events in coronary artery disease. Circulation 1993; 87:1,781–1,791.

Constantinides P. Infiltrates of activated mast cells at the site of coronary atheromatous erosion or rupture in myocardial infarction. Circulation 1995; 92:1,083.

Davies MJ. Stability and instability: two faces of coronary atherosclerosis. Circulation 1996; 94:2,013–2,020.

Falk E, Shah PK, Fuster V. Coronary plaque disruption. Circulation 1995; 92:657–671.

Farb A, Burke AP, Tang AL, Liang Y, Mannan P, Smialek J, Virmani R. Coronary plaque erosion without rupture into a lipid core. Circulation 1996; 93:1,354–1,363.

Farb A, Tang AL, Burke AP, Sessums L, Liang Y, Virmani R. Sudden coronary death. Frequency of active coronary lesions, inactive coronary lesions, and myocardial infarction. Circulation 1995; 92:1,701–1,709.

Fuster V, Badimon L, Badimon JJ, Chesebro JH. The pathogenesis of coronary artery disease and the acute coronary syndromes. New Engl J Med 1992; 326:242–318.

Gould KL. *Coronary artery stenoses and reversing heart disease.* A textbook of coronary pathophysiology, quantitative coronary arteriography, PET perfusion imaging, and reversal of coronary artery disease. Second edition. Lippincott Raven, Philadelphia, 1998.

Gould KL. Reversal of coronary atherosclerosis. Clinical promise as the basis for noninvasive management of coronary artery disease. Circulation 1994; 90:1,558–1,571.

Havel RJ, Rapaport E. Drug Therapy. New Engl J Med 1995; 332:1,491–1,498.

Kendall MJ, Lynch, KP, Hjalmarson, Hjalmarson A, Kjekshus J. ß-blockers and sudden cardiac death. Ann Int Med 1995; 123:358–367.

Kovanen PT, Kaartinen M, Paavonen T. Infiltrates of activated mast cells at the site of coronary atheromatous erosion or rupture in myocardial infarction. Circulation 1995; 92:1,084–1,088.

Libby P. Molecular bases of the acute coronary syndromes. Circulation 1995; 91:2,844–2,850.

Loree HM, Kamm RD, Stringfellow RG, Lee RT. Effects of fibrous cap thickness on peak circumferential stress in model atherosclerotic vessels. Circ Res 1992; 71:850–858.

Mann JM, Davies MJ. Vulnerable plaque; relation of charcteristics to degree of stenosis in human coronary arteries. Circulation 1996; 94:928–931.

Navab M, Fogelman AM, Berliner JA, Territo MC, Demer LL, Frank JS, Watson

AD, Edwards PA, Lusis AJ. Pathogenesis of atherosclerosis. Am J Cardiol 1995; 76:18C–23C.

Richardson PD, Davies MJ, Born GVR. Influence of plaque configuration and stress distribution on fissuring of coronary atherosclerotic plaques. Lancet 1989; 2:941–944.

Shah PK, Falk E, Badimon JJ, Fernandez-Ortiz A, Mailhac A, Villareal-Levy G, Fallon JT, Regnstrom J, Fuster V. Human monocyte-derived macrophages induce collagen breakdown in fibrous caps of atherosclerotic plaques. Potential role of matrix-degrading metalloproteinases and implications for plaque rupture. Circulation 1995; 92:1,565–1,569.

Steinberg D. Oxidative modification of LDL and atherogenesis. Circulation 1997; 95:1,062–1,071.

van der Wal AC, Becker AE, van der Loos CM, Das PK. Site of intimal rupture or erosion of thrombosed coronary atherosclerotic plaques is characterized by an inflammatory process irrespective of the dominant plaque morphology. Circulation 1994; 89:36–44.

Dysfunctional Arteries—A Time Bomb

Andrews HE, Bruckdorfer KR, Dunn RC, Jacob M. Low-density lipoproteins inhibit endothelium-dependent relaxation in rabbit aorta. Nature 1987; 327:237–239.

Armstrong ML, Heistad DD, Marcus ML, Piegors DJ, Abboud FM. Hemodynamic sequelae of regression of experimental atherosclerosis. J Clin Invest 1983; 71:104–113.

Benzuly KH, Padgett RC, Kaul S, Piegors DJ, Armstrong ML, Heistad DD. Functional improvement precedes structural regression of atherosclerosis. Circulation 1994; 89:1,810–1,818.

Bou-Holaigah I, Rowe PC, Kan J, Calkins H. The relationship between neurally mediated hypotension and the chronic fatigue syndrome. JAMA 1995; 274:961–967.

Braun S, Boyko V, Behar S, Reicher-Reiss H, Shotan A, Schlesinger Z, Rosenfeld T, Palant A, Friedensohn A, Laniado S, Goldbourt U. Calcium antagonists and mortality in patients with coronary artery disease: a cohort study of 11,575 patients. J Am Coll Cardiol 1996; 28:7–11.

Cannon RO III. The sensitive heart. A syndrome of abnormal cardiac pain perception. JAMA 1995; 273:883–887.

Casino PR, Kilcoyne CM, Quyyumi AA, Hoeg JM, Panza JA. Investigation of decreased availability of nitric oxide precursor as the mechanism responsible for impaired endothelium-dependent vasodilation in hypercholesterolemic patients. J Am Coll Cardiol 1994; 23:844–850.

Chilian WM, Dellsperger KC, Layne SM, Eastham CL, Armstrong MA, Marcus ML, Heistad DD. Effects of atherosclerosis on the coronary microcirculation. Am J Physiol 1990; 258 (Heart Circ Physio 27):H529–H539.

Cohen RA, Zitnay KM, Haudenschild CC, Cunningham LD. Loss of selective endothelial cell vasoactive functions caused by hypercholesterolemia in pig coronary arteries. Circ Res 1988; 63:903–910.

El-Tamini H, Mansour M, Wargovich TJ, Hill JA, Kerensky RA, Conti R, Pepine CJ. Constrictor and dilator responses to intracoronary acetylcholine in adjacent segments of the same coronary artery in patients with coronary artery disease. Circulation 1994; 89:45–51.

Frank MW, Harris KR, Ahlin KA, Klocke FJ. Endothelium-derived relaxing factor (nitric oxide) has a tonic vasodilating action on coronary collateral vessels. J Am Coll Cardiol 1996; 27:658–663.

Giugliano D, Marfella R, Coppola L, Verrazzo G, Acampora R, Giunta R, Nappo F, Lucarelli C, D'Onofrio F. Vascular effects of acute hyperglycemia in humans are reversed by L-arginine; evidence for reduced availability of nitric oxide during hyperglycemia. Circulation 1997; 95:1,783–1,790.

Glagov S, Weisenberg E, Zarins CK, et al. Compensatory enlargement of human atherosclerotic coronary arteries. N Engl J Med 1987; 316:1,371–1,375.

Gordon JB, Ganz P, Nabel EG, Fish RD, Zehedi J, Mudge GH, Alexander RW, Selwyn A. Atherosclerosis influences the vasomotor response of epicardial coronary arteries to exercise. J Clin Invest 1989; 83:1,946–1,952.

Harrison DG. Endothelial dysfunction in the coronary microcirculation: a new clinical entity or an experimental finding. J Clin Invest 1993; 91:1–2.

Harrison DG, Armstrong ML, Freiman PC, Heistad DD. Restoration of endothelium-dependent relaxation by dietary treatment of atherosclerosis. J Clin Invest 1987; 80:1,801–1,811.

Hodgson JM, Marshall JJ. Direct vasoconstriction and endothelium-dependent vasodilation; mechanisms of acetylcholine effects on coronary flow and arterial diameter in patients with nonstenotic coronary arteries. Circulation 1989; 79:1,043–1,051.

Kaufmann P, Vassalli G, Utzinger U, Hess OM. Coronary vasomotion during dynamic exercise: influence of intravenous and intracoronary nicardipine. J Am Coll Cardiol 1995; 26:624–631.

Krantz DS, Kop WJ, Gabbay FH, Rozanski A, Barnard M, Klein J, Pardo Y, Gottdiener JS. Circadian variation of ambulatory myocardial ischemia. Circulation 1996; 93:1,364–1,371.

Kugiyama K, Yasue H, Okumura K, Ogawa H, Fujimoto K, Nakao K, Yoshimura M, Motoyama T, Inobe Y, Kawano H. Nitric oxide activity is deficient in spasm arteries of patients with coronary spastic angina. Circulation 1996; 94:266–272.

Kuo L, Davis MJ, Cannon S, Chilian WM. Pathophysiological conseqences of atherosclerosis extend into the coronary microcirculation; restoration of endothelium-dependent responses by L-Arginine. Circ Res 1992; 70:465–476.

Kuo L, Davis MJ, Chilian WM. Longitudinal gradients for endothelium-dependent and -independent vascular responses in the coronary microcirculation. Circulation 1995; 92:518–525.

Ludmer PL, Selwyn AP, Shook TL, Wayne RR, Mudge GH, Alexander W, Ganz P. Paradoxical vasoconstriction induced by acetylcholine in atherosclerotic coronary arteries. New Engl J Med 1986; 315:1,046–1,051.

Mancini GBJ, Henry GC, Macaya C, O'Neill BJ, Pucillo AL, Carere RG, Wargovich TJ, Mudra H, Lüscher TF, Klibaner MI, Haber HE, Uprichard ACG, Pepine CJ, Pitt B. Angiotensin-converting enzyme inhibition with quinapril improves endothelial vasomotor dysfunction in patients with coronary artery disease. Circulation 1996; 94:258–265.

Penny WF, Rockman H, Long J, Bhargava V, Carrigan K, Ibriham A, Shabetal R, Ross J, Peterson KL. Heterogeneity of vasomotor response to acetylcholine along the human coronary artery. J Am Coll Cardiol 1995; 25:1,046–1,055.

Quyyumi AA, Dakak N, Andrews NP, Gilligan DM, Panza JA, Cannon RO. Contribution of nitric oxide to metabolic coronary vasodilation in the human heart. Circulation 1995; 92:320–326.

Quyyumi AA, Dakak N, Mulcahy D, Andrews NP, Husain S, Panza J, Cannon RO. Nitric oxide activity in the atherosclerotic human coronary circulation. J Am Coll Cardiol 1997; 29:308–317.

Radice M, Giudici V, Pusineri E, Breghi L, Nicoli T, Peci P, Giani P, DeAmbroggi L. Different effects of acute administration of aminophylline and nitroglycerin on exercise capacity in patients with syndrome X. Am J Cardiol 1995; 78:88–90.

Reddy KG, Nair RV, Sheehan HM, Hodgson JM. Evidence that selective endothelial dysfunction may occur in the absence of angiographic or ultrasound atherosclerosis in patients with risk factors for atherosclerosis. J Am Coll Cardiol 1994; 23:833–843.

Schächinger V, Zeiher AM. Quantitative assessment of coronary vasoreactivity in humans in vivo. Circulation 1995; 92:2087–2094.

Selke FW, Armstrong ML, Harrison DG. Endothelium-dependent vascular relaxation is abnormal in the coronary microcirculation of atherosclerotic primates. Circulation 1990; 81:1,586–1,593.

Shimokaw H, Vanhoutte PM. Dietary cod liver oil improves endothelium-dependent responses in hypercholesterolemic and atherosclerotic porcine coronary arteries. Circulation 1988; 78:1,421–1,430.

Shircore AM, Mack WJ, Selzer RH, Lee PL, Azen SP, Alaupovic P, Hodis HN. Compensatory vascular changes of remote coronary segments in response to lesion progression as observed by sequential angiography from a controlled clinical trial. Circulation 1995; 92:2,411–2,418.

Small DM, Bond MG, Waugh D, Prack M, Sawyer JK. Physiochemical and histological changes in the arterial wall of nonhuman primates during progression and regression of atherosclerosis. J Clin Invest 1984; 73:1,590–1,605.

Takahashi M, Yui Y, Yasumoto H, Aoyama T, Morishita H, Hattori R, Kawai C. Lipoproteins are inhibitors of endothelium-dependent relaxation of rabbit aorta. Am J Physiol 1990; 258:H1–H8.

Tanner FC, Noll G, Boulanger CM, Luescher TF. Oxidized low-density lipoproteins inhibit relaxations of porcine coronary arteries. Role of scavenger receptor and endothelium-derived nitric oxide. Circulation 1991; 83:2,012–2,020.

Tawakol A, Omland T, Gerhard M, Wu JT, Creager MA. Hyperhomocyst(e)inemia is associated with impaired endothelium-dependent vasodilation in humans. Circulation 1997; 95:1,119–1,121.

Tomita T, Ezaki M, Miwa M, Nakamura K, Inoue Y. Rapid and reversible inhibition by low-density lipoprotein of the endothelium-dependent relaxation to hemostatic substances in porcine coronary arteries. Circ Res 1990; 66:18–27.

Treasure CB, Klein JL, Weintraub WS, Talley JD, Stillabower ME, Kosinski AJ, Zhang J, Boccuzzi SJ, Cedarholm JC, Alexander RW. Beneficial effects of cholesterol-lowering therapy on the coronary endothelium in patients with coronary artery disease. N Engl J Med 1995; 332:481–487.

Uren NG, Marraccini P, Gistri R, deSilva R, Camici PG. Altered coronary vasodilator reserve and metabolism in myocardium subtended by normal arteries in patients with coronary artery disease. J Am Coll Cardiol 1993; 22:650–658.

Verbeuren TJ, Jordaens FH, Zonnekeyn LL, Van Hove CE, Coene MC, Herman AG. Effect of hypercholesterolemia on vascular reactivity in the rabbit. Circ Res 1986; 58:552–564.

Zeiher AM, Drexler H, Wollschlager H, Just H. Endothelial dysfunction of the coronary microvasculature is associated with impaired coronary blood flow regulation in patients with early atherosclerosis. Circulation 1991; 84.1,984–1,992.

Zeiher AM, Drexler H, Wollschlager H, Just H. Modulation of coronary vasomotor tone: progressive endothelial dysfunction with different early stages of coronary atherosclerosis. Circulation 1991; 83:391–401.

Zeiher AM, Krause T, Schächinger V, Minners J, Moser E. Impaired endothelium-dependent vasodilation of coronary resistance vessels is associated with exercised-induced myocardial ischemia. Circulation 1995; 91:2,345–2,352.

Narrowed Arteries and Swirling Flow

Albro PC, Gould KL, Westcott RJ, Hamilton GW, Ritchie JL, Williams DL. Noninvasive assessment of coronary stenoses by myocardial imaging during pharmacologic coronary vasodilation. III. Clinical trial. Am J Cardiol 1978; 42:751–760.

DeBruyne B, Bartunek J, Sys SU, Heyndrickx GR. Relation between myocardial fractional flow reserve calculated from coronary pressure measurements and exercise-induced myocrdial ischemia. Circulation 1995; 92:39–46.

De Bruyne B, Baudhuin T, Melin JA, Pijls NHJ, Sys SU, Boll A, Paulus WJ, Heyndrickx GR, Wijns W. Coronary flow reserve calculated from pressure measurements in humans, validation with positron emission tomography. Circulation 1994; 89:1,013–1,022.

Di Mario C, de Feyter PJ, Slager CJ, de Jaegere P, Roelandt JRTC, Serruys PW. Intracoronary blood flow velocity and transstenotic pressure gradient using sensor-tip pressure and Doppler guidewires. Cath Cardiovasc Diagn 1993; 28:311–319.

Ferro G, Duilio C, Spinelli L, Liucci GA, Mazza F, Indolfi C. Relation between diastolic perfusion time and coronary artery stenosis during stress-induced myocardial ischemia. Circulation 1995; 92:342–347.

Gould KL. Assessment of coronary stenoses by myocardial perfusion imaging during pharmacologic coronary vasodilatation. IV. Limits of stenosis detection by idealized, experimental, cross-sectional myocardial imaging. Am J Cardiol 1978; 42:761–768.

Gould KL. *Coronary artery stenoses and reversing heart disease.* A textbook of coronary pathophysiology, quantitative coronary arteriography, PET perfusion imaging, and reversal of coronary artery disease. Second edition. Lippincott Raven, Philadelphia, 1998.

Gould, KL. Identifying and measuring severity of coronary artery stenosis—quantitative coronary arteriography and positron emission tomography. Circulation 1988; 78:237–245.

Gould KL. Noninvasive assessment of coronary stenoses by myocardial imaging during coronary vasodilation. I. Physiologic principles and experimental validation. Am J Cardiol 1978; 41:267–278.

Gould KL, Kelley KO. Experimental validation of quantitative coronary arteriography for determining pressure-flow characteristics of coronary stenoses. Circulation 1982; 66:930–937.

Gould KL, Kirkeeide RL. Quantitation of coronary artery stenosis in vivo. Circ Res 1985; 57:341–353.

Gould, KL, Kirkeeide RL, Buchi M. Coronary flow reserve as a physiologic measure of stenosis severity. *Part I.* Relative and absolute coronary flow reserve during changing aortic pressure and cardiac workload. *Part II.* Determination from arteriographic stenosis dimensions under standardized conditions. J Am Coll Cardiol 1990; 15:459–474.

Gould KL, Lipscomb K, Hamilton GW. A physiologic basis for assessing critical coronary stenosis: instantaneous flow response and regional distribution during coronary hyperemia as measures of coronary flow reserve. Am J Cardiol 1974; 33:87–94.

Gould KL, Schelbert H, Phelps M, Hoffman E. Noninvasive assessment of coronary stenoses by myocardial perfusion imaging during pharmacologic coronary vasodilation. V. Detection of 47% diameter coronary stenosis with intravenous 13NH4+ and emission computer tomography in intact dogs. Am J Cardiol 1979; 43:200–208.

Gould KL, Westcott JR, Hamilton GW. Noninvasive assessment of coronary stenoses by myocardial imaging during coronary vasodilation II. Clinical methodology and feasibility. Am J Cardiol 1978; 41:279–289.

Kern MJ, Anderson HV. A symposium: the clinical applications of the intracoronary Doppler guidewire flow velocity in patients: understanding blood flow beyond the coronary stenosis. Am J Cardiol 1993; 71:1D–70D.

Kirkeeide RL, Gould KL, Parsel L. Assessment of coronary stenoses by myocardial imaging during coronary vasodilation. VII. Validation of coronary flow reserve as a single integrated measure of stenosis severity accounting for all its geometric dimensions. J Am Coll Cardiol 1986; 7:103–113.

Pijls NHJ, van Son AM, Kirkeeide RL, De Bruyne B, Gould KL. Experimental basis of determining maximum coronary, myocardial, and collateral blood flow by pressure measurement for assessing functional stenosis severity before and after percutaneous transluminal coronary angioplasty. Circulation 1993; 87:1,354–1,367.

Schelbert HR, Wisenberg G, Phelps ME, Gould KL, Eberhard H, Hoffman EJ, Gormesm A, Kuhl DE. Noninvasive assessment of coronary stenosis by myocardial imaging during pharmacologic coronary vasodilation. VI. Detection of coronary artery disease in man with intravenous N-13 ammonia and positron computed tomography. Am J Cardiol 1982; 49:1,197–1,207.

Serruys PW, Di Mario C, Meneveau N, de Jaegere P, Strikwerda S, de Feyter PJ, Emanuelsson H. Intracoronary pressure and flow velocity from sensor tip guidewire. A new methodological comprehensive approach for the assessment of coronary hemodynamics before and after interventions. Am J Cardiol 1993; 71:41D–53D.

Wilson RF. Assessment of the human coronary circulation using a Doppler catheter. Am J Cardiol 1991; 67:44D–56D.

How Prevalent Is Coronary Atherosclerosis?

American Heart Association. *Heart and stroke facts: 1994 statistical supplement.* Dallas, Texas.

Davis DL, Gregg ED, Hoel DG. Decreasing cardiovascular disease and increasing cancer among whites in the United States from 1973 through 1987, good news and bad news. JAMA 1994; 271:431–437.

Enos WF, Holmes RH, Beyer J. Coronary disease among United States soldiers killed in action in Korea. JAMA 1953; 152:1,090–1,093.

Guide to Clinical Preventive Services. *Report of the U.S. Preventive Services Task Force. An assessment of the effectiveness of 169 interventions.* Ed. Michael Fisher. William and Wilkins, Baltimore, 1989, pp. 3–11.

Joseph A, Ackerman D, Talley JD, Johnstone J, Kupersmith J. Manifestations of coronary atherosclerosis in young trauma victims—an autopsy study. J Am Coll Cardiol 1993; 22:459–467.

Kannel WB, Abbott RD. Incidence and prognosis of unrecognized myocardial infarction. An update on the Framingham Study. N Engl J Med 1984; 311:1,144–1,147.

Lown B. Sudden cardiac death: the major challenge confronting contemporary cardiology. Am J Cardiol 1979; 43:313–328.

McNamara JJ, Molot MA, Stremple JF, Cutting RT. Coronary artery disease in combat casualties in Viet Nam. JAMA 1971; 216:1,185–1,187.

Midwall J, Ambrose J, Pichard A, Abedin Z, Herman MV. Angina pectoris before and after myocardial infarction. Chest 1982; 81:681–686.

Olofsson BO, Bjerle P, Aberg T, Osterman G, Jacobson KA. Prevalence of coronary artery disease in patients with valvular heart disease. Acta Med Scand 1985; 218:365–371.

Reunanen A, Aromaa A, Pyorala K, Punsar S, Maatela J, Knekt P. The Social

Insurance Institution's coronary heart disease study: baseline data and 5-year mortality experience. Acta Med Scand Suppl 1983; 673:67–81.

Strong JP. Coronary atherosclerosis in soldiers: a clue to the natural history of atherosclerosis in the young. JAMA 1986; 256:2,863–2,866.

Risk Factors and Coronary Heart Disease

Adams MR, Nakagomi A, Keech A, Robinson J, McCredie R, Bailey BP, Freedman SB, Celermajer DS. Carotid intima-media thickness is only weakly correlated with the extent and severity of coronary artery disease. Circulation 1995; 92:2,127–2,134.

Ambrose JA, Tannenbaum MA, Alexopoulos D, et al. Angiographic progression of coronary artery disease and the development of myocardial infarction. J Am Coll Cardiol 1988; 12:56–62.

Atger V, Giral P, Simon A, Cambillau M, Levenson J, Gariepy J, Megnien JL, Moatti N. High-density lipoprotein subfractions as markers of early atherosclerosis. Am J Cardiol 1995; 75:127–131.

Azen SP, Mack WJ, Cashin-Hemphill L, LaBree L, Shircore AM, Selzer RH, Blankenhorn DH, Hodis HN. Progression of coronary artery disease predicts clinical coronary events. Circulation 1996; 93:34–41.

Boushey CJ, Beresford SAA, Omenn GS, Motulsky AG. A quantitative assessment of plasma homocysteine as a risk factor for vascular disease. Probable benefits of increasing folic acid intakes. JAMA 1995; 274:1,049–1,057.

Buchwald H, Matts JP, Fitch LL, Campos CT, Sanmarco ME, Amplatz K, Castaneda-Zuniga WR, Hunter DW, Pearce MB, Bissett JK, et al. Changes in sequential coronary arteriograms and subsequent coronary events: program on the surgical control of the hyperlipidemias (POSCH) group. JAMA 1992; 268:1,429–1,433.

Burchfiel CM, Laws A, Benfante R, Goldberg RJ, Hwang L-J, Chiu D, Rodriguez BL, Curb JD, Sharp DS. Combined effects of HDL cholesterol, triglyceride, and total cholesterol concentrations on 18-year risk of atherosclerotic disease. Circulation 1995; 92:1,430–1,436.

Burke AP, Farb A, Malcom GT, Liang YH, Smialek J, Virmani R. Coronary risk factors and plaque morphology in men with coronary disease who died suddenly. New Engl J Med 1997; 336:1,276–1,282.

Corti MC, Guralnik JM, Salive ME, Ferrucci L, Pahor M, Wallace RB, Hennekens CH. Serum iron level, coronary artery disease, and all-cause mortality in older men and women. Am J Cardiol 1997; 79:120–127.

Corti MC, Guralnik JM, Salive ME, Harris T, Ferrucci L, Glynn RJ, Havlik RJ. Clarifying the direct relation between total cholesterol levels and death from coronary heart disease in older persons. Ann Int Med 1997; 126:753–760.

Corti MC, Guralnik JM, Salive ME, Harris T, Field TS, Wallace RB, Berkman LF, Seeman TE, Glynn RJ, Hennekens CH, Havlik RJ. HDL cholesterol predicts coronary heart disease mortality in older persons. JAMA 1995; 274:539–544.

Dalery K, Lussier-Cacan S, Selhub J, Davignon J, Latour Y, Genest J. Homocysteine and coronary artery disease in French Canadian subjects: relation with vitamins B_{12}, B_6, pyridoxal phosphate, and folate. Am J Cardiol 1995; 75:1,107–1,111.

Ernst E, Resch KL. Fibrinogen as a cardiovascular risk factor: a meta-analysis and review of the literature. Ann Int Med 1993; 118:956–963.

Fielding CJ, Havel RJ, Todd KM, Yeo KE, Schloetter MC, Weinberg V, Frost PH. Effects of dietary cholesterol and fat saturation on plasma lipoproteins in an ethnically diverse population of healthy young men. J Clin Invest 1995; 95:611–618.

Frost PH, Davis BR, Burlando AJ, Curb JD, Guthrie GP, Isaacsohn JL, Wassertheil-Smoller S, Wilson AC, Stamler J. Coronary heart disease risk factors in men and women aged 60 years and older. Circulation 1996; 94:26–34.

Glueck CJ, Shaw P, Lang JE, Tracy T, Sieve-Smith L, Wang Y. Evidence that homocysteine is an idependent risk factor for atherosclerosis in hyperlipidemic patients. Am J Cardiol 1995; 75:132–136.

Kannel WB, D'Agostino RB, Belander AJ, Silbershatz H, Tofler GT. Long-term influence of fibrinogen on initial and recurrent cardiovascular events in men and women. Am J Cardiol 1996; 78:90–92.

Lamarche B, Tchernof A, Moorjani S, Cantin B, Dagenais GR, Lupien PJ, Despres JP. Small, dense low-density lipoprotein particles as a predictor of the risk of ischemic heart disease in men; prospective results from the Quebec cardiovascular study. Circulation 1997; 95:69–75.

Lien WP, Lai LP, Shyu KG, Hwang JJ, Chen JJ, Lei MH, Cheng JJ, Huang PJ, Tsai KS. Low-serum, high-density lipoprotein cholesterol concentration is an important coronary risk factor in Chinese patients with low serum levels of total cholesterol and triglyceride. Am J Cardiol 1996; 77:1,112–1,115.

Miller M, Seidler A, Kwiterovich PO, Pearson TA. Long-term predictors of subsequent cardiovascular events with coronary artery disease and "desirable" levels of plasma total cholesterol. Circulation 1992; 86:1,165–1,170.

Nygård O, Vollset SE, Refsum H, Stensvold I, Tverdal A, Nordrehaug JE, Ueland PM, Kvåle G. Total plasma homocysteine and cardiovascular risk profile. The Hordaland Homocysteine Study. JAMA 1995; 274:1,526–1,533.

O'Donnell CJ, Ridker PM, Glynn RJ, Berger K, Ajani U, Manson JE, Hennekens CH. Hypertension and borderline isolated systolic hypertension increase risks of cardiovascular disease and mortality in male physicians. Circulation 1997; 95:1,132–1,137.

Paunio M, Heinonen OP, Virtamo J, Klag MJ, Manninen V, Albanes D, Comstock GW. HDL cholesterol and mortality in Finnish men with special reference to alcohol intake. Circulation 1994; 90:2,902–2,918.

Perry IJ, Refsum H, Morris RW, Ebrahim SB, Ueland PM, Shaper AG. Prospective study of serum total homocysteine concentration and risk of stroke in middle-aged British men. Lancet 1995; 346:1,395–1,398.

Siscovick DL, Raghunathan TE, King I, Weinmann S, Wicklund KG, Albright J, Bovbjerg V, Arbogast P, Smith H, Kushi LH, Cobb LA, Copass MK, Psaty BM, Lemaitre R, Retzlaff B, Childs M, Knopp RH. Dietary intake and cell membrane levels of long-chain n-3 polyunsaturated fatty acids and the risk of primary cardiac arrest. JAMA 1995; 274:1,363–1,367.

Sniderman A, Pedersen T, Kjekshus. Putting low-density lipoproteins at center stage in atherogenesis. Am J Cardiol 1997; 79:664–667.

Verschuren WMM, Jacobs DR, Bloemberg BP, Kromhout D, Menotti A, Aravanis C, Blackburn H, Buzina R, Dontas AS, Fidanza F, Karvonen MJ, Nedeljkovi S, Nissinen A, Toshima H. Serum total cholesterol and long-term coronary heart disease mortality in different cultures. Twenty-five-year follow-up of the Seven Countries Study. JAMA 1995; 274:131–136.

Waters D, Craven TE, Lespérance J. Prognostic significance of progression of coronary atherosclerosis. Circulation 1993; 87:1,067–1,075.

Welty FK, Mittleman MA, Wilson PWF, Sutherland PA, Matheney TH, Lippinska I, Muller JE, Levy D, Tofler GH. Hypobetalipoproteinemia is associated with low levels of hemostatic risk factors in the Framingham offspring population. Circulation 1997; 95:825–830.

Women and Heart Disease

Chairman BR, Bourassa MG, Davis K, et al. Angiographic prevalence of high-risk coronary artery disease in patient subsets (CASS). Circulation 1981; 64:360–367.

Connor EB. Sex differences in coronary heart disease; why are women so superior? The 1995 Ancel Keys lecture. Circulation 1997; 95:252–264.

Cox JL, Teskey RJ, Lalonde LD, Illes SE. Noninvasive testing in women presenting with chest pain: evidence for diagnostic uncertainty. Canadian Journal of Cardiology 1995; II:885–890.

Guiteras VP, Chaitman BR, Waters DD, et al. Diagnostic accuracy of exercise ECG lead systems in clinical subsets of women. Circulation 1982; 65:1,465–1,474.

Hansen CL, Crabbe D, Rubin S. Lower diagnostic accuracy of thallium-201 SPECT myocardial perfusion imaging in women: an effect of smaller chamber size. J Am Coll Cardiol 1996; 28:1,214–1,219.

Hung J, Chairman BR, Lam J, et al. Noninvasive diagnostic test choices for the evaluation of coronary artery disease in women: a multivariate comparison of cardiac fluoroscopy, exercise electrocardiography, and exercise thallium myocardial perfusion scintigraphy. J Am Coll Cardiol 1984; 4:8–16.

Johansson S, Bergstrand R, Schlossman D, et al. Sex differences in cardioangiographic findings after myocardial infarction. Eur Heart J 1984; 5:374–381.

Kushi LH, Fee RM, Folsom AR, Mink PJ, Anderson KE, Sellers TA. Physical activity and mortality in postmenopausal women. JAMA 1997; 277:1,287–1,292.

Lerner DJ, Kannel WB. Patterns of coronary heart disease morbidity and mortality in the sexes: a 26-year follow-up of the Framingham population. Am Heart J 1986; 111:383–390.

Marcus ML, Harrison DG, White CW, McPherson DD, Wilson RF, Kerber KE. Assessing the physiologic significance of coronary obstructions in patients: importance of diffuse undetected atherosclerosis. Prog Cardiovasc Dis 1988; 31:39–56.

O'Connor NJ, Morton JR, Birkmeyer JD, Olmstead EM, O'Connor GT, for the Northern New England Cardiovascular Disease Study Group. Effect of Coronary Artery Diameter in patients undergoing coronary bypass surgery. Circulation 1996; 93:652–655.

Roger VL, Pellikka PA, Bell MR, Chow CWH, Bailey KR, Seward JB. Sex and test verification bias; impact on the diagnostic value of exercise echocardiography. Circulation 1997; 95:405–410.

Schrott HG, Bittner V, Vittinghoff E, Herrington DM, Hulley S, for the HERS Research Group. Adherence to National Cholesterol Education Program treatment goals in postmenopausal women with heart disease. The Heart and Estrogen/Progestin Replacement Study (HERS). JAMA 1997; 277: 1,281–1,286.

Sketch MH, Mohiuddin SM, Lynch JD, et al. Significant sex differences in the correlation of electrocardiographic exercise testing and coronary arteriograms. Am J Cardiol 1975; 36:169–173.

Wackers FJTH. Artifacts in planar and SPECT myocardial perfusion imaging. Am J Card Imag 1992; 6:42–58.

Waters DD, Szlachcic J, Bonan R, et al. Comparative sensitivity of exercise, cold pressor, and ergonovine testing in provoking attacks of variant angina in patient with active disease. Circulation 1983; 67:310.

Weiner DA, Ryan TJ, McCabe CH, et al. Exercise stress testing. Correlations among history of angina, ST-segment response, and prevalence of coronary artery diseases in the Coronary Artery Surgery Study (CASS). New Engl J Med 1979; 301:230–235.

Cholesterol Lowering—Does It Work?

Alpert JS, Cheitlin MD, Roberts J. Update in cardiology. Ann Int Med 1996; 125:40–46.

Andrews TC, Raby K, Barry J, Naimi C, Allred E, Ganz P, Selwyn AP. Effect of cholesterol reduction on myocardial ischemia in patients with coronary disease. Circulation 1997; 95:324–328.

Blankenhorn DH. Angiographic trials testing the efficacy of cholesterol lowering in reducing progression or inducing regression of coronary atherosclerosis. Coronary Art Dis 1991; 2:875–879.

Blankenhorn DH, Azren S, Kramsch DM, et al., and the MARS Research Group. Coronary angiographic changes with lovastatin therapy. Ann Int Med 1993; 119:969–976.

Blankenhorn DH, Nessim SA, Johnson RL, Sanmarco ME, Azen SP, Cashin-Hemphill L. Beneficial effects of combined colestipol-niacin therapy on coronary atherosclerosis and coronary venous bypass grafts. JAMA 1987; 257:3,233–3,240.

Brown GB, Albers JJ, Fisher LD, Schaefer SM, Lin JT, Kaplan CA, Zhao XQ,

Bisson BD, Fitzpatrick VF, Dodge HT. Niacin or Lovastatin, combined with Colestipol regresses coronary atherosclerosis and prevents clinical events in men with elevated apolipoprotein B. New Engl J Med 1990, 323:1,289–1,298.

Buchwald H, Campos CT, Boen JR, Nguyen PA, Williams SE. Disease-free intervals after partial ileal bypass in patients with coronary heart disease and hypercholesterolemia: report from the program on the surgical control of the hyperlipidemias (POSCH). J Am Coll Cardiol 1995; 26:351–357.

Buchwald H, Vargo RL, et al. Effect of partial ileal bypass surgery on mortality and morbidity from coronary heart disease in patients with hypercholesterolemia. New Engl J Med 1990; 323:946–955.

Byington RP, Furberg CD, Crouse III JR, Espeland MA, Bond MG. Pravastatin, lipids, and atherosclerosis in the carotid arteries (PLAC-II). Am J Cardiol 1995; 76:54C–59C.

Byington RP, Jukema W, Salonen JT, Pitt B, Bruschke AV, Hoen H, Furberg CD, Mancini J. Reduction in cardiovascular events during pravastatin therapy. Pooled analysis of clinical events of the pravastatin atherosclerosis intervention program. Circulation 1995; 92:2,419–2,425.

Cashin-Hemphill L, Mack WJ, Pogoda JM, Sanmarco ME, Azen SP, Blankenhorn DH. Beneficial effects of colestipol-niacin on coronary atherosclerosis. JAMA 1990; 264:3,013–3,017.

The Clinical Quality Improvement Network (CQIN) Investigators. Low incidence of assessment and modification of risk factors in acute care patients at high risk for cardiovascular events, particularly among females and the elderly. Am J Cardiol 1995; 76:570–573.

Cohen MV, Byrne M-J, Levine B, Gutowski T, Adelson R. Low rate of treatment of hypercholesterolemia by cardiologists in patients with suspected and proven coronary artery disease. Circulation 1991; 83:1,294–1,304.

Davidson MH, Stein EA, Dujovne CA, Hunninghake DB, Weiss SR, Knopp RH, Illingworth DR, Mitchel YB, Melino MR, Zupkis RV, Dobrinska MR, Amin RD, Tobert JA. The efficacy and six-week tolerability of simvastatin 80 and 160 mg/day. Am J Cardiol 1997; 79:38–42.

De Divitiis M, Rubba P, Somma S, Liguori V, Galderisi M, Montefusco S, Carreras G, Greco V, Carotenuto A, Iannuzzo G, de Divitiis O. Effects of short-term reduction in serum cholesterol with simvastatin in patients with stable angina pectoris and mild to moderate hypercholesterolemia. Am J Cardiol 1996; 78:763–768.

De Groot E, Jukema W, van Boven AJ, Reiber JHC, Zwinderman AH, Lie KI, Ackerstaff RA, Bruschke AVG, on behalf of the REGRESS study group. Effect of pravastatin on progression and regression of coronary atherosclerosis and vessel wall changes in carotid and femoral arteries: a report from the regression growth evaluation statin study. Am J Cardiol 1995; 76:40C–46C.

Denke MA, Winker MA. Cholesterol and coronary heart disease in older adults. No easy answers. JAMA 1995; 274:575–577.

Ericsson CG, Hamsten A, Nisson J, Grip L, Svane B, deFaire U. Angiographic assessment of effects of bezafibrate on progression of coronary artery disease in young male postinfarction patients. Lancet 1996; 347:849–853.

Feher MD, Foxton J, Banks D, Lant AF, Wray LR. Long-term safety of statin-fibrate combination treatment in the management of hypercholesterolemia in patients with coronary artery disease. ACC Current J Review 1995; 74:14–17.

Ferguson JJ. Meeting highlights. American College of Cardiology 45th Annual Scientific Session. Circulation 1996; 94:1–5.

Furberg CD, Adams HP, Applegate WB, et al. Effect of lovastatin on early carotid atherosclerosis and cardiovascular events. Circulation 1994; 90:1,679–1,687.

Furberg CD, Pitt B, Byington RP, Park J-S, McGovern ME, for the PLAC I and PLAC II investigators. Reduction in coronary events during treatment with pravastatin. Am J Cardiol 1995; 76:60C–63C.

Gillman MW, Cupples LA, Gagnon D, Posner BM, Ellison RC, Castelli WP, Wolf PA. Protective effect of fruits and vegetables on development of stroke in men. JAMA 1995; 273:1,113–1,117.

Gould KL. Noninvasive management of coronary artery disease by vigorous reversal treatment; CPC conference at the University of Texas Medical School at Houston. Lancet 1995; 346:750–753.

Gould KL, Martucci JP, Goldberg DI, Hess MJ, Edens RP, Latifi R, Dudrick SJ. Short-term cholesterol lowering decreases size and severity of perfusion abnormalities by positron emission tomography after dipyridamole in patients with coronary artery disease. Circulation 1994; 89:1,530–1,538.

Gould KL, Ornish D, Kirkeeide R, Brown S, Stuart Y, Buchi M, Billings J, Armstrong W, Ports T, Scherwitz L. Improved stenosis geometry by quantitative coronary arteriography after vigorous risk factor modification. Am J Cardiol 1992; 69:845–853.

Gould K, Ornish D, Scherwitz L, Brown S, Edens RP, Hess MJ, Mullani N, Bolomey L, Dobbs F, Armstrong WT, Merritt T, Ports T, Sparler S, Billings J. Changes in myocardial perfusion abnormalities by positron emission tomography after long-term, intense risk factor modification. JAMA 1995; 274:894–901.

Haskell WL, Alderman EL, Fair JM, Maron JD, Mackey SF, Superko HR, Williams PT, Johnstone IM, Champagne MA, Krauss RM, Farquhar JW. Effects of intensive multiple risk factor reduction on coronary atherosclerosis and clinical cardiac events in men and women with coronary artery disease, the Stanford coronary risk intervention project (SCRIP). Circulation 1994; 89:975–990.

Jukema JW, Bruschke AVG, van Boven AJ, Reiber HC, Bal ET, Zwinderman AH, Jansen H, Boerma GJM, van Rappard FM, Lie KI. Effects of lipid lowering by pravastatin on progression and regression of coronary artery disease in symptomatic men with normal to moderately elevated serum cholesterol levels. The regression growth evaluation statin study (REGRESS). Circulation 1995; 91:2,528–2,540.

Kane JP, Malloy MJ, Ports TA, Philips NR, Diehl JC, Havel RJ. Regression of coronary atherosclerosis during treatment of familial hypercholesterole-mia with combined drug regimens. JAMA 1990; 264:3,007–3,012.

Lacoste L, Lam JYT, Hung J, Letchacovski G, Solymoss CB, Waters D. Hyperlipi-demia and coronary disease. Correction of the increased thrombogenic potential with cholesterol reduction. Circulation 1995; 92:3,172–3,177.

LaRosa JC, Cleeman JI. Cholesterol lowering as a treatment for established coro-nary heart disease. Circulation 1992; 85:1,229–1,234.

MAAS Investigators. Effects of simvastatin on coronary atheroma. Lancet 1994; 344:633–638.

Marcelino JJ, Feingold KR. Inadequate treatment with HMG-CoA reductase in-hibitors by health care providers. Am J Med 1996; 100:605–610.

Nawrocki JW, Weiss SR, Davidson MH, Sprecher DL, Schwartz SL, Lupien PJ, Jones PH, Haber HE, Black DM. Reduction of LDL cholesterol by 25% to 60% in patients with primary hypercholesterolemia by atorvastatin, a new HMG-CoA reductase inhibitor. Arteriosclerosis, Thrombosis and Vascular Biology 1995; 15:678–682.

O'Driscoll GO, Green D, Taylor RR. Simvastatin, an HGM-coenzyme A reduc-tase inhibitor, improves endothelial function within 1 month. Circulation 1997; 95:1,126–1,131.

Ornish DM, Scherwitz LW, Brown SE, Billings JH, Armstrong WT, Ports TA, McLanahan SM, Kirkeeide RL, Brand RJ, Gould KL. Can lifestyle changes reverse atherosclerosis? Lancet 1990; 336:129–133.

Pasternak RC, Brown LE, Stone PH, Silverman DI, Gibson CM, Sacks FM, for the Harvard atherosclerosis reversibility project (HARP) study group. Ef-fect of combination therapy with lipid-reducing drugs in patients with coronary heart disease and "normal" cholesterol levels. Ann Int Med 1996; 125:529–540.

Pedersen TR, Kjekshus J, Berg K, Olsson AG, Wilhelmsen L, Wedel H, Pyörälä K, Miettinen T, Haghfelt T, Fœrgeman O, Thorgeirsson G, Jönsson B, Schwartz JS. Cholesterol lowering and the use of healthcare resources. Cir-culation 1996; 93:1,796–1,802.

Pitt B, Mancini GBJ, Ellis SG, Rosman HS, Park J-S, McGovern ME. Pravastatin limitation of atherosclerosis in the coronary arteries (PLAC I): reduction in atherosclerosis progression and clinical events. J Am Coll Cardiol 1995; 26:1,133–1,139.

Probstfield JL, Margitic SE, Byington RP, Espeland MA, Furberg CD, for the ACAPS research group. Results of the primary outcome measure and clini-cal events from the asymptomatic carotid artery progression study. Am J Cardiol 1995:76:47C–53C.

Sacks FM, Pfeffer MA, Moye L, Rouleau JL, Rutherford JD, Cole TG, Brown L, Warnica JW, Arnold JMO, Wun CC, Davis BR, Braunwald E, for the cho-lesterol and recurrent events trial investigators. The effect of pravastatin on coronary events after myocardial infarction in patients with average cho-lesterol levels. New Engl J Med 1996; 335:1,001–1,009.

Salonen R, Nyyssönen K, Porkkala E, Rummukainen J, Belder R, Park J-S, Salo-nen JT. Kuopio atherosclerosis prevention study (KAPS). A population-based primary preventive trial of the effect of LDL lowering on atherosclerotic progress in carotid and femoral arteries. Circulation 1995; 92: 1,758–1,764.

Salonen R, Nvyssönen K, Porkkala-Sarataho E, Salonen JT. The Kuopio atherosclerosis prevention study (KAPS). Effect of pravastatin treatment on lipids, oxidation resistance of lipoproteins, and atherosclerotic progression. Am J Cardiol 1995; 76:34C–39C.

Scandinavian Simvastatin Survival Study (4S). Randomised trial of cholesterol lowering in 4,444 patients with coronary heart disease. Lancet 1994; 344:1,383–1,389.

Scandinavian Simvastatin Survival Study Group. Baseline serum cholesterol and treatment effect in the Scandinavian simvastatin survival study (4S). Lancet 1995; 345:1,274–1,275.

Schectman G, Hiatt J. Dose-response characteristics of cholesterol-lowering drug therapies: implications for treatment. Ann Int Med 1996; 125:990–1,000.

Schuler G, Hambrecht R, Schlierf G, Grunze M, Methfessel S, Hauer K, Kubler W. Myocardial perfusion and regression of coronary artery disease in patients on a regimen of intensive physical exercise and low-fat diet. J Am Coll Cardiol 1992; 19:34–42.

Schuler G, Hambrecht R, Schlierf G, Niebauer J, Hauer K, Neumann J, Hoberg E, Drinkmann A, Bacher F, Grunze M, Kubler W. Regular physical exercise and low-fat diet: effects on progression of coronary artery disease. Circulation 1992; 86:1–11.

Second report of the expert panel on detection, evaluation, and treatment of high blood cholesterol in adults (adult treatment panel II), National Cholesterol Education Program. Circulation 1994; 89:1,329–1,445.

Shepherd J, Cobbe SM, Ford I, Isles CG, Lorimer AR, MacFarlane PW, McKillop JH, Packard CJ, for the West of Scotland Coronary Prevention Study Group. Prevention of coronary heart disease with pravastatin in men with hypercholesterolemia. New Engl J Med 1995; 333:1,301–1,307.

Singh RB, Rastogi SS, Verna R, et al. Randomised controlled trial of cardioprotective diet in patients with recent acute myocardial infarction: results of one year follow up. Br Med J 1992; 304:1,015–1,019.

Smith SC. Risk-reduction therapy: the challenge to change. Circulation 1996; 93:2,205–2,211.

Stafford RS, Blumenthal D, Pasternak RC. Variations in cholesterol management practices of U.S. physicians. J Am Coll Cardiol 1997; 29:139–146.

Stewart BF, Brown BG, Zhao XQ, Hillger LA, Sniderman AD, Dowdy A, Fisher LD, Albers JJ. Benefits of lipid-lowering therapy in men with elevated apolipoprotein B are not confined to those with very high low-density lipoprotein cholesterol. J Am Coll Cardiol 1994; 23:899–906.

Tamai O, Matsuoka H, Itabe H, Wada Y, Kohno K, Imaizumi T. Single LDL apheresis improves endothelium-dependent vasodilatation in hypercholesterolemic humans. Circulation 1997; 95:76–82.

Tamura A, Mikuriya Y, Nasu M, and the coronary artery regression study (CAS) group. Effect of pravastatin (10mg/day) on progression of coronary ather-osclerosis in patients with serum total cholesterol levels from 160 to 220 mg/dl and angiographically documented coronary artery disease. Am J Cardiol 1997; 79:893–896.

van Boven AJ, Jukema JW, Zwinderman AH, Crijns HJGM, Lie KI, Bruschke AVG. Reduction of transient myocardial ischemia with pravastatin in addition to the conventional treatment in patients with angina pectoris. Circulation 1996; 94:1,503–1,505.

Vogel RA. Coronary risk factors, endothelial function, and atherosclerosis: a review. Clin Cardiol 1997; 20:426–432.

Waters D, Higginson L, Gladstone P, et al. Effects of monotherapy with an HMG-CoA reductase inhibitor on the progression of coronary atherosclerosis as assessed by serial quantitative arteriography. Circulation 1994; 89:959–968.

Waters D, Higginson L, Gladstone P, Boccuzzi SJ, Cook T, Lespérance J. Effects of cholesterol lowering on the progression of coronary atherosclerosis in women. Circulation 1995; 92:2,404–2,410.

Watts GF, Lewis B, Brunt JN, Lewis ES, Coltart DJ, Smith LD, Mann JI, Swan AV. Effects on coronary artery disease of lipid-lowering diet, or diet plus cholestryramine, in the St. Thomas Atherosclerosis Regression Study (STARS). Lancet 1992; 339:563–569.

The West of Scotland Coronary Prevention Study Group. Baseline risk factors and their association with outcome in the west of Scotland coronary prevention study. Am J Cardiol 1997; 79:756–762.

Yusuf S, Anand S. Cost of prevention; the case of lipid lowering. Circulation 1996; 93:1,774–1,776.

Zhao XQ, Grown BG, Hillger L, et al. Effects of intensive lipid-lowering therapy on the coronary arteries of asymptomatic subjects with elevated apolipoprotein B. Circulation 1993; 88:2,744–2,753.

Can Cholesterol Levels Be Too Low?

Iribarren C, Reed DM, Burchfiel CM, Dwyer JH. Serum total cholesterol and mortality. Confounding factors and risk modification in Japanese-American men. JAMA 1995; 273:1,926–1,932.

Iribarren C, Reed DM, Chen R, Yano K, Dwyer JH. Low serum cholesterol and mortality. Which is the cause and which is the effect? Circulation 1995; 92:2,396–2,403.

Kuller LH, Shaten J, Neaton JD, Cutler JA. Traumatic deaths in the Multiple Risk Factor Intervention Trial. Circulation Suppl I 1992; 86:I–64.

National Task Force on the Prevention and Treatment of Obesity. Very low-calorie diets. JAMA 1993; 270:967–974.

Vartiainen E, Puska P, Pekkanen J, Tuomilehto J, Lönnqvist, Ehnholm C. Serum cholesterol concentration and mortality from accidents, suicide, and other violent causes. Br Med J 1994; 309:445–447.

Waters D, Lespérance J, Gladstone P, Boccuzzi SJ, Cook T, Hudgin R, Krip G,

Higginson L. Effects of cigarette smoking on the angiographic evolution of coronary atherosclerosis. Circulation 1996; 94:614–621.

Weidner G, Connor SL, Hollis JF, Connor WE. Improvements in hostility and depression in relation to dietary change and cholesterol lowering. The Family Heart Study. Ann Int Med 1992; 117:820–823.

Wysowski DK, Gross TP. Deaths due to accidents and violence in two recent trials of cholesterol-lowering drugs. Arch Int Med 1990; 150:2,169–2,172.

Yusuf S, Anand S. Cost of prevention. The case of lipid lowering. Circulation 1996; 93:1,774–1,776.

Smoking and Death

Benowitz NL, Fitzgerald GA, Wilson M, Zhang Q. Nicotine effects on eicosanoid formation and hemostatic function: comparison of transdermal nicotine and cigarette smoking. J Am Coll Cardiol 1993; 22:1,159–1,167.

Borland R, Pierce JP, Burns DM, Gilpin E, Johnson M, Bal D. Protection from environmental tobacco smoke in California. The case for a smoke-free workplace. JAMA 1992; 268:749–752.

Czernin J, Sun K, Brunken R, Böttcher M, Phelps M, Schelbert H. Effect of acute and long-term smoking on myocardial blood flow and flow reserve. Circulation 1995; 91:2,891–2,897.

Fiore MC, Jorenby DE, Baker TB, Kenford SL. Tobacco dependence and the nicotine patch. JAMA 1992; 268:2,687–2,694.

Gabbay FH, Krantz DS, Kop WJ, Hedges SM, Klein J, Gottdiener JS, Rozanski A. Triggers of myocardial ischemia during daily life in patients with coronary artery disease: physical and mental activities, anger and smoking. J Am Coll Cardiol 1996; 27:585–592.

Glantz SA, Parmley WW. Passive and active smoking. A problem for adults. Circulation 1996; 94:596–598.

Glantz SA, Parmley WW. Passive smoking and heart disease. JAMA 1995; 273:1,047–1,053.

Hung J, Lam JYT, Lacoste L, Letchacovski G. Cigarette smoking acutely increases platelet thrombus formation in patients with coronary artery disease taking aspirin. Circulation 1995; 92:2,432–2,436.

Kawachi I, Colditz GA, Speizer FE, Manson JE, Stampfer MJ, Willett WC, Hennekens CH. A prospective study of passive smoking and coronary heart disease. Circulation 1997; 95:2,374–2,379.

Kawachi I, Colditz GA, Stampfer MJ, Willett WC, Manson JE, Rosner B, Hunter DJ, Hennekens CH, Speizer FE. Smoking cessation in relation to total mortality rates in women. A Prospective Cohort Study. Ann Int Med 1993; 119:992–1,000.

McGinnis JM, Foege WH. Actual causes of death in the United States. JAMA 1993; 270:2,207–2,212.

Rosenberg L, Palmer JR, Shapiro S. Decline in the risk of myocardial infarction among women who stop smoking. N Engl J Med 1990; 322:213–217.

Sugiishi M, Takatsu F. Cigarette smoking is a major risk factor for coronary spasm. Circulation 1993; 87:76–79.

Siegel M. Involuntary smoking in the restaurant workplace. A review of employee exposure and health effects. JAMA 1993; 270:490–493.

Steenland K, Thun M, Lally C, Heath C. Environmental tobacco smoke and coronary heart disease in the American Cancer Society CPS-II cohort. Circulation 1996; 94:622–628.

Tønneson P, Nørregaard J, Simonsen K, Säwe U. A double-blind trial of a 16-hour transdermal nicotine patch in smoking cessation. N Engl J Med 1991; 325:311–315.

Wannamethee SG, Shaper G, Whincup PH, Walker M. Smoking cessation and the risk of stroke in middle-aged men. JAMA 1995; 274:155–160.

Wells AJ. Passive smoking as a cause of heart disease. J Am Coll Cardiol 1994; 24:546–554.

Willett WC, Green A, Stampfer MJ, et al. Relative and absolute excess risks of coronary heart disease among women who smoke cigarettes. N Engl J Med 1987; 317:1,303–1,309.

Yuan JM, Ross RK, Wang XL, Gao YT, Henderson BE, Yu MC. Morbidity and mortality in relation to cigarette smoking in Shanghai, China. JAMA 1996; 275:1,646–1,650.

Zeiher AM, Schächinger V, Minners J. Long-term cigarette smoking impairs endothelium-dependent coronary arterial vasodilator function. Circulation 1995; 92:1,094–1,100.

Excess Body Weight and Survival

Després JP, Moorjani S, Lupien PJ, Tremblay, Nadeau A, Bourchard C. Regional distribution of body fat, plasma lipoproteins, and cardiovascular disease. Arteriosclerosis 1990; 10:497–511.

Jousilahti P, Tuomilehto J, Vartiainen E, Pekkanen J, Puska P. Body weight, cardiovascular risk factors, and coronary mortality. Circulation 1996; 93:1,372–1,379.

Katzel LI, Bleecker ER, Colman EG, Rogus EM, Sorkin JD, Goldberg AP. Effects of weight loss vs aerobic exercise training on risk factors for coronary disease in healthy, obese, middle-aged and older men—a randomized controlled trial. JAMA 1995; 274:1,915–1,921.

Lavie CJ, Milani RV. Effects of cardiac rehabilitation, exercise training, and weight reduction on exercise capacity, coronary risk factors, behavioral characteristics, and quality of life in obese coronary patients. Am J Cardiol 1997; 79:397–401.

Lee IM, Manson JE, Hennekens CH, Paffenbarger RS. Body weight and mortality. A 27-year follow-up of middle-aged men. JAMA 1993; 270:2,823–2,828.

Leibel RL, Rosenbaum M, Hirsch J. Changes in energy expenditure resulting from altered body weight. N Engl J Med 1995; 332:621–628.

Manson JE, Willett WC, Stampfer MJ, Colditz GA, Hunter DJ, Hankinson SE,

Hennekens CH, Speizer FE. Body weight and mortality among women. N Engl J Med 1995; 333:677–685.

Pi-Sunyer FX. Medical hazards of obesity. Ann Int Med 1993;119:655–660.

Willett WC, Manson JE, Stampfer MJ, Colditz GA, Rosner B, Speizer FE, Hennekens CH. Weight, weight change, and coronary heart disease in women. Risk within the "normal" weight range. JAMA 1995; 273:461–465.

Physical Fitness and Survival

Blair SN, Kohl HW, Barlow CE, Paffenbarger RS, Gibbons LW, Macera CA. Changes in physical fitness and all-cause mortality. A prospective study of healthy and unhealthy men. JAMA 1995; 273:1,093–1,098.

Czernin J, Barnard J, Sun KT, Krivokapich J, Nitzsche E, Dorsey D, Phelps ME, Schelbert HR. Effects of short-term cardiovascular conditioning and low-fat diet on myocardial blood flow and flow reserve. Circulation 1995; 92:197–204.

Dubach P, Myers J, Dziekan G, Goebbels U, Reinhart W, Vogt P, Ratti R, Muller P, Miettunen R, Buser P. Effect of exercise training on myocadial remodeling in patients with reduced left ventricular function after myocardial infarction; application of magnetic resonance imaging. Circulation 1997; 95:2,060–2,067.

Fletcher GF, Balady G, Blair SN, Blumenthal J, Caspersen C, Shaitman B, Epstein S, Froelicher ESS, Froelicher VD, Pina IL, Pollock ML. Statement on exercise: benefits and recommendations for physical activity programs for all Americans. Circulation 1996; 94:857–862.

Ginsburg GS, Agil A, O'Toole M, Rimm E, Douglas PS, Rifai N. Effects of a single bout of ultraendurance exercise on lipid levels and susceptibility of lipids to peroxidation in triathletes. JAMA 1996; 276:221–225.

Hambrecht R, Niebauer J, Marburger C, Grunze M, Kälberer B, Hauer K, Schlierf G, Kübler W, Schuler G. Various intensities of leisure time physical activity in patients with coronary artery disease: effects on cardiorespiratory fitness and progression of coronary atherosclerotic lesions. J Am Coll Cardiol 1993; 22:468–477.

Kimura Y, Kubota M, Yamazaki S. Comparable effects of jogging and weight training exercise on plasma lipids and hormone levels in middle-aged men. Physiologist 1996; 39(5):A-5.

Lee IM, Hsieh CC, Paffenbarger RS. Exercise intensity and longevity in men. The Harvard Alumni Health Study. JAMA 1995; 273:1,179–1,184.

Niebauer J, Hambrecht R, Velich T, Marburger C, Hauer K, Kreuzer J, Zimmermann R, von Hodenberg E, Schlierf G, Schuler G, Kübler W. Predictive value of lipid profile for salutary coronary angiographic changes in patients on a low-fat diet and physical exercise program. Am J Cardiol 1996; 78:163–167.

NIH Consensus Development Panel on Physical Activity and Cardiovascular Health. Physical activity and cardiovascular health. JAMA 1996; 276:241–246.

Pate RR, Pratt M, Blair SN, Haskell WL, Macera CA, Bouchard C, Buchner D, Ettinger W, Heath GW, King AC, Kriska A, Leon AS, Marcus BH, Morris J, Paffenbarger RS, Patrick K, Pollock ML, Rippe JM, Sallis J, Wilmore JH. Physical activity and public health. A recommendation from the Centers for Disease Control and Prevention and the American College of Sports Medicine. JAMA 1995; 273:403–407.

Standard Exercise Tests—True or False Answers?

Bodenheimer MM. Risk stratification in coronary disease: a contrary viewpoint. Ann Int Med 1992; 116:927–936.

Bogaty P, Dagenais GR, Cantin B, Alain P, Rouleau JR. Prognosis in patients with strongly positive exercise electrocardiogram. Am J Cardiol 1989; 64: 1,284–1,288.

Bungo MW, Leland OS. Discordance of exercise thallium testing with coronary arteriography in patients with atypical presentation. Chest 1983; 83:112–116.

Diamond GA. Suspect specificity. J Am Coll Cardiol 1990; 16:1,017–1,021.

Fleg JL, Gerstenblith G, Zonderman AB, Becker LC, Weisfeldt ML, Costa PT, Lakatta EG. Prevalence and prognostic significance of exercise-induced silent myocardial ischemia detected by thallium scintigraphy and electrocardiography in asymptomatic volunteers. Circulation 1990; 81:428–436.

Gould KL. Agreement on the accuracy of thallium stress testing. J Am Coll Cardiol 1990; 16:1,022–1,023.

Gould KL. How accurate is thallium exercise testing? J Am Coll Cardiol 1989; 14:1,487–1,490.

Kloner RA, Shook T, Przyklenk K, Davis VG, Junio L, Matthews RV, Burstein S, Gibson CM, Poole WK, Cannon CP, McCabe CH, Braunwald E. Previous angina alters in-hospital outcome in TIMI 4. A clinical correlate to preconditioning? Circulation 1995; 91:37–47.

Koistinen MJ, Huikuri HV, Pirttiaho H, Linnaluoto MK, Takkunen JT. Evaluation of exercise electrocardiography and thallium tomographic imaging in detecting asymptomatic coronary artery disease in diabetic patients. British Heart Journal 1990; 63:7–11.

Krone RJ, Gregory JJ, Freedland KE, Kleiger RE, Wackers FJT, Bodenheimer MM, Benhorin J, Schwartz RG, Parker JO, Van Voorhees L, Moss AJ. Limited usefulness of exercise testing and thallium scintigraphy in evaluation of ambulatory patients several months after recovery from an acute coronary event: implications for management of stable coronary heart disease. J Am Coll Cardiol 1994; 24:1,274–1,281.

Mangano DT, London MJ, Tubau JF, Browner WS, Hollenber M, Krupski W, Layoug EL, Massi B. Dipyridamole thallium 201-scintigraphy as a perioperative screening test, a reexamination of its predictive potential. Circulation 1991; 84:493–502.

Mulcahy D, Husain S, Zalor G, Rehman A, Andrews NP, Schenke WH, Geller NL, Quyyumi A. Ischemia during ambulatory monitoring as a prognostic indicator in patients with stable coronary artery disease. JAMA 1997; 277: 318–324.

Nolewajka AJ, Kostuk WJ, Howard J, Rechnitzer PA, Cunningham DA. 201-Thallium stress myocardial imaging: an evaluation of fifty-eight asymptomatic males. Clin Cardiol 1981; 4:134–138.

Schwartz RS, Jackson WG, Celio PV, Richardon LA, Hickman JR. Accuracy of exercise 201 TI myocardial scintigraphy in asymptomatic young men. Circulation 1993; 87:165–172.

von Arnim T. Prognostic significance of transient ischemic episodes: response to treatment shows improved prognosis. J Am Coll Cardiol 1996; 28:20–24.

How Accurate Is the Coronary Arteriogram?

Cianflone D, Ciccirillo F, Buffon A, Trani C, Scabbia EV, Finocchiaro ML, Crea F. Comparison of coronary angiographic narrowing in stable angina pectoris, unstable angina pectoris, and in acute myocardial infarction. Am J Cardiol 1995; 76:215–219.

Dupouy P, Larrazet F, Ghalid A, Rande JLD, Geschwind HJ. Is intravascular ultrasound a new standard for coronary artery imaging? J Intervent Cardiol 1993; 6:321–330.

Escaned J, Baptista J, De Mario C, Haase J, Ozaki Y, Linker DT, de Feyter PJ, Roelandt JRTC, Serruys PW. Circulation 1996; 94:966–972.

Fleming RM, Kirkeeide RL, Smalling RW, Gould KL, Stuart Y. Patterns in visual interpretation of coronary arteriograms as detected by quantitative coronary arteriography. J Am Coll Cardiol 1991; 18:945–951.

Gould KL. *Coronary artery stenoses and reversing heart disease.* A textbook of coronary pathophysiology, quantitative coronary arteriography, PET perfusion imaging, and reversal of coronary artery disease. Second edition. Lippincott Raven, Philadelphia, 1998.

Hodgson JM, Reddy KG, Suneja R, Nair RN, Lesnefsky EJ, Sheehan HW. Intracoronary ultrasound imaging: correlation of plaque morphology with angiography, clinical syndrome, and procedural results in patients undergoing coronary angioplasty. J Am Coll Cardiol 1993; 21:35–44.

Marcus ML, Harrison DG, White CW, McPherson DD, Wilson RF, Kerber KE. Assessing the physiologic significance of coronary obstructions in patients: importance of diffuse undetected atherosclerosis. Prog Cardiovasc Dis 1988; 31:39–56.

Mintz GS, Painter JA, Pichard AD, Kent KM, Satler LF, Popma JJ, Chuang YC, Bucher TA, Sokolowicz LE, Leon MB. Atherosclerosis in angiographically "normal" coronary artery reference segments: an intravascular ultrasound study with clinical correlations. J Am Coll Cardiol 1995; 25: 1,479–1,485.

Mintz GS, Popma JL, Augusto DP, Kent KM, Satler LF, Chuang YC, DeFalco RA, Leon MB. Limitations of angiography in the assessment of plaque distribution in coronary artery disease; a systematic study of target lesion eccentricity in 1,446 lesions. Circulation 1996; 93:924–931.

Porter TR, Sears T, Xie F, Michela A, Mata H, Welse D, Shurmur S. Intravascular ultrasound study of angiographically mildly diseased coronary arteries. J Am Coll Cardiol 1993; 22:1,858–1,865.

St. Goar FG, Pinto FJ, Alderman EL, Fitzgerald PJ, Stadius ML, Popp RL. Intravascular ultrasound imaging of angiographically normal coronary arteries: an in vivo comparison with quantitative angiography. J Am Coll Cardiol 1991; 18:952–958.

St. Goar FG, Pinto JF, Alderman EL, Fitzgerald PJ, Stinson EB, Billingham ME, Path FRC, Popp RL. Detection of coronary atherosclerosis in young adult hearts using intravascular ultrasound. Circulation 1992; 86:756–763.

Seiler C, Kirkeeide RL, Gould KL. Basic structure-function relations of the epicardial coronary vascular tree—the basis of quantitative coronary arteriography for diffuse coronary artery disease. Circulation 1992; 85:1,987–2,003.

Seiler C, Kirkeeide RL, Gould KL. Measurement from arteriograms of regional myocardial bed size distal to any point in the coronary arterial tree for assessing anatomic area at risk. J Am Coll Cardiol 1993; 21:783–797.

Topol EJ, Nissen SE. Our preoccupation with coronary luminology. The dissociation between clinical and angiographic findings in ischemic heart disease. Circulation 1995; 92:2,333–2,342.

Tuzcu EM, Hobbs RE, Rincon G, Bott-Silverman C, DeFranco AC, Robinson K, McCarthy PM, Stewart RW, Guyer S, Nissen SE. Occult and frequent transmission of atherosclerotic coronary disease with cardiac transplantation. Insights from intravascular ultrasound. Circulation 1995; 91:1,706–1,713.

White CW, Wright CB, Doty DB, Hiratza LF, Eastham CL, Harrison DG, Marcus ML. Does the visual interpretation of the coronary arteriogram predict the physiological significance of a coronary stenosis? N Engl J Med 1984; 310:819–824.

Yamagishi M, Miyatake K, Tamai J, Nakatani S, Koyama J, Nissen S. Intravascular ultrasound detection of atherosclerosis at the site of focal vasospasm in angiographically normal or minimally narrowed coronary segments. J Am Coll Cardiol 1994; 23:352–357.

High Tech for the Heart—Positron Emission Tomography (PET)

Beanlands RSB, Musik O, Melon P, Sutor R, Sawada S, Muller D, Bondie D, Hutchins GD, Schwaiger M. Noninvasive quantification of regional myocardial flow reserve in patients with coronary atherosclerosis using nitrogen-13 ammonia positron emission tomography. J Am Coll Cardiol 1995; 26:1,465–1,475.

Czernin J, Barnard J, Sun KT, Krivokapich J, Nitzsche E, Dorsey D, Phelps ME, Schelbert HR. Effect of short-term cardiovascular conditioning and low-fat diet on myocardial blood flow and flow reserve. Circulation 1995; 92:197–204.

Demer LL, Gould KL, Goldstein RA, Kirkeeide RL. Diagnosis of coronary artery disease by positron emission tomography: comparison to quantitative coronary arteriography in 193 patients. Circulation 1989; 79:825–835.

Demer LL, Gould KL, Goldstein RA, Kirkeeide RL. Noninvasive assessment of coronary collaterals in man by PED imaging. J Nuc Med 1990; 31:259–270.

DiCarli M, Czernin J, Hoh CK, Gerbaudo VH, Brunken RC, Huang S-C, Phelps ME, Schelbert HR. Relation among stenosis severity, myocardial blood flow, and flow reserve in patients with coronary artery disease. Circulation 1995; 91:1,944–1,951.

Gould KL. Clinical cardiac positron emission tomography: State of the art. Circulation 1991; 84:I-22–I-36.

Gould KL. *Coronary artery stenoses*. A textbook of coronary pathophysiology, quantitative coronary arteriography, PET perfusion imaging, and reversal of coronary artery disease. Second edition. Chapman Hall, New York, 1998.

Gould KL. PET perfusion imaging and nuclear cardiology. J Nuc Med 1991; 32:579–606.

Gould KL, Goldstein RA, Mullani N, Kirkeeide R, Wong G, Smalling R, Fuentes F, Nishikawa A, Matthews W. Noninvasive assesment of coronary stenoses by myocardial imaging during pharmacologic coronary vasodilation VIII. Feasibility of 3D cardiac positron imaging without a cyclotron using generator produced Rb-82. J Am Coll Cardiol 1986; 7:775–792.

Gould KL, Martucci JP, Goldberg DI, Hess, MJ, Edens RP, Latifi R, Dudrick, SJ. Short-term cholesterol lowering decreases size and severity of perfusion abnormalities by positron emission tomography after dipyridamole in patients with coronary artery disease. A potential noninvasive marker of healing coronary endothelium. Circulation 1994; 89:1,530–1,538.

Gould KL, Ornish D, Scherwitz L, Brown S, Edens RP, Hess MJ, Mullani N, Bolomey L, Dobbs F, Armstrong WT, Merritt T, Ports T, Sparler S, Billings J. Changes in myocardial perfusion abnormalities by positron emission tomography after long-term, intense risk factor modification. JAMA 1995; 274:894–901.

Hicks K, Ganti G, Mullani N, Gould KL. Automated quantitation of 3D cardiac PET for routine clinical use. J Nuc Med 1989; 30:1,787–1,797.

Krivokapich J, Czernin J, Schelbert HR. Dobutamine positron emission tomography: absolute quantitation of rest and dobutamine myocardial blood flow and correlation with cardiac work and percent diameter stenosis in patients with and without coronary artery disease. J Am Coll Cardiol 1996; 28:565–572.

Nasher PJ, Brown RE, Oskarsson H, Winniford MD, Rossen JD. Maximal coronary flow reserve and metabolic coronary vasodilation in patients with diabetes mellitus. Circulation 1995; 91:635–640.

Yoshida K, Mullani N, Gould KL. Coronary flow and flow reserve by PET simplified for clinical applications using rubidium-82 or nitrogen-13-ammonia. J Nuc Med 1996; 37:1,701–1,712.

Other Tests—What Do They Show?

Agatston AS, Janowitz WR, Hildner FJ, Zusmer NR, Viamonte M, Detrano R. Quantification of coronary artery calcium using ultrafast computed tomography. J Am Coll Cardiol 1990; 15:827–832.

Bormann JL, Stanford W, Stenberg RG, Winniford MD, Berbaum KS, Talman CL, Galvin JR. Ultrafast computed tomographic detection of coronary artery calcification as an indicator of stenosis. Am J Card Imag 1992; 6:191–196.

Budoff MJ, Georgiou D, Brody A, Agatston AS, Kenneth J, Wolfkiel C, Stanford W, Shields P, Lewis RJ, Janowitz WR, Rich S, Brundage BH. Ultrafast computed tomography as a diagnostic modality in the detection of coronary artery disease. A multicenter study. Circulation 1996; 93:898–904.

Detrano R, Hsiai T, Wang S, Puentes G, Fallavolllita J, Shields P, Stanford W, Wolfkiel C, Georgiou D, Budoff M, Reed J. Prognostic value of coronary calcification and angiographic stenoses in patients undergoing coronary angiography. J Am Coll Cardiol 1996; 27:285–290.

Devries S, Wolfkiel C, Fusman B, Bakdash H, Ahmed A, Levy P, Chomka E, Kondos G, Zajac E, Rich S. Infuence of age and gender on the presence of coronary calcium detected by ultrafast computed tomography. J Am Coll Cardiol 1995; 25:76–82.

Devries S, Wolfkiel C, Shah V, Chomka E, Rich S. Reproducibility of the measurement of coronary calcium with ultrafast computed tomography. Am J Cardiol 1995; 75:973–975.

Elhendy A, Geleijnse ML, Roelandt JRTC, Cornel JH, van Domburg RT, Fioretti PM. Stress-induced left ventricular dysfunction in silent and symptomatic myocardial ischemia during dobutamine stress test. Am J Cardiol 1995; 75:1,112–1,115.

Fallavollitta JA, Brody A, Bunnell IL, Kumar K, Canty JM. Fast computed tomography detection of coronary calcification in the diagnosis of coronary artery disease; comparison with angiography in patients 50 years old. Circulation 1994; 89:285–290.

Fusman B, Wolfkiel CJ. Ultrafast computed tomography for detection of coronary artery calcification. Am J Card Imag 1995; 9:206–212.

Goel M, Honye J, Nakamura S, Hagar J, Burn C, Huwe S, Eisenberg H, Tobis J. Significance of coronary calcification by ultrafast computed tomography: comparison with intravascular ultrasound. Circulation Supp I 1992; 86: I–476.

Kajinami K, Seki H, Takekoshi N, Mabuchi H. Noninvasive prediction of coronary atherosclerosis by quantification of coronary artery calcification using electron beam computed tomography: comparison with electrocardiographic and thallium exercise stress test results. J Am Coll Cardiol 1995; 26:1,209–1,221.

Kaufmann RB, Peyser PA, Sheedy PF, Rumberger JA, Schwartz RS. Quantification of coronary artery calcium by electron beam computed tomography for determination of severity of angiographic coronary artery disease in younger patients. J Am Coll Cardiol 1995; 25:626–632.

Manning WJ, Atkinson DJ, Grossman W, Paulin S, Edelman RR. First-pass nuclear magnetic resonance imaging studies using gadolinium-DTPA in patients with coronary artery disease. J Am Coll Cardiol 1991; 18:959–965.

Poncelet BP, Wedeen VJ, Weisskoff RM, Cohen MS, Holmvang G, Brady TJ, Kantor HL. Quantification of the LAD coronary flow with magnetic resonance echo-planar imaging. Circulation Supp I 1992; 86:I–476.

Poncelet BP, Weisskoff RM, Wedeen VJ, Brady TJ, Kantor K. Time of flight quantification of coronary flow with echo-planar MRI. Magn Reson Med 1993; 30:447–457.

Rumberger JA, Sheedy PF, Breen JF, Schwartz RS. Coronary calcium, as determined by electron beam computed tomography, and coronary disease on arteriogram. Effect of patient's sex on diagnosis. Circulation 1995; 91: 1,363–1,367.

van der Wall, E, Vliegen HW, de Roos A, Bruschke AVG. Magnetic resonance imaging in coronary artery disease. Circulation 1995; 92:2,723–2,739.

Weiss RM, Otoadese EA, Noel MP, DeJong SC, Heery SD. Quantitation of absolute regional myocardial perfusion using cine computed tomography. J Am Coll Cardiol 1994; 23:1,186–1,193.

Wong, ND, Detrano RC, Abrahamson D, Tobis JM, Gardin JM. Coronary artery screening by electron beam computed tomography. Facts, controversy, and future. Circulation 1995; 92:632–636.

Does Coronary Bypass Surgery Prolong Your Life?

Arai AE, Grauer SE, Anselone CG, Pantely GA, Bristow JD. Metabolic adaptation to a gradual reduction in myocardial blood flow. Circulation 1995; 92:244–252.

Caracciolo EA, Davis KB, Sopko G, Kaiser GC, Corley SD, Schaff H, Taylor HA, Chaitman BR. Comparison of surgical and medical group survival in patients with left main equivalent coronary artery disease. Long-term CASS experience. Circulation 1995; 91:2,335–2,344.

CASS Principal Investigators and Their Associates. Coronary Artery Surgery Study (CASS): a randomized trial of coronary artery bypass surgery. Circulation 1983; 68:939–950.

Davies RF, Goldberg D, Forman S, Pepine CJ, Knatterud GL, Geller N, Sopko G, Pratt C, Deanfield J, Conti R. Asymptomatic cardiac ischemia pilot (ACIP) study two-year follow-up; outcomes of patients randomized to initial strategies of medical therapy versus revascularization. Circulation 1997; 95:2,037–2,043.

European Carotid Surgery Trialists' Collaborative Group. Endarterectomy for moderate symptomatic carotid stenosis: interim results from the MRC European carotid surgery trial. Lancet 1996; 347:1,591–1,593.

Gould KL. Does positron emission tomography improve patient selection for coronary revascularization? J Am Coll Cardiol 1992; 20:556–568.

Gould KL, Haynie M, Hess MJ, Yoshida K, Mullani N, Smalling RW. Myocardial metabolism of fluorodeoxyglucose compared to cell membrane integrity for the potassium analogue Rb-82 for assessing viability and infarct size in man by PET. J Nuc Med 1991; 32:1–9.

Hariharan R, Bray M, Ganim R, Doenst T, Goodwin G, Taegtmeyer H. Fundamental limitations of [^{18}F]2-deoxy-2-fluoro-d-glucose for assessing myocardial glucose uptake. Circulation 1995; 91:2,435–2,444.

Hueb WA, Bellotti G, DeOliveira SA, Arie S, DeAlbuquerque CP, Jatene AD, Pileggi F. The medicine, angioplasty, or surgery study (MASS): a prospective, randomized trial of medical therapy, balloon angioplasty, or bypass surgery for single proximal left anterior descending artery stenoses. J Am Coll Cardiol 1995; 26:1,600–1,605.

Lee KS, Marwick TH, Cook SA, Go RT, Fix JS, James KB, Sapp SK, MacIntyre WJ, Thomas JD. Prognosis of patients with left ventricular dysfunction, with and without viable myocardium after myocardial infarction. Relative efficacy of medical therapy and revascularization. Circulation 1994; 90:2,687–2,694.

Merhige M, Garza D, Sease D, Rowe RW, Tewson T, Emran A, Bolomey L, Gould KL. Quantitation of the critically ischemic zone at risk during acute coronary occlusion using PET. J Nuc Med 1991; 32:1,581–1,586.

Qureshi U, Nagueh SF, Afridi I, Vaduganathan P, Blaustein A, Verani MS, Winters WL, Zoghbi WA. Dobutamine echocardiography and quantitative rest-redistribution ^{201}Tl tomography in myocardial hibernation; relation of contractile reserve to ^{201}Tl uptake and comparative prediction of recovery function. Circulation 1997; 95:626–635.

Roach GW, Kanchuger M, Mangano CM, Newman M, Nussmeier N, Wolman R, Aggarwal A, Marschall K, Graham SH, Ley C, Ozanne G, Mangano DT. Adverse cerebral outcomes after coronary bypass surgery. N Engl J Med 1996; 335:1,857–1,863.

Schelbert HR. Different roads to the assessment of myocardial viability. Circulation 1995; 91:1,894–1,895.

Scott SM, Deupree RH, Sharma GVRK, Luchi RJ. VA study of unstable angina. 10-year results show duration of surgical advantage for patients with impaired ejection fraction. Circulation 1994; 90:II-120–II-123.

Tamaki N, Kawamoto M, Tadamura E, Magata Y, Yonekura Y, Nohara R, Sasayama S, Nishimura K, Ban T, Konishi J. Prediction of reversible ischemia after revascularization. Perfusion and metabolic studies with positron emission tomography. Circulation 1995; 91:1,697–1,705.

Tardiff BE, Califf RM, Morris D, Bates E, Woodlief LH, Lee KL, Green C, Rutsch W, Betriu A, Aylward P, Topol EJ. Coronary revascularization surgery after myocardial infarction: impact of bypass surgery on survival after thrombolysis. J Am Coll Cardiol 1997; 29:240–249.

The VA Coronary Artery Bypass Surgery Cooperative Study Group. Eighteen-year follow-up in the veterans affairs cooperative study of coronary artery bypass surgery for stable angina. Circulation 1992; 86:121–130.

Vanoverschelde JLJ, Wijns W, Borgers M, Heyndrickx G, Depré C, Flameng W, Melin JA. Chronic myocardial hibernation in humans; from bedside to bench. Circulation 1997; 95:1,961–1,971.

vom Dahl J, Muzik O, Wolfe ER, Allman C, Hutchins G, Schwaiger M. Myocardial rubidium-82 tissue kinetics assessed by dynamic positron emission tomography as a marker of myocardial cell membrane integrity and viability. Circulation 1996; 93:238–245.

Winslow CM, Kosecoff JB, Chassin M, Kanouse DE, Brook RH. The appropriateness of performing coronary artery bypass surgery. JAMA 1988; 260: 505–509.

Yoshida K, Gould KL. Quantitative relation of myocardial infarct size and myocardial viability by positron emission tomography to left ventricular ejection fraction and 3-year mortality with and without revascularization. J Am Coll Card 1993; 22:984–997.

Yusuf S, Zucker D, Peduzzi P, Fisher LD, Takaro T, Kennedy JW, Davis K, Killip T, Passamani E, Norris R, Morris C, Mathur V, Varnauskas E, Chalmers TC. Effect of coronary artery bypass graft surgery on survival: overview of 10-year results from randomised trials by the Coronary Artery Bypass Graft Surgery Trialists Collaboration. Lancet 1994; 344:563–570.

Balloon Dilation of Narrowed Coronary Arteries

Anderson HV, Vignale SJ, Benedict CR, Willerson JR. Restenosis after coronary angioplasty. J Intervent Cardiol 1993; 6:189–202.

Bauters C, McFadden EP, Lablanche JM, Quandalle P, Bertrand ME. Restenosis rate after multiple percutaneous transluminal coronary angioplasty procedures at the same site. Circulation 1993; 88:969–974.

Coronary angioplasty versus medical therapy for angina: the second randomized intervention treatment of angina (RITA-2) Trial. Lancet 1997; 350:461–468.

Fleming RM, Kirkeeide RL, Smalling RW, Gould KL, Stuart Y. Patters in visual interpretation of coronary arteriograms as detected by quantitative coronary arteriography. J Am Coll Cardiol 1991; 4:257–260.

Frye RL. President's page: does it really make a difference? J Am Coll Cardiol 1992; 19:468–470.

Gould KL. Can percutaneous transluminal coronary angioplasty be considered successful for managing coronary artery disease? J Intervent Cardiol 1991; 4:257–260.

Gould KL. Invasive procedures in acute myocardial infarction. Are they beneficial? JAMA 1994; 272:891–893.

Gould, KL. Quantitative analysis of coronary artery restenosis after coronary angioplasty—has the rose lost its bloom? J Am Coll Cardiol 1992; 19: 946–947.

Mark DB, Nelson CL, Califf RM, Harrell FE, Lee KL, Jones RH, Fortin DF, Stack RS, Glower DD, Smith LR, DeLong ER, Smith PK, Reves JG, Jollis JG, Tcheng JE, Muhlbaier LH, Lowe JE, Phillips HR, Pryor DB. Continuing evolution of therapy for coronary artery disease. Initial results from the era of angioplasty. Circulation 1994; 89:2,015–2,025.

Rensing BJ, Hermans WRM, Vos J, Tijssen JBP, Rutch W, Danchin N, Heyndricks BR, Mast EG, Wijna W, Serruys PW. Luminal narrowing after percutaneous transluminal coronary angioplasty. Circulation 1993; 88: 975–985.

Ritchie JL, Phillips KA, Luft HS. Coronary angioplasty. Statewide experience in California. Circulation 1993; 88:2,735–2,743.

Topol EJ, Ellis SG, Cosgrove DM, Bates ER, Muller DWM, Schork NJ, Schork MA, Loop FD. Analysis of coronary angioplasty practice in the United States with an insurance claims data base. Circulation 1993; 87:1,489–1,497.

Toward fewer procedures and better outcomes. (Editorial) JAMA 1993; 269: 794–796.

Chest Pain: Reversal? Balloon? Bypass?

Bogarty P, Dagenais GR, Cantin B, Alain P, Rouleau JR. Prognosis in patients with a strongly positive exercise electrocardiogram. Am J Cardiol 1989; 64:1,284–1,288.

Cannon RO. The sensitive heart. A syndrome of abnormal cardiac pain perception. JAMA 1995; 273:883–887.

Gandhi MM, Wood DA, Lampe FC. Characteristics and clinical significance of ambulatory myocardial ischemia in men and women in the general population presenting with angina pectoris. J Am Coll Cardiol 1994; 23:74–81.

Little WC, Braden G, Applegate RJ. Angiographic evaluation of the extent and progression of coronary artery disease: limitations of "lumenology." Council Newsletter, Clin Cardiol spring 1995. Ed. BJ Gersh.

Little WC, Downes TR, Applegate RJ. The underlying coronary lesion in myocardial infarction: implications for coronary angiography. Clin Cardiol 1991; 14:868–874.

Miller TD, Christian TF, Taliercia CP, Zinsmeister AR, Gibbons RJ. Severe exercise-induced ischemia does not identify high risk patients with normal left ventricular function and one- or two-vessel coronary artery disease. J Am Coll Cardiol 1994; 23:219–224.

Quyyumi AA, Panza JA, Diodata JG, Callahan TS, Bonow RO, Epstein SE. Prognostic implications of myocardial ischemia during daily life in low-risk patients with coronary artery disease. J Am Coll Cardiol 1993; 21:700–708.

Costs of Reversal Treatment, Balloon Dilation, and Bypass Surgery

Gould KL. PET, PTCA, and economic priorities. Clin Cardiol 1990; 13:153–164.

Gould KL, Goldstein RA, Mullani NA. Economic analysis of clinical positron emission tomography of the heart with rubidium-82. J Nuc Med 1989; 30:707–717.

Hamilton VH, Racicot FE, Zowall H, Coupal L, Grover SA. The cost-effectiveness of HMG-CoA reductase inhibitors to prevent coronary heart disease. Estimating the benefits of increasing HDL-C. JAMA 1995; 273:1,032–1,038.

Johannesson M, Jönsson B, Kjekshus J, Olsson AG, Pedersen TR, Wedel H. Cost effectiveness of simvastatin treatment to lower cholesterol levels in patients with coronary heart disease. N Engl J Med 1997; 336:332–336.

Patterson RE, Eisner RL, Horowitz SF. Comparison of cost-effectiveness and utility of exercise ECG, single photon emission computed tomography, positron emission tomography, and coronary angiography for diagnosis of coronary artery disease. Circulation 1995; 91:54–65.

Pederson TR, Kjekshus J, Berg K, Olsson AG, Wilhelmsen L, Wedel H, Pyrälä K, Miettinen T, Haghfelt T, Fœrgeman O, Thorgeirsson G, Jönsson B, Schwartz S. Cholesterol lowering and the utilization of healthcare resources: results of the Scandinavian Simvastatin Survival Study (4S). Circulation 1996; 93:1,796–1,802.

Topol EJ, Ellis SG, Cosgrove DM, Bates ER, Muller DWM, Schork NJ, Schork MA, Loop FD. Analysis of coronary angioplasty practice in the United States with an insurance claims data base. Circulation 1993; 87:1,489–1,497.

Wittels EH, Hay JW, Gotto AM. Medical costs of coronary artery diseases in the United States. Am J Cardiol 1990; 65:432–440.

Types of Food—Fat, Protein, and Carbohydrate

Anderson JW, Johnstone BM, Cook-Newell ME. Meta-analysis of the effects of soy protein intake on serum lipids. N Engl J Med 1995; 333:176–282.

Assmann G, Schulte H, von Eckardstein A. Hypertriglyceridemia and elevated lipoprotein (a) are risk factors for major coronary events in middle-aged men. Am J Cardiol 1996; 77:1,179–1,184.

Bakhit RM, Klein BP, Essex-Sorlie D, Ham JO, Erdman JW, Potter SM. Intake of 25 g of soybean protein with or without soybean fiber alters plasma lipids in men with elevated cholesterol concentrations. Journal of Nutrition 1994; 124:213–222.

Bender DA, Bender AE. *Nutrition.* A reference handbook. Oxford University Press, Oxford, 1997, pp. 131–133.

Bosaeus I, Belfrage L, Lindgren C, Andersson H. Olive oil instead of butter increases net cholesterol excretion from the small bowel. European Journal of Clinical Nutrition 1992; 46:111–115.

Bosello O, Cominancini L, Zocca I, Garbin U, Compri R, Davoli A, Brunetti L. Short- and long-term effects of hypocaloric diets containing proteins of different sources on plasma lipids and apoproteins of obese subjects. Annals of Nutrition and Metabolism 1988; 32:206–214.

Brown AJ, Roberts DCK. Moderate fish oil intake improves lipemic response to a standard fat meal; a study in 25 healthy men. Arteriosclerosis and Thrombosis 1991; 11:457–466.

Burr ML, Fehily AM, Gilbert JF, Rogers S, Holliday RM, Sweetnam PM, Elwood

PC, Deadman NM. Effects of changes in fat, fish, and fibre intakes on death and myocardial reinfarction: diet and reinfarction trial (DART). Lancet 1989; Sept 30:757–760.

Carroll KK. Review of clinical studies on cholesterol-lowering response to soy protein. Journal of American Dietetic Association 1991; 91:820–827.

Daviglus ML, Stamler J, Orencia AJ, Dyer AR, Liu K, Greenland P, Walsh MK, Morris D, Shekelle RB. Fish consumption and the 30-year risk of fatal myocardial infarction. N Engl J Med 1997; 336:1,046–1,053.

de Lorgeril M, Renaud S, Mamelle N, Salen P, Martin JL, Monjaud I, Guidollet J, Touboul P, Delaye J. Mediterranean alpha-linolenic acid-rich diet in secondary prevention of coronary heart disease. Lancet 1994; 343:1,454–1,459.

de Lorgeril M, Salen P, Martin JL, Mamelle N, Monjaud I, Touboul P, Delaye J. Effect of a Mediterranean type of diet on the rate of cardiovascular complications in patients with coronary artery disease. J Am Coll Cardiol 1996; 28:1,103–1,108.

Drexel H, Amann FW, Beran J, Rentsch K, Candinas R, Muntwyler J, Luethy A, Gasser T, Follath F. Plasma triglycerides and three lipoprotein cholesterol fractions are independent predictors of the extent of coronary atherosclerosis. Circulation 1994; 90:2,230–2,235.

Dupont J. Vegetable oils, in *Encyclopaedia of food science, food technology, and nutrition*. Edited by R Macrae, RK Robinson, MJ Sadler. Academic Press, New York, 1993, pp. 4,711–4,713.

Fumeron F, Brigant L, Ollivier V, de Prost D, Driss F, Darcet P, Bard MJ, Parra HJ, Fruchart JC, Apfelbaum M. N-3 polyunsaturated fatty acids raise low-density lipoproteins, high-density lipoprotein 2, and plaminogen-activator inhibitor in healthy young men. American Journal of Clinical Nutrition 1991; 54:1,188–1,122.

Gaddi A, Ciarrocchi A, Matteucci A, Rimondi S, Ravaglia G, Descovich GC, Sirtori CR. Dietary treatment for familial hypercholesterolemia—differential effects of dietary soy protein according to the apolipoprotein E phenotypes[1-3]. American Journal of Clinical Nutrition 1991; 53:1,191–1,196.

Gillman MW, Cupples LA, Gagnon D, Posner BM, Ellison RC, Castelli WP, Wolf PA. Protective effect of fruits and vegetables on development of stroke in men. JAMA 1995; 273:1,113–1,117.

Ginsberg HN, Barr SL, Gilbert A, Karmally W, Deckelbaum R, Kaplan K, Ramakrishnan R, Holleran S, Dell RB. Redution of plasma cholesterol levels in normal men on an American Heart Asssocation Step 1 diet or a Step 1 diet with added monounsaturated fat. N Engl J Med 1990; 322:574–579.

Gould KL. Essential fatty acids. Circulation 1997 (In Press).

Gould KL. Letter to the editor. JAMA 1996; 275:1,402–1,403.

Gould KL, Ornish D, Kirkeeide R, Brown S, Stuart Y, Buchi M, Billings J, Armstrong WW, Ports T, Scherwitz L. Improved stenosis geometry by quantitative coronary arteriography after vigorous risk factor modification. Am J Cardiol 1992; 69:845–853.

Green P, Fuch J, Schoenfeld N, Leibovici L, Lurie Y, Beigel Y, Rotenberg Z, Mamet R, Budowski P. Effects of fish oil ingestion on cardiovascular risk factors in hyperlipidemic subjects in Israel: a randomized, double blind, crossover trial. Journal of Clinical Nutrition 1990; 52:1,118–1,124.

Hammond EG, Johnson LA, Murphy PA. Soya beans, properties and analysis, in *Encyclopaedia of food science, food technology, and nutrition*. Edited by R Macrae, RK Robinson, MJ Sadler. Academic Press, New York, 1993, pp. 4,223–4,225.

Harris WS. Fish oils and plasma lipid and lipoprotein metabolism in humans: a critical review. Journal of Lipid Research 1989; 30:785–807.

Harris WS, Windsor SL, Dujovne CA. Effects of four doses of n-3 fatty acids given to hyperlipidemic patients for six months. Journal of the American College of Nutrition 1991; 10:220–227.

Haskell WL, Alderman EL, Fair JM, Maron DJ, Mackey SF, Superko R, Williams PT, Johnston IM, Champagne MA, Krauss RM, Farquhar JW. Effects of intensive multiple risk factor reduction on coronary atherosclerosis and clinical cardiac events in men and woman with coronary artery disease. The Stanford Coronary Risk Intervention Project (SCRIP). Circulation 1994; 89:975–990.

Hermann W, Biermann J, Kostner GM. Comparison of effects of N-3 to N-6 fatty acids on serum level of lipoprotein(a) in patients with coronary artery disease. Am J Cardiol 1995; 76:459–462.

Holvoet P, Collen D. Lipid lowering and enhancement of fibrinolysis with niacin. Circulation 1995; 92:698–699.

Inagaki M, Harris WS. Changes in lipoprotein composition in hypertriglyceridemic patients taking cholesterol-free fish oil supplements. Atherosclerosis 1990; 82:237–246.

Karpe F, Steiner G, Uttelman K, Olivecrona T, Amsten A. Postprandial lipoproteins and progress of coronary atherosclerosis. Atherosclerosis 1994; 106: 83–97.

Kearney MT, Charlesworth A, Cowley AJ, Macdonald IA. William Heberden revisited: postprandial angina—interval between food and exercise and meal composition are important determinants of time to onset of ischemia and maximal exercise tolerance. J Am Coll Cardiol 1997; 29:302–307.

Lee TH, Hoover RL, Williams JD. Effect of dietary enrichment with eicosapentaneoic acid and docosahexanoic acid on in vitro neutrophil and monocyte leukotriene generation and neutrophil function. New Engl J Med 1985; 312:1,217–1,224.

Lindgren FT, Adamson GL, Shore VG, Nelson GJ, Schmidt PC. Effect of a salmon diet on the distribution of plasma lipoproteins and apolipoproteins in normolipidemic adult men. Lipids 1991; 26:97–101.

Luostarinen R, Siegbahn A, Saldeen T. Effect of dietary fish oil supplemented with different doses vitamin E on neutrophil chemotaxis in healty volunteers. Nutrition Research 1992; 12:1,419–1,430.

Meinertz H, Nilausen K, Faergeman O. Effects of dietary proteins on plasma lipoprotein levels in normal subjects: interaction with dietary cholesterol. Journal of Nutritional Science and Vitaminology 1990; 36:S157–S164.

Meinertz H, Nilausen K, Faergeman O. Soy protein and casein in cholesterol-enriched diets: effects on plasma lipoproteins in normolipidemic subjects. American Journal of Clinical Nutrition 1989; 50:786–793.

Mensink RP, Katan MB. Effect of dietary fatty acids on serum lipids and lipoproteins. Arteriosclerosis and Thrombosis 1992; 12:911–919.

Mori TA, Vandongen R, Beilin LJ, Burke V, Morris J, Ritchie J. Effects of varying dietary fat, fish, and fish oils on blood lipids in a randomized controlled trial in men at risk of heart disease. American Journal of Clinical Nutrition 1994; 59:1,060–1,068.

Mori TA, Vandongen R, Mahaniain F, Douglas A. Plasma lipid levels and platelet and neutrophil function in patients with vascular disease following fish oil and oil supplementation. Metabolism 1992; 41:1,059–1,067.

O'Keefe Jr. JD, Harris WS, Nelson J, Windsor SL. Effects of pravastatin with niacin or magnesium on lipid levels and postprandial lipemia. Am J Cardiol 1995; 76:480–484.

Ornish D, Brown SE, Scherwitz LW, Billings JH, Armstrong WT, Ports TA, McLanahan SM, Kirkeeide RL, Brand RJ, Gould KL. Can lifestyle changes reverse coronary heart disease? The Lifestyle Heart Trial. Lancet 1990; 336:129–133.

Patsch JR, Miesenböck G, Hopferwieser T, Mühlberger V, Knapp E, Dunn JK, Gotto AM, Patsch W. Relation of triglyceride metabolism and coronary artery disease. Studies in the postprandial state. Arteriosclerosis and Thrombosis 1992; 12:1,336–1,345.

Phillips NR, Waters D, Havel RJ. Plasma lipoproteins and progression of coronary artery disease evaluated by angiography and clinical events. Circulation 1993; 88:2,762–2,770.

Prasad RBN. Walnuts and pecans, in *Encyclopaedia of food science, food technology, and nutrition.* Edited by R Macrae, RK Robinson, MJ Sadler. Academic Press, New York, 1993, pp. 4,828–4,834.

Quinn TG, Alderman EL, McMillan A, Haskel W, for the SCRIP Investigators. Development of new coronary atherosclerotic lesions during a 4-year multifactor risk reduction program: the Stanford Coronary Risk Intervention Project (SCRIP). J Am Coll Cardiol 1994; 24:900–908.

Rapp JH, Connor WE, Lin DS, Porter JM. Dietary eicosapentaenoic acid and docosahexaneoic acid from fish oil. Their incorporation into advanced human atherosclerotic plaques. Arteriosclerosis and Thrombosis 1991; 11:903–911.

Recommended Dietary Allowances, 10th edition; subcommittee on the 10th edition of the RDAs, Food and Nutrition Board Commission on Life Sciences, National Research Council. National Academy Press, Washington, D.C. 1989.

Rimm EB, Ascherio A, Giovannucci E, Spiegelman D, Stampfer MJ, Willett WC. Vegetable, fruit, and cereal fiber intake and risk of coronary heart disease among men. JAMA 1996; 275:447–451.

Rodriguez BL, Sharp DS, Abbott RD, Burchfiel CM, Masaki K, Chyou PH, Huang B, Yano K, Curb JD. Fish intake may limit the increase in risk of coronary heart disease morbidity and mortality among heavy smokers. Circulation 1996; 94:952–956.

Sacks FM. More on chewing the fat. The good fat and the good cholesterol. New Engl J Med 1991; 325:1,740–1,741.

Salomaa V, Rasi V, Pekkanen J, Jauhiainen M, Vahtera E, Pietinen P, Korhone H, Kuulasmaa K, Ehnholm C. The effects of saturated fat and n-6 polyunsaturated fat on postprandial lipemia and hemostatic activity. Atherosclerosis 1993; 103:1–11.

Sanders T. Essential fatty acids, in *Encyclopaedia of food science, food technology, and nutrition*. Edited by R Macrae, RK Robinson, MJ Sadler. Academic Press, New York, 1993, pp. 1,651–1,654.

Schectman G, Kaul S, Cherayil GD, Lee M, Kissebah A. Can the hypotriglyceridemic effect of fish oil concentrate be sustained? Ann Int Med 1989; 110:346–352.

Schuler G, Hambrecht R, Schlierf G, Niebauer J, Hauer K, Neumann J, Hoberg E, Drinkmann A, Bacher F, Grunze M, Kübler W. Regular physical exercise and low-fat diet. Effects on progression of coronary artery disease. Circulation 1992; 86:1–11.

Siguel E. Letter to the editor. Circulation 1997 (In Press).

Siguel E. A new relationship between total/high density lipoprotein cholesterol and polyunsaturated fatty acids. Lipids 1996; 31:S51–S56.

Siguel EN, Chee KM, Gong J, Schaefer EJ. Criteria for essential fatty acid deficiency in plasma as assessed by capillary column gas-liquid chromatography. Clinical Chemistry 1987; 33:1,869–1,873.

Siguel EN, Lerman RH. Altered fatty acid metabolism in patients with angiographically documented coronary artery disease. Metabolism 1994; 43:982–993.

Siguel EN, Maclure M. Relative activity of unsaturated fatty acid metabolic pathways in humans. Metabolism 1987; 36:664–669.

Singh RB, Rastogi SS, Verma R, Laxmi B, Singh R, Ghosh S, Niaz MA. Randomised controlled trial of cardioprotective diet in patients with recent acute myocardial infarction: results of one year follow up. Br Med J 1992; 304:1,015–1,019.

Siscovick DS, Raghunathan TE, King I, Weinmann S, Wicklund KG, Albright J, Bovbjerg V, Arbogast P, Smith H, Kushi LH, Cobb LA, Copass MK, Psaty BM, Lemaitre R, Retzlaff B, Childs M, Knopp RH. Dietary intake and cell membrane levels of long-chain n-3 polyunsaturated fatty acids and the risk of primary cardiac arrest. JAMA 1995; 274:1,363–1,367.

Skartien AH, Lyberg-Beckmann S, Holme I, Hjermann I, Prydz I. Effect of alteration in triglyceride levels on factor VII-phospholipid complexes in plasma. Arteriosclerosis Nov–Dec 1989; 9:798–801.

Snyder HE. Soya beans, in *Encyclopaedia of food science, food technology, and nutrition*. Edited by R Macrae, RK Robinson, MJ Sadler. Academic Press, New York, 1993, pp. 4,215–4,218.

Spiller GA, Jenkins DJA, Cragen LN, Gates JE, Bosello O, Berra K, Rudd C, Stevenson M, Superko R. Effect of a diet high in monounsaturated fat from almonds on plasma cholesterol and lipoproteins. Journal of the American College of Nutrition 1992; 11:126–130.

Sprecher DL, Harris BV, Goldberg AC, Anderson EC, Bayuk LM, Russell BS, Crone DS, Quinn C, Bateman J, Kuzmak BR, Allgood LD. Efficacy of psyllium in reducing serum cholesterol levels in hypercholesterolemic patients on high or low-fat diets. Ann Int Med. 1993; 119:545–554.

Stacpoole, PW, Alig J, Ammon 'L, Crockett SE. Dose-response effects of dietary marine oil on carbohydrate and lipid metabolism in normal subjects and patients with hypertriglyceridemia. Metabolism 1989; 38:946–956.

Superko HR, Orr JR, Krauss RM. Reduction of small, dense LDL by gemfibrozil in LDL subclass pattern B. Circulation 1995; 92:1–250(abst).

Szuhaj BF. Phospholipids, in *Encyclopaedia of food science, food technology, and nutrition*. Edited by R Macrae, RK Robinson, MJ Sadler. Academic Press, New York, 1993, pp. 3,553–3,558.

Tornvall P, Båvenholm P, Landou C, deFaire U, Hamsten A. Relation of plasma levels and composition of apolipoproteinB-containing lipoproteins to angiographically defined coronary artery disease in young patients with myocardial infarction. Circulation 1993; 88:2,180–2,189.

Turini ME, Powell WS, Behr SR, Holub BJ. Effects of a fish-oils and vegetable-oil formula on aggregation and ethanolamin-containing lysophospholipid generation in activated human platelets and on leukotriene production in stimulated neutrophils. American Journal of Clinical Nutrition 1994; 60:717–724.

Uiterwaal CSPM, Grobbee DE, Witteman JCM, van Stiphout WAHJ, Krauss XH, Havekes LM, de Bruijn AM, van Tol A, Hofman A. Postprandial triglyceride response in young adult men and familial risk for coronary atherosclerosis. Ann Int Med 1994; 121:576–583.

Vogel RA, Corretti MC, Plotnick GD. Effect of a single high-fat meal on endothelial function in healthy subjects. Am J Cardiol 1997; 79:350–354.

Von Schacky C, Kiefl R, Marcus AJ, Broekman MJ, Kaminski VE. Dietary n-3 fatty acids accelerate catabolism of leukotriene B4 in human granulocytes. Biochimica Biophysica Acta 1993; 1166:20–24.

Warshafsky S, Kamer RS, Sivak SL. Effect of garlic on total serum cholesterol. A meta-analysis. Ann Int Med 1993; 119:599–605.

Watts GF, Lewis B, Brunt JNH, Lewis ES, Coltart DJ, Smith LDR, Mann JI, Swan AV. Effects on coronary artery disease of lipid-lowering diet, or diet plus cholestyramine, in the St. Thomas atherosclerosis regression study (STARS). Lancet 1992; 339:563–569.

Wolfe BM, Giovannetti PM. High protein diet complements resin therapy of familial hypercholesterolemia. Clinical Investigative Medicine 1992; 15:349–359.

Wolfe BM, Giovannetti PM. Short-term effects of substituting protein for carbohydrate in the diets of moderately hypercholesterolemic human subjects. Metabolism 1991; 40:338–343.

Antioxidant Vitamins and Aspirin

Anderson TJ, Meredith IT, Yeung AC, Frei B, Selwyn AP, Ganz P. The effect of cholesterol-lowering and antioxidant therapy on endothelium-dependent coronary vasomotion. New Engl J Med 1995; 332:488–493.

Chamiec T, Herbaczyska-Cedro K, Ceremuyski L, with Klosiewicz-Wasek B, Wasek W. Effects of antioxidant vitamins C and E on signal-averaged electrocardiogram in acute myocardial infarction. Am J Cardiol 1996; 77:237–241.

Garber AM, Browner WS, Hulley SB. Review: cholesterol lowering reduces mortality in high-risk, middle-aged men. Ann Int Med 1996; 124:518–531.

Garcia-Dorado D, Théroux P, Tornos P, Sambola A, Oliveras J, Santos M, Soler JS. Previous aspirin use may attenuate the severity of the manifestation of acute ischemic syndromes. Circulation 1995; 92:1,743–1,748.

Goldstein RE, Andrews M, Hall WJ, Moss AJ. Marked reduction in long-term cardiac deaths with aspirin after a coronary event. J Am Coll Cardiol 1996; 28:326–330.

Heitzer T, Just H, Munzel T. Antioxidant vitamin C improves endothelial dysfunction in chronic smokers. Circulation 1996; 94:6–9.

Hodis HN, Mack WJ, LaBree L, Cashin-Hemphill L, Sevanian A, Johnson R, Azen SP. Serial coronary angiographic evidence that antioxidant vitamin intake reduces progression of coronary artery atherosclerosis. JAMA 1995; 273:1,849–1,854.

Jialal I, Grundy SM. Effect of combined supplementation with alpha-tocopherol, ascorbate, and beta carotene on low-density lipoprotein oxidation. Circulation 1993; 88:2,780–2,786.

Knekt P, Färvinen R, Reunanen A, Maatela J. High dietary intake of flavinoids was associated with decreased mortality. Br Med J 1996; 312:478–481.

Kritchevsky SB, Shimakawa T, Tell GS, Dennis B, Carpenter M, Eckfeldt JH, Preacher-Ryan H, Heiss G. Dietary antioxidants and carotid artery wall thickness—the ARIC study. Circulation 1995; 92:2,142–2,150.

Levine GN, Frei B, Koulouris SN, Gerhard MD, Keaney Jr. JF, Vita JA. Ascorbic acid reverses endothelial vasomotor dysfunction in patients with coronary artery disease. Circulation 1996; 93:1,107–1,113.

Meydani SN, Meydani M, Blumberg JB, Leka LS, Siber G, Loszewski R, Thompson C, Pedrosa MC, Diamond RD, Stollard D. Vitamin E supplementation and in vivo immune response in healthy elderly subjects. JAMA 1997; 277:1,380–1,386.

Miwa K, Miyagi Y, Igawa A, Nakagawa K, Inoue H. Vitamin E deficiency in variant angina. Circulation 1996; 94:14–18.

Morris DL, Kritchevsky SB, Davis CE. Serum carotenoids and coronary heart disease; the lipid research clinics coronary primary prevention trial and follow-up study. JAMA 1994; 272:1,439–1,441.

Rapola JM, Virtamo J, Haukka JK, et al. Vitamin E was associated with a decreased risk for angina pectoris. JAMA 1996; 275:693–698.

Reilly M, Delanty N, Lawson JA, FitzGerald GA. Modulation of oxidant stress in vivo in chronic cigarette smokers. Circulation 1996; 94:19–25.

Singh RB, Ghosh S, Niaz MA, Singh R, Beegum R, Chibo H, Shoumin Z, Postiglione A. Dietary intake, plasma levels of antioxidant vitamins, and oxidative stress in relation to coronary artery disease in elderly subjects. Am J Cardiol 1995; 76:1,233–1,238.

Singh RB, Niaz MA, Rastogi SS, Rastogi S. Usefulness of antioxidant vitamins in suspected acute myocardial infarction (the Indian experiment of infarct survival-3). Am J Cardiol 1996; 77:232–236.

Sohal RS, Weindruch R. Oxidative stress, caloric restriction, and aging. Science 1996; 273:59–63.

Stephens NG, Parsons A, Schofield PM, Kelly F, Cheeseman K, Mitchinson MJ, Brown MJ. Randomised controlled trial of vitamin E in patients with coronary disease: Cambridge Heart Antioxidant study (CHAOS). Lancet 1996; 347:781–786.

Stephens NG, Parsons A, Schofield PM, Kelly F, Cheeseman K, Mitchinson MJ, Brown MJ. Vitamin E reduced the risk for cardiovascular events in coronary atherosclerosis. Cambridge Heart Antioxidant Study. Lancet 1996; 347:781–786.

Ting HH, Timimi FK, Boles KS, Creager SJ, Ganz P, Creager MA. Vitamin C improves endothelium-dependent vasodilation in patients with non-insulin-dependent diabetes mellitus. J Clin Invest 1996; 97:22–28.

Estrogens and Coronary Heart Disease

Col NF, Eckman MH, Karas RH, Pauker SG, Goldberg RJ, Ross EM, Orr RK, Wong JB. Patient-specific decisions about hormone replacement therapy in postmenopausal women. JAMA 1997; 277:1,140–1,147.

Guetta V, Cannon RO. Cardiovascular effects of estrogen and lipid-lowering therapies in postmenopausal women. Circulation 1996; 93:1,928–1,937.

Lieberman EH, Gerhard MD, Uehata A, Walsh BW, Selwyn AP, Ganz P, Yeung AC, Creager MA. Estrogen improves endothelium-dependent, flow-mediated vasodilation in postmenopausal women. Ann Int Med 1994; 121:936–941.

Manolio TA, Furberg CD, Shemanski L, Psaty BM, O'Leary DH, Tracy RP, Bush TL. Associations of postmenopausal estrogen use with cardiovascular disease and its risk factors in older women. Circulation 1993; 88:2,163–2,171.

Reis SE, Gloth ST, Blumenthal RS, Resar JR, Zacur HA, Gerstenblith G, Brinker JA. Ethinyl estradiol acutely attenuates abnormal coronary vasomotor sresponse to acetylcholine in postmenopausal women. Circulation 1994; 89:52–60.

Rosano GMC, Sarrel PM, Poole-Wilson PA, Collins P. Beneficial effect of oestrogen on exercise-induced myocardial ischaemia in women with coronary artery disease. Lancet 1993; 342:133–136.

Samaan SA, Crawford MH. Estrogen and cardiovascular function after menopause. J Am Coll Cardiol 1995; 26:1,403–1,410.

Stanford JL, Weiss NS, Voigt LF, Daling JR, Habel LA, Rossing MA. Combined estrogen and progestin hormone replacement therapy in relation to risk of breast cancer in middle-aged women. JAMA 1995; 274:137–142.

The Writing Group for the PEPI Trial. Effects of estrogen or estrogen/progestin regimens on heart disease risk factors in postmenopausal women. The post-menopausal estrogen/progestin interventions (PEPI) trial. JAMA 1995; 273:199–208.

Stress Management

Barefoot JC, Helms MJ, Mark DB, Blumenthal JA, Califf RM, Haney TL, O'Connor CM, Siegler IC, Williams RB. Depression and long-term mortality risk in patients with coronary artery disease. Am J Cardiol 1996; 78:613–617.

Barefoot JC, Schroll M. Symptoms of depression, acute myocardial infarction, and total mortality in a community sample. Circulation 1996; 93:1,976–1,980.

Bou-Holaigah I, Rowe PC, Kan J, Calkins H. The relationship between neurally mediated hypotension and the chronic fatigue syndrome. JAMA 1995; 274:961–967.

Carney RM, Freedland KE, Sheline YI, Weiss ES. Depression and coronary heart disease: a review for cardiologists. Clin Cardiol 1997; 20:196–200.

Carney RM, Saunders RD, Freedland KE, Stein P, Rich MW, Jaffe AS. Association of depression with reduced heart rate variability in coronary artery disease. Am J Cardiol 1995; 76:562–564.

Dakak N, Quyyumi AA, Eisenhofer G, Goldstein DS, Cannon RO. Sympathetically mediated effects of mental stress on the cardiac microcirculation of patients with coronary artery disease. Am J Cardiol 1995; 76:125–130.

Denollet J, Sys SU, Stroobant N, Rombouts H, Gillebert TC, Brutsaert DL. Personality as independent predictor of long-term mortality in patients with coronary heart disease. Lancet 1996; 347:417–421.

Frasure-Smith N, Lespérance F, Talajic M. Depression and 18-month prognosis after myocardial infarction. Circulation 1995; 91:999–1,005.

Gullette ECX, Blumenthal JA, Babyak M, Jang W, Waugh RA, Frid DJ, O'Connor CM, Morris JJ, Krantz DS. Effects of mental stress on myocardial ischemia during daily life. JAMA 1997; 277:1,521–1,526.

Hlatky MA, Lam LC, Lee KL, Clapp-Channing NE, Williams RB, Pryor DB, Califf RM, Mark DB. Job strain and the prevalence and outcome of coronary artery disease. Circulation 1995; 92:327–333.

Jiang W, Babyak M, Krantz DS, Waugh RA, Coleman RE, Hanson MM, Frid DJ, McNulty S, Morris JJ, O'Connor CM, Blumenthal JA. Mental stress-induced myocardial ischemia and cardiac events. JAMA 1996; 275:1,621–1,656.

Kawachi I, Sparrow D, Spiro A, Vokonas P, Weiss ST. A prospective study of anger and coronary heart disease. Circulation 1996; 94:2,090–2,095.

Kubansky LD, Kawachi I, Spiro A, Weiss ST, Vokonas PS, Sparrow D. Is worrying bad for your heart? A prospective study of worry and coronary heart disease in the normative aging study. Circulation 1997; 95:818–824.

Lichodziejewska B, Klos J, Rezler J, Grudzka K, Dluziewska M, Budaj A, Ceremuzynski L. Clinical symptoms of mitral valve prolapse are related to hypomagnesemia and attenuated by magnesium supplementation. Am J Cardiol 1997; 79:768–772.

Mittleman MA, Maclure M, Sherwood JB, Mulry RP, Tofler GH, Jacobs SC, Friedman R, Benson H, Muller JE, for the Determinants of Myocardial Infarction Onset Study investigators. Triggering of acute myocardial infarction onset by episodes of anger. Circulation 1995; 92:1,720–1,725.

O'Connor NJ, Manson JE, O'Connor GT, Buring JE. Psychosocial risk factors and nonfatal myocardial infarction. Circulation 1995; 92:1,458–1,464.

Weidner G, Connor SL, Hollis JF, Connor WE. Improvements in hostility and depression in relation to dietary change and cholesterol lowering. The Family Heart Study. Ann Int Med 1992; 117:820–823.

Zehender M, Meinertz T, Faber T, Caspary A, Jeron AN, Bremm K, Just H, for the MAGICA investigators. J Am Coll Cardiol 197; 29:1,028–1,034.

Index

achiness, muscle, 174, 201–202

addictive behavior, and cholesterol lowering, 67, 68

adenosine, in stress testing, 94–95

age, 45
  and benefit of cholesterol lowering, 54, 55t
  and CAD, 43, 44, 44t

alcohol, 154, 199–200

alcoholism, and cholesterol lowering, 67, 68

alpha-linoleic acid, 159. *See also* fatty acids

alternatives, to reversal treatment, 205–206

alternative treatment modalities
  cost-effectiveness of, 121
  scientifically based, 130–131

American Heart Association, 120
  dietary guidelines of, xxiii, 13, 58, 164
  fat guidelines of, 144–145
  vs. Gould Guidelines, 129

anatomy of heart, 3, 4f

anger, and atherosclerosis, 189. *See also* stress

angina. *See also* chest pain
  coronary bypass surgery for, 102, 103f
  due to coronary heart disease, 180–182
  effect of triglycerides on, 193
  exertional, 180
  management of, 181
  mechanisms for, 181
  progressive, 182
  resting, 181

second randomized intervention treatment of (RITA-2), 104, 113, 121

angiogram, coronary, 25. *See also* arteriogram
  accuracy of, 81–85
  after exercise testing, 80

angioplasty, balloon, 108. *See also* balloon dilation

angiotensin converting enzyme (ACE) inhibitors, 134

antianginal drugs, and reversal treatment, 193

antioxidant vitamins
  action of, 172
  daily doses of, 173

antismoking lawsuits, 69

aorta, 3, 4f, 7, 9f

aortic valve, 7, 9f

appetite, suppression of, 138, 155. *See also* hunger

arachinoids, 159

arrhythmias
  defined, 17
  monitoring of, 18

arteries. *See also* coronary arteries
  definitive diagnosis of dysfunctional, 78
  hardening of, 10, 131

arteriogram, coronary, xvii–xviii, xxi, 25
  accuracy of, 81–85
  clinical application of, 82
  compared with PET, 37–40
  costs of, 120t
  limitations of, 26, 34, 38–39, 48, 89–90, 119t

About the Author

Dr. Gould was born and raised in rural south Alabama, graduating from Mc-Cally Military Academy followed by Oberlin College, where he received a physics degree, and then entered medical school. After receiving his M.D. degree and completing medical residency at the University of Seattle in Washington, Dr. Gould spent two years in the Epidemic Intelligence Service based in Hawaii, focusing on leprosy and measles in island populations of the South Pacific. He returned to Seattle for cardiology training under Dr. Robert Bruce, the developer of the treadmill test, pursued research on coronary artery disease, and achieved the rank of associate professor in 1976. In 1979 he moved to the University of Texas as professor and director of the Division of Cardiology, and founding director of the Positron Diagnostic and Research Center. Dr. Gould stepped aside from administrative duties in 1987 to focus clinically and scientifically on PET imaging and quantitative coronary arteriography for identifying coronary artery disease, measuring its severity, and reversing it by vigorous risk-factor modification. This effort has evolved into a full-time clinical and research commitment to the comprehensive noninvasive management of coronary artery disease, both prevention and reversal, without invasive procedures at reduced cardiac care costs with improved outcomes.

Dr. Gould received the International George von Hevesy Prize for Research in 1978, the George E. Brown Memorial Lectureship of the American Heart Association in 1990, numerous teaching awards in both basic science and clinical cardiology, and has been honored nationally by membership in the Association of American Physicians, the American Society of Clinical Investigation, and the Board of Trustees of the American College of Cardiology. He is currently associate editor of *Circulation* and on the editorial boards of the major cardiovascular journals. He is past chairman of the Council on Circulation of the American Heart Association and past president of the Houston Cardiology Society. Dr. Gould published the first and only textbook, *Coronary Artery Stenosis and Reversing Heart Disease*, on quantifying coronary artery narrowing, coronary blood flow, and cardiac PET imaging. The second edition was recently published. Throughout these several careers Dr. Gould has received twenty-six years of continuous competitive research grant funding from the National Institutes of Health, the American Heart Association, and the Veterans Administration Career Development program.

Currently, Dr. Gould is a professor of medicine and director of the Weatherhead PET Center for Preventing and Reversing Atherosclerosis at the University of Texas Medical School in Houston, established by an endowment from Albert and Celia Weatherhead of Cleveland, Ohio. He is also associated with the President Bush Center for Cardiovascular Health of Hermann Hospital and the University of Texas Medical School.